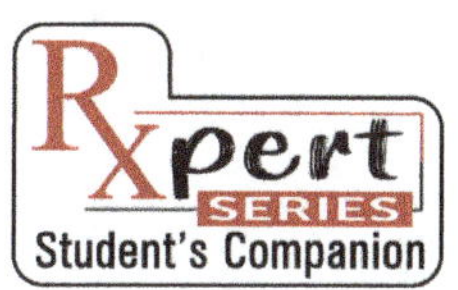

Pharmaceutical Biotechnology

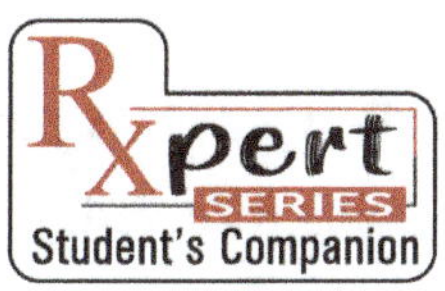

Pharmaceutical Biotechnology

Dr. Ravi Kumar Maddali

M.Pharm., Ph.D., PDF (USA).

Principal
Geethanjali College of Pharmacy
Cheeryal(V), Keesara (M), Medchal,
Malkajgiri District, Telangana State 501 301.

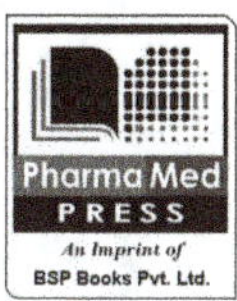

PharmaMed Press
An imprint of BSP Books Pvt. Ltd.
4-4-309/316, Giriraj Lane,
Sultan Bazar, Hyderabad - 500 095.

Published by

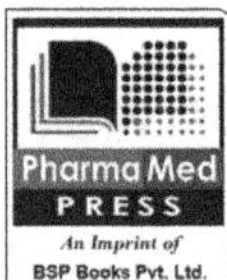

PharmaMed Press

An imprint of BSP Books Pvt. Ltd.

4-4-309/316, Giriraj Lane, Sultan Bazar, Hyderabad - 500 095.
Phone: 040-23445688; Fax: 91+40-23445611
E-mail: info@pharmamedpress.net
www.bspbooks.net/www.pharmamedpress.net

ISBN: 978-93-95039-21-5 (Hardback)

PREFACE

The main aim of this book is to present entire concept in Pharmaceutical Biotechnology as per the PCI syllabus to the students in single book with at least a minimal skill in biological sciences and technology. The primary emphasis is on scientific applications in the fields of genetic engineering, medicine and fermentation technology which leading to a new biological revolutions in diagnosis, preventions and cure of diseases, new and cheaper pharmaceutical drugs, vaccines and antibiotics.

This book was written with a series of learning objectives in mind. After reading this book, the student should be able to:

1. Explain about the basics of biotechnology, enzyme immobilization, biosensors, production of enzymes, protein engineering and genetic engineering.

2. Summarize the rDNA technology, interferon, vaccines, hormones and types of immunity.

3. Outline various structures of immunoglobulins, MHC, hypersensitivity reactions and hybridoma technology.

4. Explain the concept of immune blotting techniques, genetic organization of eukaryotes, prokaryote, microbial genetics and microbial biotransformation.

5. Discuss about the mutations, fermentation methods, design and large scale production, Production of antibiotics and vitamins.

This book is primarily intended for the undergraduate students of pharmacy and the allied professions. However, graduate students in Biotechnology, Microbiology, Medicine, Medical Biotechnology, Pharmaceutical Biotechnology, Cellular Biotechnology, Fermentation Biotechnology, Food Biotechnology, and Bioinformatics.

I believe this book titled "Pharmaceutical Biotechnology" will be a book of choice for students, and Faculty in their academic persuit. Valued suggestions and comments are welcomed to refine the material and incorporate the suggestions in the future editions of this book.

-Author

CONTENTS

CHAPTER 2

CARRIER, VECTORS, RESERVOIRS

CHAPTER 3

IMMUNOGENICITY

CHAPTER 4

MICROBIAL GENETICS

CHAPTER 5

FERMENTATION AND FERMENTATION PRODUCTS

CHAPTER 1

INTRODUCTION TO BIOTECHNOLOGY

LEARNING OBJECTIVES

After studying the chapter the students familiarize themselves with the following concepts:

- *Introducing the subject Biotechnology and significance in various Fields in Pharmaceutical Industry.*
- *Basic Concepts on Biosensors Principles*
- *Protein Engineering*
- *Genetic Engineering*

Biotechnology is a multidisciplinary subject that combines biological sciences with engineering technologies to change live organisms and biological systems in order to create products that advance healthcare, medicine, agriculture, food, medicines, and environmental control. R&D in Biological Sciences and Industrial Processes are the two primary categories of biotechnology. The biological sciences section is concerned with research and development in areas such as microbiology, cell biology, genetics, and molecular biology, among others, in order to better understand disease occurrence and treatment, agricultural development, food production, environmental protection, and so on. In biological sciences, the majority of R&D is done in the laboratory. The industrial processes section is concerned with the large-scale manufacture of medications, vaccines, biofuels, and pharmaceuticals employing biochemical processes and techniques.

1.1 History of Biotechnology

The origins of biotechnology can be traced back to zymotechnology, which began with a focus on brewing procedures for beer. However, by the end of World War I, zymotechnology had expanded to address bigger industrial concerns, and the potential of industrial fermentation had given rise to biotechnology. Microbial fermentations are the oldest biotechnological processes, as evidenced by a Babylonian tablet dating from around 6000 B.C. that was discovered in 1881 and described the creation of beer.

Leavened bread was first made with the help of yeast around 4000 B.C. In the third millennium B.C., the Sumerians were able to brew up to twenty different types of beer. The first vinegar production company was developed in France near Orleans in the 14th century.

With his newly developed microscope, Antony Van Leeuwenhoek examined yeast cells for the first time in 1680. Louis Pasteur first mentioned lactic acid fermentation by microbes in 1857.

By the end of the nineteenth century, a great number of enterprises and groups of scientists had been active in the field of biotechnology, and Germany and France had created large-scale sewage purification systems using bacteria.

Delbruck, Heyduck, and Hennerberg found the large-scale application of yeast in the food business between 1914 and 1916. Bacteria were used to produce acetone, butanol, and glycerine within the same time period.

Alexander Fleming developed penicillin in 1920, and large-scale production of the antibiotic began in 1944.

A timeline of modern biotechnology's development

500 B.C.: In China, the first antibiotic, mouldy soybean curds, is put to use to treat boils.

A.D.100: The first insecticide is produced in China from powdered chrysanthemums.

1761: English surgeon Edward Jenner pioneer's vaccination, inoculating a child with a viral smallpox vaccine.

1870: Breeders crossbreed cotton, developing hundreds of varieties with superior qualities.

1870: The first experimental corn hybrid is produced in a laboratory.

1911: American pathologist Peyton Rous discovers the first cancer-causing virus.

1928: Scottish scientist Alexander Fleming discovers penicillin.

1933: Hybrid corn is commercialized.

1942: Penicillin is mass-produced in microbes for the first time.

1950s: The first synthetic antibiotic is created.

1951: Artificial insemination of livestock is accomplished using frozen semen.

1958: DNA is made in a test tube for the first time.

1978:   Recombinant human insulin is produced for the first time.

1979:   Human growth hormone is synthesized for the first time.

1980:   Smallpox is globally eradicated following 20-year mass vaccination effort.

1980:   The U.S. Supreme Court approves the principle of patenting organisms, which allows the Exxon oil company to patent an oil-eating microorganism.

1981:   Scientists at Ohio University produce the first transgenic animals by transferring genes from other animals into mice.

1982:   The first recombinant DNA vaccine for livestock is developed.

1982:   The first biotech drug, human insulin produced in genetically modified bacteria, is approved by FDA. Genentech and Eli Lilly developed the product.

1985:   Genetic markers are found for kidney disease and cystic fibrosis.

1986:   The first recombinant vaccine for humans, a vaccine for hepatitis B, is approved.

1986:   Interferon becomes the first anticancer drug produced through biotech.

1988:   The first pest-resistant corn, Bt corn, is produced.

1990:   The first successful gene therapy is performed on a 4-year-old girl suffering from an immune disorder.

1992:   FDA approves bovine somatotropin (BST) for increased milk production in dairy cows.

1993:   FDA approves Betaseron®, the first of several biotech products that have had a major impact on multiple sclerosis treatment.

1994:   The first breast cancer gene is discovered.

1994:   The Americas are certified polio-free by the International Commission for the Certification of Polio Eradication.

1995:   Gene therapy, immune-system modulation and recombinantly produced antibodies enter the clinic in the war against cancer.

1996:   A gene associated with Parkinson's disease is discovered.

1996:   The first genetically engineered crop is commercialized.

1997: A sheep named Dolly in Scotland becomes the first animal cloned from an adult cell.

1998: FDA approves Herceptin®, a pharmacogenomic breast cancer drug for patients whose cancer overexpresses the HER2 receptor.

1999: A diagnostic test allows quick identification of Bovine Spongicorm Encephalopathy (BSE, also known as "mad cow" disease) and Creutzfeldt - Jakob disease (CJD)

2000: Kenya field-tests its first biotech crop, virus-resistant sweet potato.

2001: FDA approves Gleevec® (imatinib), a gene-targeted drug for patients with chronic myeloid leukemia. Gleevec is the first gene-targeted drug to receive FDA approval.

2002: EPA approves the first transgenic rootworm-resistant corn.

2002: The banteng, an endangered species, is cloned for the first time.

2003: China grants the world's first regulatory approval of a gene therapy product, Gendicine (Shenzhen SiBiono GenTech), which delivers the p53 gene as a therapy for squamous cell head and neck cancer.

2003: The Human Genome Project completes sequencing of the human genome.

2004: UN Food and Agriculture Organization endorse biotech crops, stating biotechnology is a complementary tool to traditional farming methods that can help poor farmers and consumers in developing nations.

2004: FDA approves the first antiangiogenic drug for cancer, Avastin®.

2005: The Energy Policy Act is passed and signed into law, authorizing numerous incentives for bioethanol development.

2006: FDA approves the recombinant vaccine Gardasil®, the first vaccine developed against human papillomavirus (HPV), an infection implicated in cervical and throat cancers, and the first preventative cancer vaccine.

2006: USDA grants Dow Agro Sciences the first regulatory approval for a plant-made vaccine.

2007:   FDA approves the H5N1 vaccine, the first vaccine approved for avian flu.

2009:   Global biotech crop acreage reaches 330 million acres.

2009:   FDA approves the first genetically engineered animal for production of a recombinant form of human antithrombin.

1.2   Scope of Biotechnology

Hereditary engineering has raised hopes for therapeutic proteins, medicines, and biological creatures such as seeds, insecticides, altered yeasts, and genetically modified human cells to treat genetic illnesses. With the introduction of gene therapy, stem cell research, cloning, and genetically modified food, the science of genetic engineering remains a hot topic of debate in today's culture.

Traditional biotechnology approaches such as plant and animal breeding, food production, fermentation products and processes, and pharmaceutical and fertiliser manufacture should all be seen as part of modern biotechnology.

1.2.1   The Key Components of Modern Biotechnology are as follows

(i)   **Genomics:** The study of all genes in a species at a molecular level.

(ii)   **Bioinformatics:** The application of information technology to evaluate and manage enormous data sets resulting from gene sequencing or related procedures, involving the assembling of data from genomic analysis into accessible formats.

(iii) **Transformation:** Incorporation of one or more genes providing potentially valuable features into plants, animals, fish, or tree species.

(iv)   Organisms with enhanced genetics

(v)   Organisms that have been genetically changed (GMO).

(vi)   Living organisms that have been changed (LMO).

(vii) **Molecular breeding:** Using marker-assisted selection (MAS) to identify and evaluate useful features in breeding programmes;

(viii) **Diagnostics:** Using molecular characterization to enable more accurate and faster pathogen identification; and

(ix) **Vaccine technology:** the use of modern immunology to the development of recombinant deoxyribonucleic acid (rDNA) vaccines for improved disease management in cattle and fish.

Biotechnology encompasses a spectrum of technologies, ranging from old biotechnology's long-established and commonly utilised procedures to unique and rapidly evolving modern biotechnology techniques (Fig.1.1).

During the 1970s, scientists developed novel technologies for exact recombination of parts of deoxyribonucleic acid (DNA), the biological material that determines hereditary features in all living cells, and for transferring portions of DNA from one organism to another. rDNA technology, often known as genetic engineering, is a set of enabling techniques.

Gradient of Biotechnologies

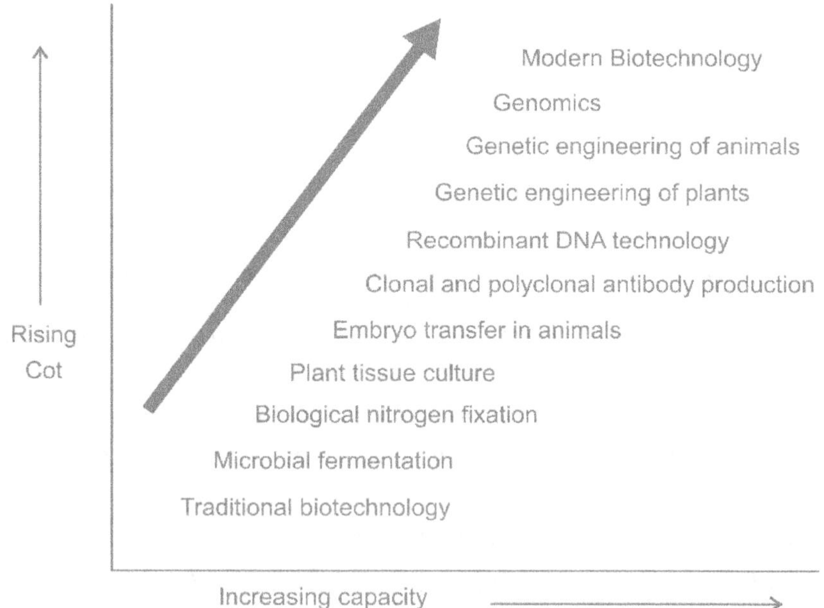

Fig. 1.1 Gradient of Biotechnologies

New techniques in rDNA technology, monoclonal and polyclonal antibodies, and new cell and tissue culture technologies are all used in modern biotechnology.

1.3 Applications of Biotechnology

(i)   Therapeutics

(ii)   Diagnostics

(iii)   Genetically modified crops for agriculture

(iv)   Processed food

(v)   Waste disposal are examples of biotechnology applications.

(vi)   Providing the best catalyst in the form of an improved organism, usually in the form of a microbe or pure enzyme

(vii)   Downstream processing technologies to purify the protein/organic molecule by engineering ideal conditions for a catalyst to work.

Agriculture and Biotechnology

There are three possibilities for increasing food production:

(i)   Agriculture based on agrochemicals.

(ii)   Genetically altered crop-based agriculture and

(iii)   Organic agriculture

Green biotechnology is the use of biotech methods in agriculture and food production. The Green Revolution was successful in raising crop yields, owing to the use of improved crop types and agrochemicals (fertilizers and pesticides).

The following are some of the benefits of using genetically engineered plants

(i)   Crops have been genetically modified to be more resistant to abiotic conditions such as cold, heat, drought, salinity, and so on.

(ii)   It has reduced crop reliance on chemical pesticides by making them pest-resistant.

(iii)   Post-harvest losses are significantly minimized.

(iv)   The early exhaustion of soil fertility is averted as plant efficiency in mineral utilization increases.

(v) The nutritional value of food generated from GM (Genetically Modified) crops has increased.

(vi) Genetic engineering has been utilised to develop custom-made plants for businesses such as starch, fuel, pharmaceuticals, and others.

Plants that are resistant to pests are grown.

(a) **Bt Cotton** is a type of cotton that has been genetically modified.

Bacillus thuringiensis, a soil bacterium, produces Cry proteins, which are harmful to insect larvae such as Tobacco budworm, armyworm, beetles, and mosquitoes. Because the alkaline pH of the gut solubilizes the crystals, the Cry proteins exist as inactive protoxins that are transformed into active toxin when swallowed by the insect. The active toxin attaches to the surface of midgut epithelial cells and causes holes to form. This induces swelling and cell lysis, resulting in the insect's death (Larva). The bacterium's genes (cry genes) producing this protein have been extracted and integrated into a variety of crop plants, including cotton, tomato, corn, rice, soybean, and others. Cry I Ac and cry II Ab control cotton bollworms, cry I Ab controls corn borer, cry III Ab controls Colorado potato beetle, and cry III Bb controls corn rootworm, respectively.

(b) **Nematode Resistance:** The nematode Meloidogyne incognita infects tobacco plants, reducing production. Using Agrobacterium as a vector, the parasite's particular genes (in the form of c DNA) are transferred into the plant. The genes are inserted in such a way that they produce both sense/coding RNA and antisense RNA (complimentary to sense/coding RNA). Because these two RNAs are complementary, they form a double-stranded RNA (ds RNA), which neutralizes the nematode's particular RNA through RNA interference. As a result, the parasite is unable to develop in the transgenic host, leaving the transgenic plant pest-free.

Biotechnology's application in medicine

The rDNA technology has been used to create more effective and safe therapeutic medications. The recombinant medicines did not cause an undesirable immune response, as is frequent with comparable compounds obtained from nonhuman sources.

(1) Insulin that has been genetically modified (Humulin)

Chain A and chain B are two short polypeptide chains connected by disulphide bridges in human insulin. Insulin is produced as a prohormone that must be converted into a mature and functioning hormone. Another polypeptide in the prohormone termed C-peptide is eliminated during maturation. In 1983, the American corporation Eli Lilly generated two DNA sequences coding for human insulin chains A and B and inserted them into plasmids of E. coli to create insulin. Disulphide bridges were used to connect the two chains that were formed.

(2) Gene therapy

Genes are injected into an individual's cells and tissues in this procedure to repair specific genetic disorders. It entails inserting a normal gene into a human or embryo to replace the gene's faulty mutant allele. Viruses that attack the host and infect it with their genetic material are all vectors. In 1990, a four-year-old girl with adenosine deaminase (ADA) deficiency received the first clinical gene therapy. In some children, bone marrow transplantation can cure ADA deficiency, however it is not totally curative. Lymphocytes were produced in a cultural and functional ADA for gene therapy. The lymphocytes are subsequently inoculated with cDNA. These lymphocytes are subsequently infused into the patient's body; the patient will need these genetically altered cells on a regular basis. It would be a permanent treatment if a functioning gene was delivered into the bone marrow cells at an early embryonic stage.

(3) Molecular diagnostics

For early diagnosis of illnesses, recombinant DNA molecules and procedures such as PCR (Polymerase Chain Reaction) are used. When the cloned gene is expressed to make recombinant proteins, it aids in the development of sensitive diagnostic tools like ELISA. The cloned genes can also be employed as 'probes' to identify complementary DNA strands. A probe is a single-stranded segment of DNA that has been labelled with a radioactive molecule and is used to hybridize with its complementary DNA to find it. After that, autoradiography is used to detect radioactivity. A approach like this can be used to detect the presence of a normal or mutant gene. PCR is used to detect HIV as well as gene mutations.

Production of Transgenic Animals

(i) Transgenic animals are those whose DNA has been modified to allow them to possess and express a foreign gene. The following are examples of how transgenic animals are used:

(ii) Transgenic animals can be produced specifically to allow researchers to investigate how genes are regulated and how they affect the body's regular functioning and development, for example. Information about the biological role of insulin-like growth factor is gathered.

(iii) The transgenic animals are engineered to act as models for human diseases in order to improve our understanding of how genes contribute to disease development.

(iv) Transgenic animals that generate useful biological products can be developed by inserting a fragment of DNA from an organism (s) that codes for that product, such as alpha-1 antitrypsin, a human protein that is used to treat emphysema. Rosie, the first transgenic cow, produced milk high in human protein (2.4g/ltr) as well as human alpha-lactalbumin, a more nutritionally balanced product for human new-borns.

(v) Transgenic mice are being generated for the purpose of assessing vaccination safety. (For example, polio vaccination).

(vi) To assess the toxicity of pharmaceuticals, transgenic animals with increased sensitivity to harmful chemicals are being produced.

Ethical Issues

When creatures are genetically modified, their consequences can be unpredictable /undesirable when they are introduced into the ecosystem. Patent issues have arisen as a result of the modification and usage of such organisms for public service. As a result, the Indian government has established an institution that is tasked with determining the legality of genetic alteration and the safety of integrating genetically modified organisms into public services. The Genetic Engineering Approval Committee is one such body (GEAC).

Biopiracy

The developed/industrialized countries are wealthy financially, but they lack biodiversity and traditional knowledge, whereas emerging and underdeveloped countries have a wealth of bioresearch and traditional knowledge. Some industrialized countries use other countries' bio resources and traditional knowledge without their permission or pay (Biopiracy). Basmati rice, which is grown in India, is known for its particular flavour and aroma. However, an American firm obtained intellectual rights to Basmati through the US copyright and trademark office, and this corporation developed a new variety of Basmati by crossing an Indian variety with semi-dwarf kinds. Some countries are currently enacting legislation to prevent such illicit use of their bioresources and traditional knowledge.

1.4   Introduction to Enzyme Biotechnology

Enzymes are biological catalysts that speed up reactions but are not consumed in the process; they can be employed over and over again as long as they are active. The term "enzyme" was coined in 1878 by German scientist Wilhelm Kuhne to describe yeast's ability to make alcohol from carbohydrates, and it is derived from the Greek words en (meaning "inside") and zume (meaning "yeast"). Many advancements were achieved in the extraction, characterisation, and commercial exploitation of enzymes in the late nineteenth and early twentieth centuries, but it wasn't until the 1920s that enzymes were crystallised, indicating that catalytic activity is related with protein molecules. For the following 60 years or so, all enzymes were thought to be proteins, but in the 1980s, it was discovered that some ribonucleic acid (RNA) molecules can also catalyse reactions. These RNAs, known as ribozymes, play a crucial function in gene expression. Biochemists developed the technology to create antibodies with catalytic characteristics throughout the same decade. These so-called 'abzymes' hold a lot of promise as new industrial catalysts and medicines. The immense catalytic activity of enzymes is likely best described by the constant kcat, often known as the turnover rate, turnover frequency, or turnover number. This constant denotes the number of substrate molecules that a single enzyme molecule may convert to product in a given amount of time (usually per minute or per second). A single molecule of carbonic anhydrase, for example, may catalyse the conversion of almost half a million molecules of its substrates, carbon dioxide (CO_2) and water (H_2O), into the product, bicarbonate (HCO_3), in less than a second—an incredible feat. Enzymes are extraordinarily potent catalysts, but they also have exceptional selectivity, catalysing the conversion of only one type (or a small number of comparable types) of substrate molecule into product molecule. Group specificity is demonstrated by some enzymes. Alkaline phosphates, for example, can remove a phosphate group from a variety of substrates (an enzyme that is typically met in first-year laboratory sessions on enzyme kinetics).

Other enzymes have substantially higher absolute specificity, which is a term used to characterise how particular they are. Glucose oxidase, for example, is almost completely selective for its substrate, -D-glucose, and has little activity with other monosaccharides. Many analytical assays and devices (biosensors) that assess a specific substrate (e.g. glucose) in a complicated mixture place a premium on specificity (e.g. a blood or urine sample).

1.4.1   Names and Classifications of Enzymes

Although individual proteolytic enzymes have the suffix -in, enzymes commonly have common names (sometimes referred to as 'trivial names') that allude to the reaction that they catalyse, with the suffix -ase (e.g. oxidase, dehydrogenase, carboxylase) (e.g. trypsin, chymotrypsin, papain). Frequently, the enzyme's common name also denotes the substrate on which it works (e.g. glucose oxidase, alcohol dehydrogenase, pyruvate decarboxylase). However, certain common names (for example, invertase, diastase, and catalase) reveal little about the substrate, product, or reaction.

The International Union of Biochemistry established the Enzyme Commission to address the growing complexity and inconsistencies in enzyme name. The first Enzyme Commission Report was released in 1961, and it outlined a method for identifying enzymes. The sixth edition, issued in 1992, had information on almost 3200 distinct enzymes, with annual supplements bringing the total to over 5000.

All enzymes are given a four-part Enzyme Commission (EC) number in this system. The enzyme lactate dehydrogenase, for example, has the EC number 1.1.1.27 and is more properly known as l–lactate: NAD+ oxidoreductase.

1.4.2   Immobilization of Enzymes

Enzymes are combined in a solution with substrates in most procedures, and they can't be economically recovered after the reaction, so they're usually thrown away. As a result, there is an incentive to use enzymes that are immobilized or insolubilized in order to keep them in a biochemical reactor for further catalysis. Enzyme immobilization is used to accomplish this.

"Enzymes physically contained or localized in a definite defined region of space with retention of their catalytic activity, and which can be used repeatedly and continuously," according to the definition of immobilized enzymes. Immobilization techniques form the foundation for a variety of biotechnology products, including diagnostics, bio-affinity chromatography, and biosensors, in addition to its use in industrial processes.

Only single immobilized enzymes were utilized at first, but from the 1970s, more complicated systems with two-enzyme reactions, cofactor regeneration, and living cells were produced. Interactions ranging from reversible physical adsorption and ionic connections to stable covalent bonds can be used to attach enzymes to the support. Although the most effective immobilization technique depends on the nature of the enzyme and the carrier, immobilization technology has become more of a question of rational design in recent years. Some features, such as catalytic activity and thermal stability, are altered as a result of enzyme immobilization. These effects have been proven and exploited in the past. For immobilizing enzymes, the concept of stabilization has been a major driving force. Furthermore, genuine molecular stabilization has been proven, such as proteins immobilized through multipoint covalent binding.

1.4.3 Enzyme Immobilization Salient Features

➤ The enzyme phase is known as the carrier phase, and it is a water insoluble but hydrophilic porous polymeric matrix, such as agarose or cellulose.

➤ Fine particulate, membranous, or microcapsule enzyme phases are all possibilities.

➤ Cross-linking allows the enzyme to bind to another enzyme.

➤ Using immobilization techniques, a unique module is created that allows fluid to readily pass through, changing the substrate into product while also allowing the catalyst to be easily removed from the product as it exits the reactor.

➤ At certain pH, ionic strength, or solvent conditions, the support or carrier used in the immobilization approach is not stable. As a result, it's possible that the enzyme component will be broken or dissolved after the reaction, releasing the enzyme component.

➤ Multiple or repetitive use of a single batch of enzymes Immobilized enzymes are usually more stable Ability to stop the reaction quickly by removing the enzyme from the reaction solution Product is not contaminated with the enzyme Easy separation of the enzyme from the product Allows development of a multienzyme reaction system Reduces effluent disposal problems.

Immobilization of enzymes has the following disadvantages

➤ It adds to the cost, and it invariably affects the stability and activity of enzymes.

➤ When one of the substrates is proven to be insoluble, the approach may not be beneficial.

➤ Certain immobilization procedures have major issues with substrate diffusion, which makes it difficult to get to the enzyme.

1.4.4   Immobilization methods for Enzymes

1. **Physical method:** Physical forces such as Vander Waals forces, hydrophobic interactions, and hydrogen bonding are used to attach enzymes to various matrices. Controlling physicochemical parameters allows the process to be reversed in nature. It consists of the methods listed below.

   (i) **Entrapment:** Physical entrapment of enzymes inside a polymer or gel matrix can immobilize them. The matrix holes are large enough to hold the enzyme while allowing the substrate and product molecules to flow through. The enzyme (or cell) is not subjected to severe binding pressures or structural distortions in this approach, known as lattice entrapment.

Changes in pH or temperature, as well as the addition of solvents, may cause some deactivation throughout the immobilization process. Polyacrylamide gel, collagen, gelatin, starch, cellulose, silicone, and rubber are some of the matrices used to entrap enzymes. This approach has multiple advantages, including simplicity, no change in intrinsic enzyme characteristics, no chemical modification, low enzyme demand,

and a variety of matrices. The following are some of the method's drawbacks: enzyme leakage, the ability to use only modest substrate/product sizes, the need for a delicate balance between the matrix's mechanical qualities and their effect on enzyme activity, and the presence of a diffusional constraint.

Enzymes can be trapped in a variety of ways

1. Inclusion of enzymes in gels

This is an enzyme entrapment within the gels.

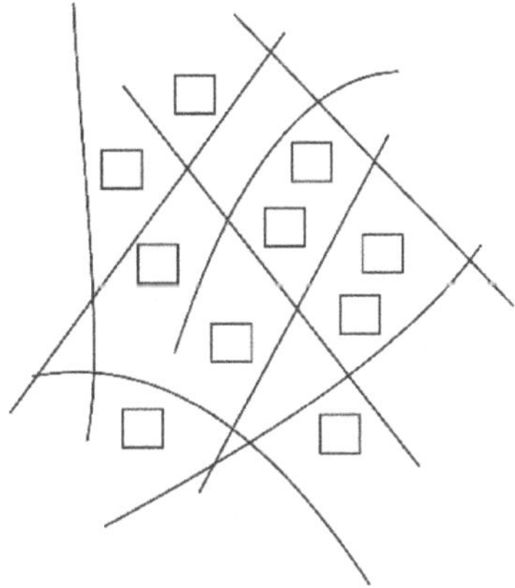

Fig. 1.2 Inclusion of enzyme in gel

2. Enzyme inclusion in fibres

The enzymes are trapped in a fibre format of the matrix

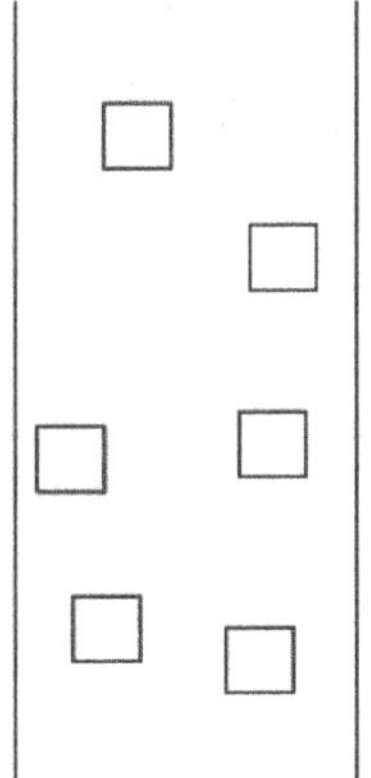

Fig. 1.3 Inclusion of enzyme in fibres

3. Enzyme inclusion in microcapsules

The enzymes are encapsulated within a microcapsule matrix in this situation. The matrix's hydrophobic and hydrophilic forms polymerize to form a microcapsule with enzyme molecules within. Enzyme entrapment is hampered by the leakage of enzymes from the matrix. For the immobilization of entire cells, most workers choose to employ the entrapment technique. In the industrial manufacture of amino acids (L-isoleucine, L-aspartic acid), L-malic acid, and hydroquinone, entrapped cells are used.

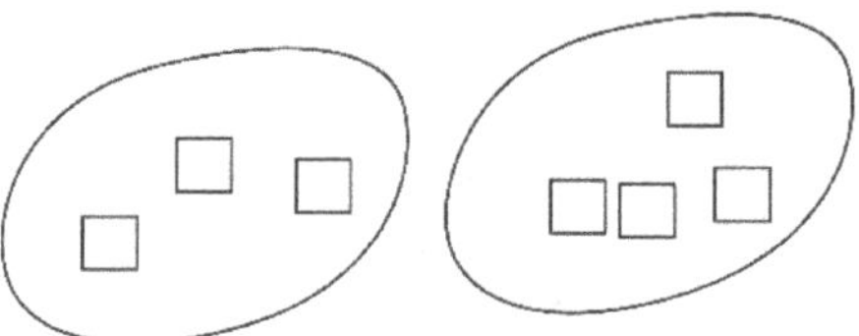

Fig. 1.4 Inclusion in microcapsules

(ii) **Adsorption:** Non-covalent linkages such as ionic or hydrophobic contacts, hydrogen bonding, and van der Waals forces attach the enzyme to the support material without any pre-activation of the support. Ceramic, alumina, activated carbon, kaolinite, bentonite, porous glass, chitosan, dextran, gelatin, cellulose, and starch are some of the organic and inorganic matrices that have been employed. pH, temperature, solvent type, ionic strength, enzyme concentration, and adsorbent concentration are all variables that must be optimized in the immobilization technique. The enzyme is applied directly to the surface (active adsorbent) without any non-adsorbed enzyme being removed during the washing process. The approach is straightforward and gentle, with a wide range of carriers available for simultaneous purification and enzyme immobilization (e.g., Asparginase on CM-cellulose) with no conformational changes. However, because a lot of parameters play a role in enzyme desorption in response to minor changes in its microenvironment, it necessitates extensive tuning. (e.g., pH, temperature, solvent, ionic strength and high substrate concentrations).

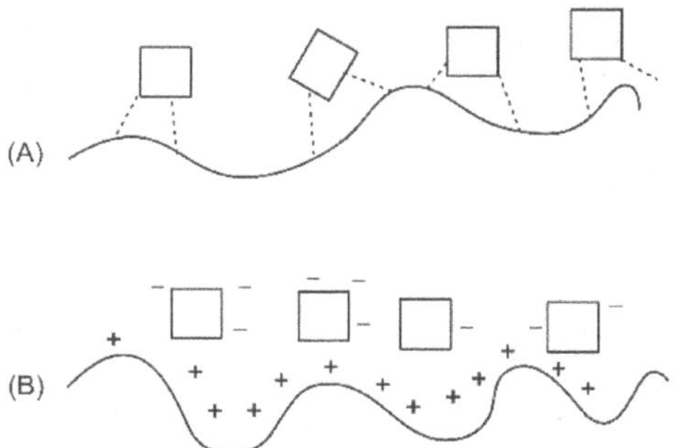

Fig. 1.5 Inclusion of Enzyme through Adsorption

(A)   Immobilized enzymes by vanderwaal forces

(B)   Immobilized enzymes by hydrogen bonds

(iii) **Microencapsulation:** Enzymes are immobilized by encapsulating them in spherical semi-permeable polymer membranes with regulated porosity (1–100m). Depending on the contents, semi-permeable membranes can be either permanent or non-permanent. Non-permanent membranes are formed of liquid surfactant, while permanent membranes are made of cellulose nitrate and polystyrene. Encapsulation of colours, medicines, and other substances is also done with these membranes. Because enzymes immobilized by encapsulation have such huge surface areas, they have a higher catalytic efficiency. Microencapsulation can be done in three different methods.

1. The construction of unique membrane reactors.

2. Emulsion formation is the second step.

3. Emulsion stabilization to create microcapsules

Recently, microencapsulation has been utilized to immobilize enzymes and mammalian cells. Microencapsulation, for example, can immobilize pancreatic cells growing in vitro. This method has also been used to successfully immobilize hybridoma cells.

2. Using Chemicals

This involves the irreversible attachment of enzymes to various matrices via covalent or ionic bonds.

(i)   **Covalent attachment:** The enzyme is attached to the matrix via covalent bonds (diazotation, amino bond, Schiff's base formation, amidation reactions, thiol-disulfide, peptide bond, and alkylation reactions). Enzyme molecules are connected to the matrix's reactive groups (e.g., hydroxyl, amide, amino, carboxyl groups) either directly or through a spacer arm, which is artificially bonded to the matrix using various chemical reactions (e.g., diazotization, etc. imine bond formation, Schiff base). Natural (e.g., glass, Sephadex, Agarose, Sepharose) or synthetic (e.g., glass, Sephadex, Agarose, Sepharose) matrices are often utilized (e.g., acrylamide, methacrylic acid, and styrene). The cost, availability, binding capacity, hydrophilicity, structural rigidity, and durability of a matrix are all factors to consider when choosing one for a certain application. Non-essential amino acids (other than active site groups) are used in this method of immobilization, resulting in minimal conformational alterations. It contributes to immobilized enzymes' increased tolerance to harsh physical and chemical environments (e.g., temperature, denaturants, organic solvents). Due to harsh immobilization circumstances and concurrence of comparable amino-groups at the active site being involved during enzyme contact with the matrix, this kind of immobilization puts more strain on the enzyme and can cause significant changes in conformational and catalytic properties.

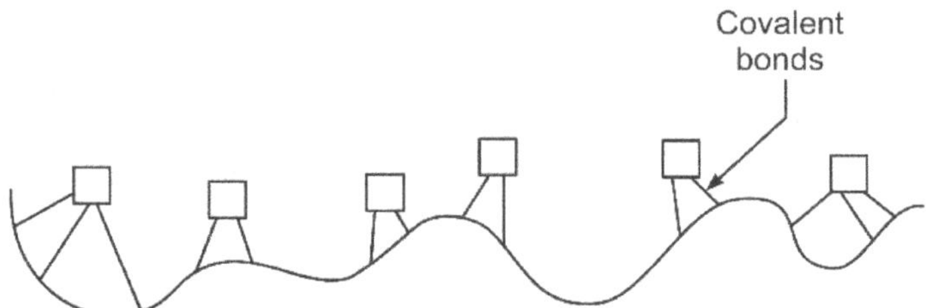

Fig. 1.6 Inclusion of Enzyme through Covalent Bonding

(ii) **Cross-Linking:** Using bi- or multi-functional reagents, a number of covalent links are formed between the enzyme and the matrix (e.g., glutardialdehyde, glutaraldehyde, glyoxal, diisocyanates, hexamethylene diisocyanate, toluene diisocyanate). Under mild conditions, lysine amino groups, cysteine sulfhydryl groups, phenolic OH groups of tyrosine, or imidazole groups of histidine are commonly employed for enzyme binding. The simplicity of this procedure is its greatest advantage. However, because to the non-regulation of the reaction, a significant amount of enzyme is lost. Furthermore, diffusion limits the effectiveness of this method of enzyme immobilization.

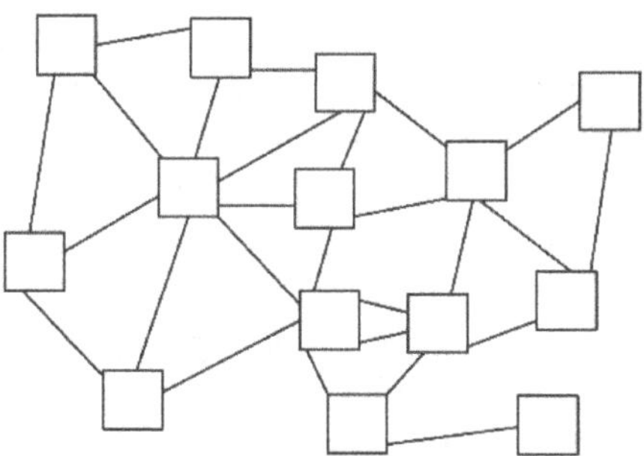

Fig. 1.7 Inclusion of Enzyme through Cross Linking

(iii) Ionic binding: Ionic interactions between enzyme molecules and a charged matrix are the basis for this method. The bigger the amount of enzyme attached to the matrix, the higher the surface charge density on the matrix. Enzyme molecules are sometimes physically adsorbed to the matrix in addition to ionic interactions. The method of enzyme immobilization is similar to that of physical adsorption, as explained before. The pH of the solution, the concentration of the enzyme, and the temperature all affect enzyme binding via ionic interactions during immobilization. Polysaccharide derivatives (e.g., diethylaminoethylcellulose, dextran, carboxymethylcellulose, chitosan), synthetic polymers (e.g., polyethylene vinyl alcohol), and inorganic materials are all often used matrices (e.g., Amberlite, alumina, silicates, bentonite, sepiolite, silica gel). Because of this approach of immobilization, only minor modifications in enzyme structure occur.

However, because there is a higher risk of enzyme detachment from the matrix under suboptimal conditions, extra attention is paid to maintaining proper ionic strength and pH of the fluid in which the immobilized enzyme conducts catalysis.

(iv) Affinity ligands: Specific ligands are employed to attach the enzyme to the matrix, such as the his-tag on the enzyme to a metal-containing matrix, the lectin-containing domain to carbohydrate moieties on the matrix, or sometimes substrate-mimicking chemical compounds. In some situations, ligands are naturally present on the enzyme; in others, they are intentionally attached by fusing a nucleotide sequence corresponding to the tag with the DNA encoding a polypeptide of the given enzyme. Due to the non-involvement of active site residues and higher immobilization efficiency due to the presence of high densities of ligands on the matrix, this method of immobilization results in minimal changes in enzyme configuration, with high stability and catalytic efficiency of the immobilized enzyme. This approach can be used to immobilize a variety of proteins, including antibodies, cytokines, streptavidin, and others. Enzymes that have been immobilized via this approach have been used in biotechnology, diagnostics, and medicine. This approach has also been utilized in animal cell culture to connect several types of mammalian cells to diverse matrices containing a range of peptides, growth factors, and cytokines to a specific binding domain located on the cell, as well as to activate them.

1.4.5   Matrices Employed in the Immobilization of Enzymes

Enzymes are either adhered to the surface of matrices or entrapped inside them by physical or chemical means during enzyme immobilization.

The following are the matrices that were utilized to immobilize enzymes:

Surface-Bound Enzymes

The chemical, biological, mechanical, and kinetic properties of immobilized enzymes are all governed by the physical and chemical properties of the matrices employed for enzyme immobilization. Biopolymer, synthetic organic polymer, hydrogels, smart polymer, or inorganic solid can all be used as the matrix.

- Biopolymers are polysaccharides that are insoluble in water (e.g., cellulose, starch, agarose, chitosan, and proteins such as gelatin and albumin).

- **Synthetic organic polymers**

  Eupergit-C (acrylic resins), Sepa beads FP-EP, Amberlite XAD-7 (porous acrylic resins), and other synthetic organic polymers are utilised for enzyme immobilisation. Eupergit-C has a 170 mm surface diameter and a 25 nm pore diameter. N,N′-methylene-bi-(methacrylamide), methacrylamide, allyl glycidyl ether, and glycidyl methacrylate are used to make it. It's hydrophilic and chemically and mechanically stable across a pH range of 0–14. It possesses a high density of oxirane moieties on its surface, which allows it to bind several enzymes via covalent connections at neutral or alkaline pH. As a result, it provides long-term operating stability throughout a broad pH range (1–12).

- Alumina, silica, zeolites, and mesoporous silicas are examples of inorganic solids (MCM-41, and SBA-15). They are known to be the most cost-effective matrix for immobilising a variety of industrial and non-industrial enzymes.

- **Smart Polymer**

  The thermostable biocompatible polymer [poly-N-isopropylacrylamide (polyNIPAM)] is the best studied example of smart polymer. PolyNIPAM has the unusual feature of existing in two states: solution when the temperature is below 32 °C and polymer when the temperature is above 32 °C.

1.4.6   Immobilized Enzymes and Cells Have a Wide Range of Applications

(i) **Application in Biomedicine:** In medicine, immobilised enzymes are used to diagnose and cure illnesses. The inborn metabolic insufficiency can be remedied by substituting waste metabolites with encapsulated enzymes (i.e., enzymes encapsulated by erythrocytes). The RBC works as a carrier for exogenous enzyme medicines, and the enzymes are biocompatible in nature, thus there is no immune response. Enzyme encapsulation through electroporation is the simplest method of immobilisation in the biomedical area, and it is a reversible procedure with the ability to renew the enzyme. When enzymes are coupled with biomaterials, biological and functional systems are created. Biomaterials are utilised to mend defects in tissue engineering applications. In biomedicine, the advantage of enzyme immobilisation is that free enzymes are devoured by cells and are not active for long periods of time, thus the immobilised enzymes remain stable, stimulating growth and repairing defects. The distribution of enzymes to oncogenic regions in cancer therapy has been improved with innovative approaches. Nanoparticles and nanospheres are frequently utilised as enzyme carriers for therapeutic drug delivery.

(ii) **Application in the food industry:** Purified enzymes are employed in the food business, but the enzymes denature throughout the purifying process. As a result of the immobilisation approach, the enzymes are stable. Syrups are made with the enzymes that have been immobilised. Immobilized beta-galactosidase is used in the manufacturing of baker's yeast to hydrolyze lactose in whey.

(iii) **Production of Biodiesel:** Biodiesel is made up of monoalkyl esters of long-chain fatty acids. Biodiesel is made by esterifying alcohol (methanol, ethanol) with triglycerides (vegetable oil, animal fat) in the presence of a catalyst. High energy consumption, glycerol recovery, and side reactions that may pollute the environment are among disadvantages of catalyst manufacture. As a result, the biological synthesis of liquid fuel with lipases is currently receiving a lot of attention and is rapidly improving. Lipase catalyses the reaction with less energy and at more benign conditions. However, lipase manufacturing is expensive, resulting in lipase immobilisation, which allows for recurrent use and stability. Because methanol inactivates lipase in the biological generation of biodiesel, the immobilisation approach is advantageous for biodiesel production.

(iv) **Wastewater Treatment:** As the consumption of fresh water and water bodies rises, they are more mixed with polluted industrial waste water, necessitating waste water treatment. Textile, paper, and leather industries are all sources of dye effluents, and the effluents are high in dye colourants. These effluents are hazardous to the environment and are carcinogenic even at low concentrations. Enzymes are being utilised to breakdown colouring materials. Preoxidases, laccase, and azo reductases are enzymes used in wastewater treatment. Extreme temperatures, low or high pH, and high ionic strength can cause these enzymes to lose their function; to alleviate this problem, immobilised enzymes are utilised.

(v) **Textile Industry:** Microbially generated enzymes are of tremendous interest in the textile industry. Cellulase, amylase, liccase, pectinase, cutinase, and other enzymes are employed in a variety of textile applications, including scouring, biopolishing, desizing, denim finishing, and wool treatment. Cellulase is one of these enzymes that has been widely employed from the beginning to the present. Instead of employing harsh chemicals that pollute the environment and harm materials, the textile industry has moved to enzyme processes. The processing of fabrics with enzymes necessitates high temperatures and elevated pH, which free enzymes are unable to handle. As a result, enzyme immobilisation for this technique can tolerate high temperatures and keep its activity for more than 5-6 cycles.

(vi) Detergent Industry: Enzymes are also used in the detergent industry to remove stains. Protease is an enzyme used in the detergent business to remove stains such as blood, egg, grass, and human sweat. Amylase is a starch-based enzyme that can be used to remove stains from potatoes, gravies, and chocolate. Lipase is an enzyme that is used to remove oil and fat stains as well as stains in cuffs and collars. For cotton-based materials, cellulase is used to increase softening, colour brightening, and soil stain removal. In today's detergent industry, biotech cleaning ingredients are frequently employed. Biobased detergents have superior cleaning properties as compared to synthetic detergents. When opposed to synthetic detergents, enzyme-based detergents can be used in lower quantities, have greater biodegradability, do not harm the environment, and operate well at low temperatures; these are the advantages of enzymes in the detergent sector.

1.4.7 Manufacture of Commercial Products

A selected list of important immobilized enzymes and their industrial applications is given in the following Table. 1.1

Table 1.1 List of Immobilized Enzymes

Immobilized enzyme	*Application(s)*
Aminoacylase	Production of L-amino acids from D, L-acyl amino acids
Glucose isomerase	Production of high fructose syrup from glucose (or starch)
Amylase	Production of glucose from starch
Invertase	Splitting of sucrose to glucose and fructose
β-Galactosidase	Splitting of lactose to glucose and galactose
Penicillin acylase	Commercial production of semi-synthetic penicillins
Aspartase	Production of aspartic acid from fumaric acid
Fumarase	Synthesis of malic acid from fumaric acid
Histidine ammonia lyase	Production of urocanic acid from histidine
Ribonuclease	Synthesis of nucleotides from RNA
Nitrilase	Production of acrylamide from acrylonitrile

Here are some specifics on the production of L-amino acids and high fructose syrup.

L-Amino Acid Production

L-amino acids (rather than D-amino acids) are essential for usage in food and feed supplements, as well as medical applications. The chemical processes used to make them produce a racemic combination of D- and L-amino acids. D, L-acyl amino acids can be formed by acylation. Aminoacylase, an immobilised enzyme (often found on DEAE sephadex), may hydrolyze D, L-acyl amino acids to generate L-amino acids.

$$\text{D, L-Acyl amino acids} \xrightarrow{\text{Aminoacylase}} \text{L-Amino acids} + \text{D, L-Acyl amino acids}$$

The unhydrolyzed D-acyl amino acids can be isolated from the free L-amino acids. The latter can be degraded into D, L-acyl amino acids and recycled using an enzyme reactor with immobilised Aminoacylase. This method produces massive amounts of L-methionine, L-phenylalanine, L-tryptophan, and L-valine all over the world.

High Fructose Syrup Production

Fructose is the sweetest of the monosaccharides, with sweetening power twice that of sucrose. Glucose is around 75% sweeter than sucrose. As a result, glucose (the most prevalent monosaccharide) cannot be used as a sweetener in place of sucrose. As a result, there is a high need for fructose, a sweet sugar that has the same calorific value as glucose or sucrose.

The quantities of glucose and fructose in high fructose syrup (HFS) are nearly equal. From a nutritional standpoint, HFS is essentially identical to sugar. In the manufacture of soft beverages and processed foods and baking, HFS is a good substitute for sugar.

Using an immobilised enzyme called glucose isomerase, high fructose syrup can be made from glucose. Hydrolysis is used to create glucose from starch-containing raw materials (wheat, potato, corn). Following that, glucose isomerase isomerizes glucose to fructose. HFS, which contains around 50% fructose, is the end product. (Note: Some publications refer to HFS as high fructose corn syrup, abbreviated as HFCS.)

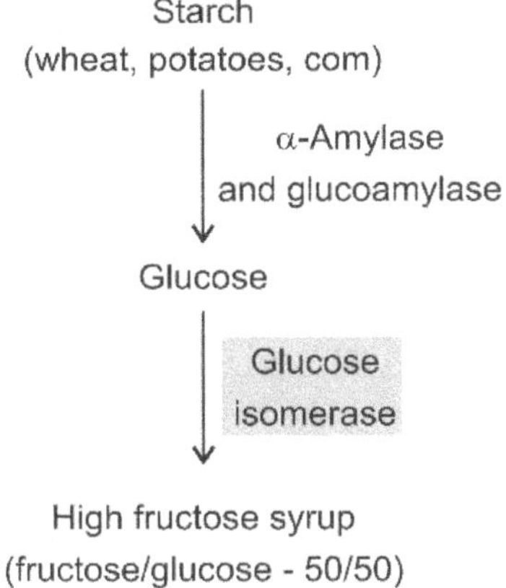

Production of high fructose syrup from starch (glucose isomerase is the immobilized enzyme)

Glucose isomerise The intracellular enzyme glucose isomerase is generated by a variety of bacteria. The ideal sources include Arthrobacter, Bacillus, and Streptomyces species. Because glucose isomerase is an intracellular enzyme, isolating it without losing its biological function necessitates the use of specialised and expensive procedures. Whole or partially fragmented cells are frequently immobilised and employed.

1.4.8   Analytical Applications of Immobilized Enzymes and Cell

In Biochemical Analysis

Immobilized enzymes (or cells) can be utilised in biochemical analysis to build precise and specialised analytical techniques for the quantification of a variety of biochemical substances.

Table 1.2 Immobilized enzymes used in analytical biochemistry

Immobilized enzyme	Substance assayed
Glucose oxidase	Glucose
Urease	Urea
Cholesterol oxidase	Cholesterol

Table 1.2 *contd…*

Immobilized enzyme	Substance assayed
Lactate dehydrogenase	Lactate
Alcohol oxidase	Alcohol
Hexokinase	ATP
Galactose oxidase	Galactose
Penicillinase	Penicillin
Ascorbic acid oxidase	Ascorbic acid
L-Amino acid oxidase	L-Amino acids
Cephalosporinase	Cephalosporin
Monoamine oxidase	Monoamine

Examples of immobilized enzymes used in analytical biochemistry

The action of the immobilised enzyme on the substrate is crucial to the analytical assay principle. The assay can be performed with a drop in substrate concentration, a rise in product level, or a change in cofactor concentration. There are two types of detection systems that are routinely used.

Thermistors are heat measuring devices that can record the heat created in a reaction catalysed by an enzyme. Potential changes in the reaction system are measured using electrode devices. An enzyme thermistor and an enzyme electrode, as well as a specialised urease electrode, are shown in the diagram below (Fig. 1.1).

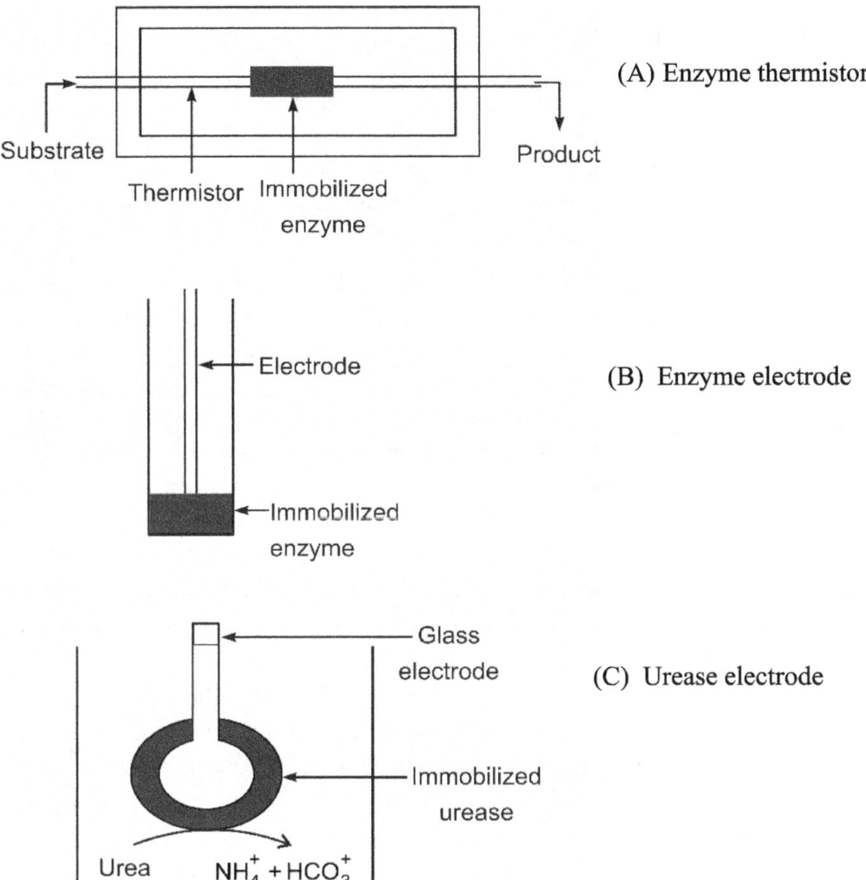

Fig. 1.8 Immobilized enzymes or cells in analytical biochemistry

In Affinity Chromatography and Purification

Immobilized enzymes can be employed in affinity chromatography and purification. It is feasible to purify a variety of chemicals using affinity, such as antigens, antibodies, and cofactors.

1.5   Biosensors

A biosensor is an analytical device which converts a biological response into an electrical signal (Fig. 1.**9**). The term 'biosensor' is often used to cover sensor devices used in order to determine the concentration of substances and other parameters of biological interest even where they do not utilize a biological system directly.

Biosensors represent a rapidly expanding field, at the present time, with an estimated 60% annual growth rate; the major impetus coming from the health-care industry (e.g. 6% of the western world are diabetic and would benefit from the availability of a rapid, accurate and simple biosensor for glucose) but with some pressure from other areas, such as food quality appraisal and environmental monitoring. Research and development in this field is wide and multidisciplinary, spanning biochemistry, bioreactor science, physical chemistry, electrochemistry, electronics and software engineering. Most of this current approach concerns potentiometric and amperometric biosensors and colorimetric paper enzyme strips. A successful biosensor must possess at least some of the following beneficial features:

1. The biocatalyst must be highly specific for the purpose of the analyses, be stable under normal storage conditions and, show good stability over a large number of assays (i.e. much greater than 100).

2. The reaction should be as independent of such physical parameters as stirring, pH and temperature as is manageable.

3. The response should be accurate, precise, reproducible and linear over the useful analytical range, without dilution or concentration. It should also be free from electrical noise.

4. If the biosensor is to be used for invasive monitoring in clinical situations, the probe must be tiny and biocompatible, having no toxic or antigenic effects. If it is to be used in fermenters it should be sterilisable. This is preferably performed by autoclaving but no biosensor enzymes can presently withstand such drastic wet-heat treatment. In either case, the biosensor should not be prone to fouling or proteolysis.

5. The complete biosensor should be cheap, small, portable and capable of being used by semi-skilled operators.

6. There should be a market for the biosensor

The biological response of the biosensor is determined by the biocatalytic membrane which accomplishes the conversion of reactant to product. Immobilised enzymes possess a number of advantageous features which makes them particularly applicable for use in such systems. They may be re-used, which ensures that the same catalytic activity is present for a series of analyses. This is an important factor in securing reproducible results and avoids the pitfalls associated with the replicate pipetting of free enzyme proportionality constant, k_L, in equation. Even if total dependence on the external diffusional rate is not achieved (or achievable), any increase in the dependence of the reaction rate on external or internal diffusion will cause a reduction in the dependence on the pH, ionic strength, temperature and inhibitor concentrations.

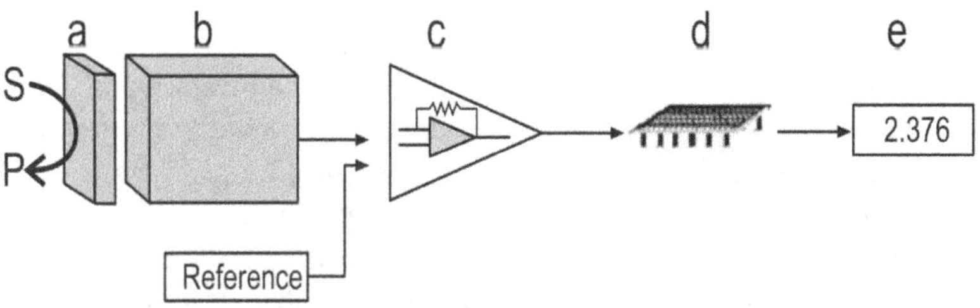

Fig. 1.9 Schematic diagram showing the main components of a biosensor. The biocatalyst (a) converts the substrate to product. This reaction is determined by the transducer (b) which converts it to an electrical signal. The output from the transducer is amplified (c) processed (d) and displayed (e).

The key part of a biosensor is the transducer (shown as the 'black box' in Fig. 1.9) which makes use of a physical change accompanying the reaction. This may be

1. The heat output (or absorbed) by the reaction (calorimetric biosensors),

2. Changes in the distribution of charges causing an electrical potential to be produced (potentiometric biosensors),

3. Movement of electrons produced in a redox reaction (amperometric biosensors),

4. Light output during the reaction or a light absorbance difference between the reactants and products (optical biosensors), or

5. Effects due to the mass of the reactants or products (piezo-electric biosensors).

There are three so-called 'generations' of biosensors;

First generation biosensors where the normal product of the reaction diffuses to the transducer and causes the electrical response, second generation biosensors which involve specific 'mediators' between the reaction and the transducer in order to generate improved response, and third generation biosensors where the reaction itself causes the response and no product or mediator diffusion is directly involved.

The electrical signal from the transducer is often low and superimposed upon a relatively high and noisy (i.e. containing a high frequency signal component of an apparently random nature, due to electrical interference or generated within the electronic components of the transducer) baseline.

The signal processing normally involves subtracting a 'reference' baseline signal, derived from a similar transducer without any biocatalytic membrane, from the sample signal, amplifying the resultant signal difference and electronically filtering (smoothing) out the unwanted signal noise. The relatively slow nature of the biosensor response considerably eases the problem of electrical noise filtration. The analogue signal produced at this stage may be output directly but is usually converted to a digital signal and passed to a microprocessor stage where the data is processed, converted to concentration units and output to a display device or data store.

1.5.1   Calorimetric Biosensors

Many enzyme catalyzed reactions are exothermic, generating heat (Table 1.3) which may be used as a basis for measuring the rate of reaction and, hence, the analyte concentration. This represents the most generally applicable type of biosensor. The temperature changes are usually determined by means of thermistors at the entrance and exit of small packed bed columns containing immobilized enzymes within a constant temperature environment (Fig. 1.10. Under such closely controlled conditions, up to 80% of the heat generated in the reaction may be registered as a temperature change in the sample stream. This may be simply calculated from the enthalpy change and the amount reacted. If a 1 mM reactant is completely converted to product in a reaction generating 100 kJ mole^{-1} then each ml of solution generates 0.1 J of heat. At 80% efficiency, this will cause a change in temperature of the solution amounting to approximately 0.02 C. This is about the temperature change commonly encountered and necessitates a temperature resolution of 0.0001 C for the biosensor to be generally useful.

Table 1.3 Heat Output (Molar enthalpies) of Enzyme Catalyzed Reactions

Reactant	Enzyme	Heat output -DH (kJ mole^{-1})
Cholesterol	Cholesterol oxidase	53
Esters	Chymotrypsin	4 - 16
Glucose	Glucose oxidase	80
Hydrogen peroxide	Catalase	100
Penicillin G	Penicillinase	67
Peptides	Trypsin	10 - 30
Starch	Amylase	8
Sucrose	Invertase	20
Urea	Urease	61
Uric acid	Uricase	49

1.5.2   Potentiometric Biosensors

Potentiometric biosensors make use of ion-selective electrodes in order to transduce the biological reaction into an electrical signal. In the simplest terms this consists of an immobilised enzyme membrane surrounding the probe from a pH-meter (Fig. 1.11), where the catalysed reaction generates or absorbs hydrogen ions (Table 1.4). The reaction occurring next to the thin sensing glass membrane causes a change in pH which may be read directly from the pH-meter's display. Typical of the use of such electrodes is that the electrical potential is determined at very high impedance allowing effectively zero current flow and causing no interference with the reaction.

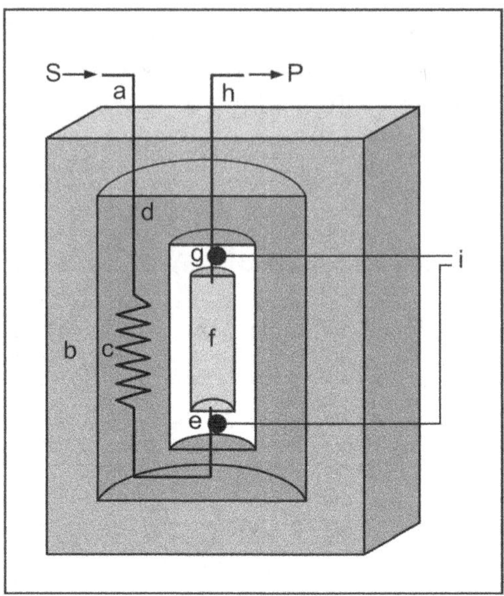

Fig. 1.10 Schematic diagram of a calorimetric biosensor. The sample stream (a) passes through the outer insulated box (b) to the heat exchanger (c) within an aluminium block (d). From there, it flows past the reference thermistor (e) and into the packed bed bioreactor (f) 1ml volume), containing the biocatalyst, where the reaction occurs. The change in temperature is determined by the thermistor (g) and the solution passed to waste (h). External electronics (l) determines the difference in the resistance, and hence temperature, between the thermistors.

There are three types of ion-selective electrodes which are of use in biosensors:

Glass electrodes for cations (e.g. normal pH electrodes) in which the sensing element is a very thin hydrated glass membrane which generates a transverse electrical potential due to the concentration-dependent competition between the cations for

1. Specific binding sites. The selectivity of this membrane is determined by the composition of the glass. The sensitivity to H^+ is greater than that achievable for NH_4^+,

2. Glass pH electrodes coated with a gas-permeable membrane selective for CO_2, NH_3 or H_2S. The diffusion of the gas through this membrane causes a change in pH of a sensing solution between the membrane and the electrode which is then determined.

3. Solid-state electrodes where the glass membrane is replaced by a thin membrane of a specific ion conductor made from a mixture of silver sulphide and a silver halide. The iodide electrode is useful for the determination of I⁻ in the peroxidase reaction (Table 1.4) and also responds to cyanide ions.

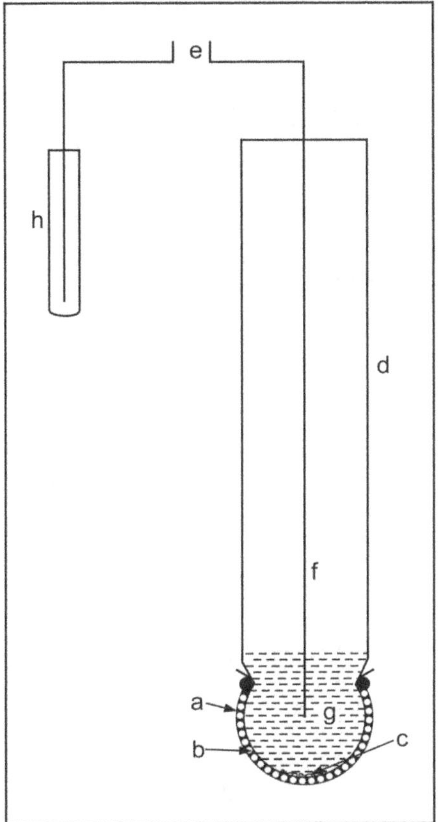

Fig. 1.11 A simple potentiometric biosensor. A semi-permeable membrane (a) surrounds the biocatalyst (b) entrapped next to the active glass membrane (c) of a pH probe (d). The electrical potential (e) is generated between the internal Ag/AgCl electrode (f) bathed in dilute HCl (g) and an external reference electrode (h)

Table 1.4 Reactions involving the Release or Absorption of Ions that may be utilized by Potentiometric Biosensors.

(a) H^+ cation,

glucose oxidase H_2O
D-glucose $+ O_2 \rightarrow$ D-glucono-1,5-lactone $+ H_2O_2 \rightarrow$ D-gluconate $+ H^+$

penicillinase
penicillin $\rightarrow$ penicilloic acid $+ H^+$

urease (pH 6.0)[a]——
$H_2NCONH_2 + H_2O + 2H^+ \rightarrow 2NH_4^+ + CO_2$

urease (pH 9.5)[b]
$H_2NCONH_2 + 2H_2O \rightarrow 2NH_3 + HCO_3^- + H^+$

lipase
neutral lipids $+ H_2O \rightarrow$ glycerol $+$ fatty acids $+ H^+$

(b) NH_4^+ cation,

L-amino acid oxidase
L-amino acid $+ O_2 + H_2O \rightarrow$ keto acid $+ NH_4^+ + H_2O_2$

asparaginase `
L-asparagine $+ H_2O \rightarrow$ L-aspartate $+ NH_4^+$

urease (pH 7.5)
$H_2NCONH_2 + 2H_2O + H^+ \rightarrow 2NH_4^+ + HCO_3^-$

(c) I^- anion,

peroxidase
$H_2O_2 + 2H^+ + 2I^- \rightarrow I_2 + 2H_2O$

(d) CN^- anion,

b-glucosidase
amygdalin $+ 2H_2O \rightarrow$ 2glucose $+$ benzaldehyde $+ H^+ + CN^-$

[a] Can also be used in NH_4^+ and CO_2 (gas) potentiometric biosensors.

[b] Can also be used in an NH_3 (gas) potentiometric biosensor.es80ll66bp

A recent development from ion-selective electrodes is the production of ion-selective field effect transistors (ISFETs) and their biosensor use as enzyme-linked field effect transistors (**ENFETs, Fig. 1.14**). Enzyme membranes are coated on the ion-selective gates of these electronic devices, the biosensor responding to the electrical potential change via the current output. Thus, these are potentiometric devices although they directly produce changes in the electric current. The main advantage of such devices is their extremely small size ($<< 0.1$ mm^2) which allows cheap mass-produced fabrication using integrated circuit technology. As an example, a urea-sensitive FET (ENFET containing bound urease with a reference electrode containing bound glycine) has been shown to show only a 15% variation in response to urea (0.05 - 10.0 mg ml^{-1}) during its active lifetime of a month. Several analytes may be determined by miniaturised biosensors containing arrays of ISFETs and ENFETs. The sensitivity of FETs, however, may be affected by the composition, ionic strength and concentrations of the solutions analyzed.

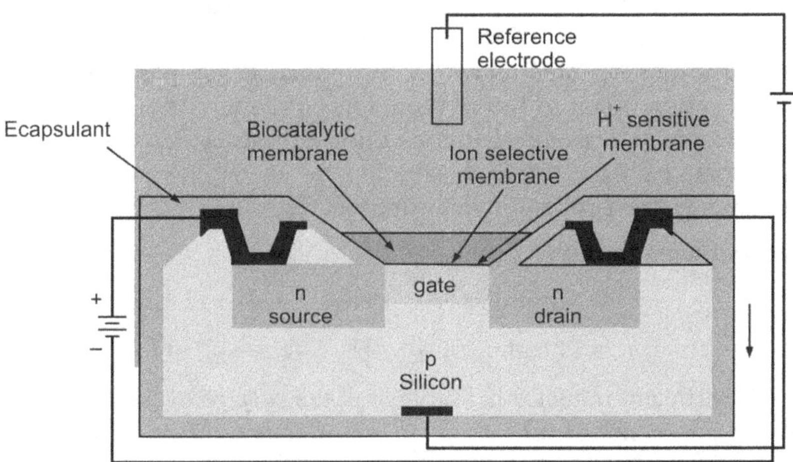

Fig. 1.12 Schematic diagram of the section across the width of an ENFET

The actual dimensions of the active area are about 500 mm long by 50 mm wide by 300 mm thick. The main body of the biosensor is a p-type silicon chip with two n-type silicon areas; the negative source and the positive drain. The chip is insulated by a thin layer (0.1 mm thick) of silica (SiO_2) which forms the gate of the FET. Above this gate is an equally thin layer of H$^+$-sensitive material (e.g. tantalum oxide), a protective ion selective membrane, the biocatalyst and the analyte solution, which is separated from sensitive parts of the FET by an inert encapsulating polyimide photopolymer. When a potential is applied between the electrodes, a current flows through the FET dependent upon the positive potential detected at the ion-selective gate and its consequent attraction of electrons into the depletion layer. This current (I) is compared with that from a similar, but non-catalytic ISFET immersed in the same solution. (Note that the electric current is, by convention, in the opposite direction to the flow of electrons).

1.5.3   Amperometric Biosensors

Amperometric biosensors function by the production of a current when a potential is applied between two electrodes. They generally have response times, dynamic ranges and sensitivities similar to the potentiometric biosensors. The simplest amperometric biosensors in common usage involve the Clark oxygen electrode (Fig. 1.13). This consists of a platinum cathode at which oxygen is reduced and a silver/silver chloride reference electrode. When a potential of -0.6 V, relative to the Ag/AgCl electrode is applied to the platinum cathode, a current proportional to the oxygen concentration is produced. Normally both electrodes are bathed in a solution of saturated potassium chloride and separated from the bulk solution by an oxygen-permeable plastic membrane (e.g. Teflon, polytetrafluoroethylene).

The following reactions occur:

$$\text{Ag anode } 4Ag^0 + 4Cl^- \rightarrow 4AgCl + 4e^-$$

$$\text{Pt cathode } O_2 + 4H^+ + 4e^- \rightarrow 2H_2O$$

The efficient reduction of oxygen at the surface of the cathode causes the oxygen concentration there to be effectively zero. The rate of this electrochemical reduction therefore depends on the rate of diffusion of the oxygen from the bulk solution, which is dependent on the concentration gradient and hence the bulk oxygen concentration. It is clear that a small, but significant, proportion of the oxygen present in the bulk is consumed by this process; the oxygen electrode measuring the rate of a process which is far from equilibrium, whereas ion-selective electrodes are used close to equilibrium conditions. This causes the oxygen electrode to be much more sensitive to changes in the temperature than potentiometric sensors. A typical application for this simple type of biosensor is the determination of glucose concentrations by the use of an immobilized glucose oxidase membrane.

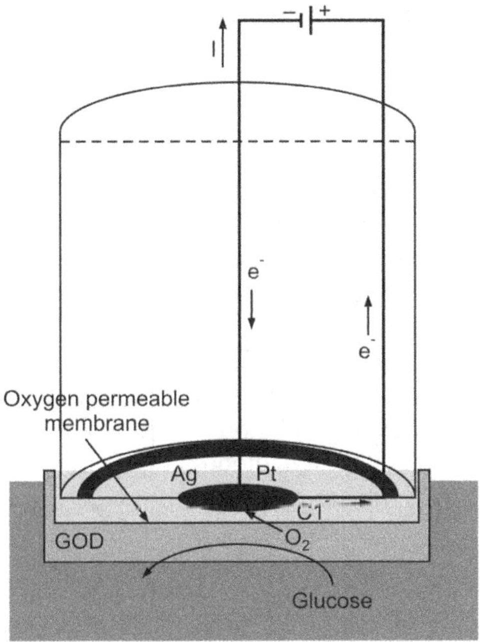

Fig. 1.13 Schematic diagram of a simple amperometric biosensor

A potential is applied between the central platinum cathode and the annular silver anode. This generates a current (I) which is carried between the electrodes by means of a saturated solution of KCl. This electrode compartment is separated from the biocatalyst (here shown glucose oxidase, GOD) by a thin plastic membrane, permeable only to oxygen. The analyte solution is separated from the biocatalyst by another membrane, permeable to the substrate(s) and product(s). This biosensor is normally about 1 cm in diameter but has been scaled down to 0.25 mm diameter using a Pt wire cathode within a silver plated steel needle anode and utilizing dip-coated membranes.

An alternative method for determining the rate of this reaction is to measure the production of hydrogen peroxide directly by applying a potential of +0.68 V to the platinum electrode, relative to the Ag/AgCl electrode, and causing the reactions:

$$\text{Pt anode } H_2O_2 \rightarrow O_2 + 2H^+ + 2e^-$$

$$\text{Ag cathode } 2AgCl + 2e^- \rightarrow 2Ag^0 + 2Cl$$

1.5.4   Optical Biosensors

There are two main areas of development in optical biosensors.

These involve determining changes in light absorption between the reactants and products of a reaction, or measuring the light output by a luminescent process. The former usually involve the widely established, if rather low technology, use of colorimetric test strips. These are disposable single-use cellulose pads impregnated with enzyme and reagents. The most common use of this technology is for whole-blood monitoring in diabetes control. In this case, the strips include glucose oxidase, horseradish peroxidase (EC 1.11.1.7) and a chromogen (e.g. *o*-toluidine or 3,3',5,5'-tetramethylbenzidine). The hydrogen peroxide, produced by the aerobic oxidation of glucose), oxidising the weakly colored chromogen to a highly coloured dye.

1.5.4.1 Peroxidase

$$\text{Chromogen(2H)} + H_2O_2 \rightarrow \text{dye} + 2H_2O$$

The evaluation of the dyed strips is best achieved by the use of portable reflectance meters, although direct visual comparison with a colored chart is often used. A wide variety of test strips involving other enzymes are commercially available at the present time. A most promising biosensor involving luminescence uses firefly luciferase (*Photinus*-luciferin 4-monooxygenase (ATP-hydrolysing), EC 1.13.12.7) to detect the presence of bacteria in food or clinical samples. Bacteria are specifically lysed and the ATP released (roughly proportional to the number of bacteria present) reacted with D-luciferin and oxygen in a reaction which produces yellow light in high quantum yield.

1.5.4.2 Luciferase

$$\text{ATP} + \text{D-luciferin} + O_2 \rightarrow \text{oxyluciferin} + \text{AMP} +$$

$$\text{pyrophosphate} + CO_2 + \text{light (562 nm)}$$

The light produced may be detected photometrically by use of high-voltage, and expensive, photomultiplier tubes or low-voltage cheap photodiode systems. The sensitivity of the photomultiplier-containing systems is, at present, somewhat greater ($< 10^4$ cells ml^{-1}, $< 10^{-12}$ M ATP) than the simpler photon detectors which use photodiodes. Firefly luciferase is a very expensive enzyme, only obtainable from the tails of wild fireflies. Use of immobilized luciferase greatly reduces the cost of these analyses.

1.5.5   Piezo-Electric Biosensors

Piezo-electric crystals (e.g. quartz) vibrate under the influence of an electric field. The frequency of this oscillation (f) depends on their thickness and cut, each crystal having a characteristic resonant frequency. This resonant frequency changes as molecules adsorb or desorb from the surface of the crystal, obeying the relationships

$$\Delta f = \frac{kf^2 \Delta m}{A}$$

Where Δf is the change in resonant frequency (Hz), Δm is the change in mass of adsorbed material (g), K is a constant for the particular crystal dependent on such factors as its density and cut, and A is the adsorbing surface area (cm^2). f = frequency of piezoelectric quartz crystal in MHz, for any piezo-electric crystal, the change in frequency is proportional to the mass of absorbed material, up to about a 2% change. This frequency change is easily detected by relatively unsophisticated electronic circuits. A simple use of such a transducer is a formaldehyde biosensor, utilizing a formaldehyde dehydrogenase coating immobilized to a quartz crystal and sensitive to gaseous formaldehyde.

The major drawbacks: These devices are the interference from atmospheric humidity and the difficulty in using them for the determination of material in solution.

Advantages: They are, however, inexpensive, small and robust, and capable of giving a rapid response.

1.5.6   Immunosensors

Biosensors may be used in conjunction with enzyme-linked immunosorbent assays (**ELISA**). The principles behind the ELISA technique are shown in Fig. 1.14. ELISA is used to detect and amplify an antigen-antibody reaction; the amount of enzyme-linked antigen bound to the immobilized antibody being determined by the relative concentration of the free and conjugated antigen and quantified by the rate of enzymic reaction. Enzymes with high turnover numbers are used in order to achieve rapid response. The sensitivity of such assays may be further enhanced by utilizing enzyme-catalyzed reactions which give intrinsically greater response; for instance, those giving rise to highly colored, fluorescent or bioluminescent products. Assay kits using this technique are now available for a vast range of analyses.

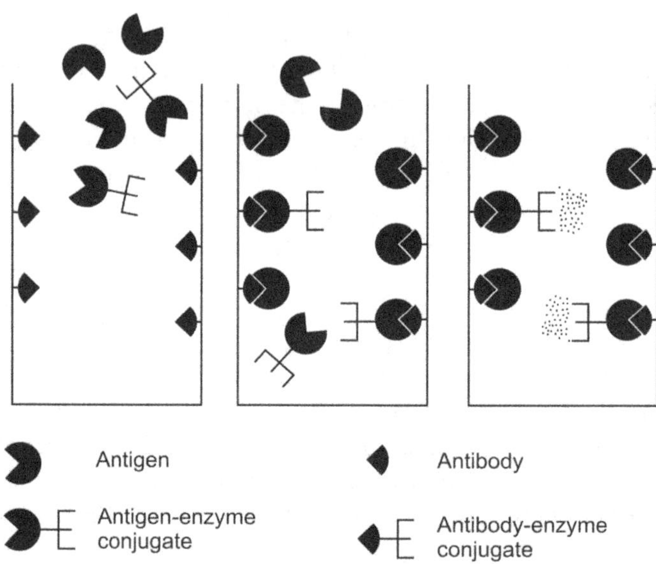

Fig. 1.14 Principles of a direct competitive ELISA. (i) Antibody, specific for the antigen of interest is immobilized on the surface of a tube. A mixture of a known amount of antigen-enzyme conjugate plus unknown concentration of sample antigen is placed in the tube and allowed to equilibrate. (ii) After a suitable period the antigen and antigen-enzyme conjugate will be distributed between the bound and free states dependent upon their relative concentrations. (iii) Unbound material is washed off and discarded. The amount of antigen-enzyme conjugate that is bound may be determined by the rate of the subsequent enzymic reaction.

Recently ELISA techniques have been combined with biosensors, to form **immunosensors**, in order to increase their range, speed and sensitivity. A simple immunosensor configuration is shown in Fig. 1.15, where the biosensor merely replaces the traditional colorimetric detection system. However more advanced immunosensors are being developed (Fig. 1.15 (b)) which rely on the direct detection of antigen bound to the antibody-coated surface of the biosensor. Piezoelectric and FET-based biosensors are particularly suited to such applications.

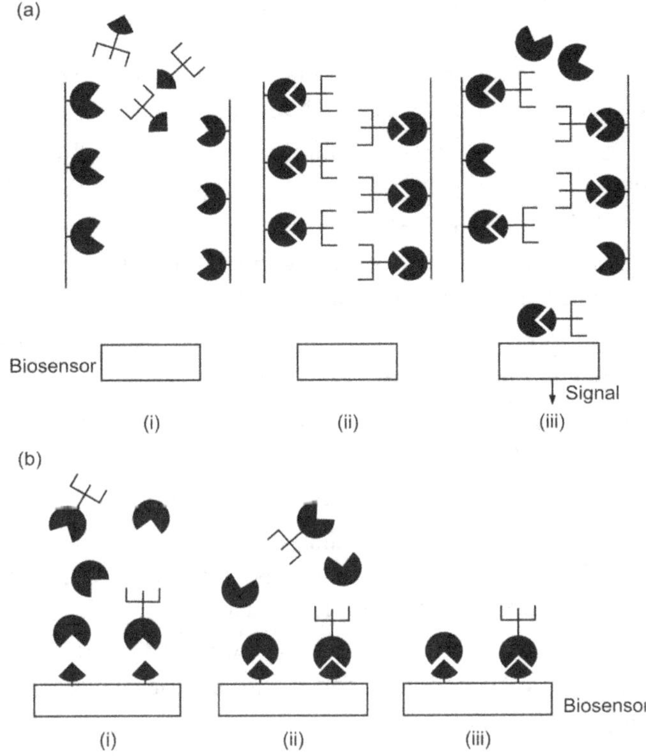

Fig. 1.15 Principles of immunosensors. (a)(i) A tube is coated with (immobilized) antigen. An excess of specific antibody-enzyme conjugate is placed in the tube and allowed to bind. (a)(ii) After a suitable period any unbound material is washed off. (a)(iii) The analyte antigen solution is passed into the tube, binding and releasing some of the antibody-enzyme conjugate dependent upon the antigen's concentration. The amount of antibody-enzyme conjugate released is determined by the response from the biosensor. (b)(i) A transducer is coated with (immobilized) antibody, specific for the antigen of interest. The transducer is immersed in a solution containing a mixture of a known amount of antigen-enzyme conjugate plus unknown concentration of sample antigen. (b)(ii) After a suitable period the antigen and antigen-enzyme conjugate will be distributed between the bound and free states dependent upon their relative concentrations. (b)(iii) Unbound material is washed off and discarded. The amount of antigen-enzyme conjugate bound is determined directly from the transduced signal.

1.5.7   Microbial Biosensors

◆ A biosensor is a device that detects, transmits and records information regarding a physiological or biochemical change.

◆ Technically, it is a probe that integrates a biological component with an electronic transducer thereby converting a biochemical signal into a quantifiable electrical response.

◆ Biosensors make use of a variety of transducers such as electrochemical, optical, acoustic and electronic.

◆ The function of a biosensor depends on the biochemical specificity of the biologically active material.

◆ The choice of the biological material will depend on a number of factors viz the specificity.

◆ storage, operational and environmental stability.

◆ Selection also depends on the analyte to be detected such as chemical compounds antigens, microbes, hormones, nucleic acids or any subjective parameters like smell and taste.

◆ Enzymes, antibodies, DNA, receptors, organelles and micro-organisms as well as animal and plant cells or tissues have been used as biological sensing elements.

◆ Some of the major attributes of a good biosensing system are its specificity, sensitivity, reliability, portability, (in most cases) ability to function even in optically opaque solutions, real-time analysis and simplicity of operation.

1.5.8   Use of Microbial Cells as Biosensing Elements

◆ Advantages of microbes as biological sensing materials in the fabrication of biosensors

◆ Present ubiquitously

◆ Able to metabolise a wide range of chemical compounds

◆ Great capacity to adapt to adverse conditions

◆ Develop the ability to degrade new molecules with time

◆ One of the ways to obviate this problem is to use permeabilised cells.

◆ Permeablisation can be achieved via Physical (freezing and thawing),

♦ Chemical (organic solvents/detergents) and

♦ Enzymatic (lysozyme, papain) approaches

♦ The most common technique uses organic solvents such as toluene, chloroform, ethanol and butanol or detergents like

N-cetyl-N, N, N-trim ethyl ammonium bromide (CTAB), Na-deoxycholate and digitonin (Patil and D'Souza, 1997).

♦ Such chemical treatment creates minute pores by removing some of the lipids from the cell membranes, thereby allowing for the free diffusion of small molecular weight substrates/products across the cell membrane while retaining most of the macromolecular compounds like the enzymes inside the cell.

♦ The Permeablisation process, however, renders the cell non-viable but can serve as an economical source of intracellular enzymes.

♦ In the case of periplasmic enzymes such as invertase and catalase in yeast (D'Souza and Nadkarni, 1980; Svitel et al., 1998) and uniease and phosphatases in bacteria (Kamath and D'Souza, 1992; Macaskie et al.,1992) whole cells can be used without Permeablisation

♦ One of the recent advances is to engineer the cell to transport the intra cellular enzyme and anchor it into the peri-plasmic space.

♦ Such an approach has been applied to obtain recombinant *Escherichia coli* cells with surface expressed oragno phosphorous hydrolase (OPH), an enzyme useful in the fabrication of biosensors for the detection of organophosphate compounds (Mulchandani et al., 1998a,b).

♦ These cells could degrade the organophosphates more efficiently (Mulchandani   et. al., 1998a,b) without the diffusional limitations otherwise observed in engineered cells expressing OPH intra-cellular (Rainina et al., 1996).

♦ The above approach is an important development in the field of microbial-biosensors as it provides a cell system with no membrane transport problems and at the same time will not affect the cellular structure and activity.

♦ This is in contrast to chemically permeabilised cells which result in loss of cell viability

♦ These types of genetic approaches may have major significance in the future, especially for sensors like BOD wherein polymers such as protein, starch, lipid etc., have to be broken down to monomers before they can be metabolised.

♦ Another limitation in using whole cells is the low specificity as compared to biosensors containing pure enzymes.

♦ This is mainly due to the unwanted side reactions catalyzed by other enzymes in a cell.

♦ Several approaches are being investigated to minimize such non-specific reactions.

♦ Permeabilisation of the cell empties it of most of the small molecular weight cofactors etc., thus minimizing the unwanted side reactions (D'Souza, 1989a).

♦ Thus a whole cell of yeast containing intracellular –galactosidase converts lactose to ethanol and CO_2 whereas the same cell on permeabilisation converts lactose only to glucose and galactose due to the loss of cofactors from the cell (Rao et al., 1988; Joshi et al.,1989).

♦ Side reactions, which can occur due to the presence of other enzymes in a cell, can also be minimised by inactivating such enzymes either by physical (heat) or chemical means when non-viable cells are used (Godboleet al., 1983; Di Paolantonio and Rechnitz,1983; D'Souza, 1989a; Riedel, 1998).

♦ Another approach that is of significance in viable cell-based biosensors is the blockage of unwanted metabolic pathways or transport systems.

♦ Thus, for the determination of glutamic acid in the presence of glucose by Bacillus subtilis, the glucose up take carrier system of the cell was blocked using a thiol inhibitor like chloromercuri benzoate and also the glycolysis was reversibly inhibited by NaF (Riedel and Scheller, 1987). .

♦ Microbial biosensors based on light emission from luminescent bacteria are being applied as a sensitive, rapid and non-invasive assay in several biological systems (Burlage and Kuo, 1994; Matrubutham and Sayler, 1998).

♦ Bioluminescent bacteria are found in nature, their habitat ranging from marine (Vibrio fischeri) to terrestrial (Photorhabdus luminescens) environments.

♦ Bioluminescent whole cell biosensors have also been developed using genetically engineered micro-organisms (GEM) for the monitoring of organic, pesticide and heavy metal contamination.

♦ The micro-organisms used in these biosensors are typically produced with a constructed plasmid in which genes that code for luciferase are placed under the control of a promoter that recognizes the analyte of interest.

♦ When such microbes metabolise the organic pollutants, the genetic control mechanism also turns on the synthesis of luciferase, which produces light that can be detected by luminometers.

♦ One approach to environmental monitoring is to detect changes in gene expression patterns induced by adverse conditions.

♦ Bacterial strains that increase light production in the presence of specific chemicals have been constructed using bioluminescence genes (lux) as reporters of transcriptional responses.

♦ A typical example is the *Pseudomonas fluorescens* HK44, a lux - based bioluminescent bio-reporter that is capable of emitting light upon exposure to naphthalene, salicylate and other substitute danalogues.

1.5.9   Immobilization of Bio Materials

♦ The basic requirement of a biosensor is that the biological material should bring the physico-chemical changes in close proximity of a transducer.

♦ Immobilisation not only helps in forming the required close proximity between the biomaterial and the transducer, but also helps in stabilising it for reuse.

♦ The biological material has been immobilised directly on the transducer or in most cases, in membranes, which can subsequently be mounted on the transducer.

♦ Biomaterials can be immobilised either through adsorption, entrapment, covalent binding, cross-linking or a combination of all these techniques (D'Souza, 1989a, 1999; Bickerstaff, 1997).

♦ *e.g.,* Covalent binding, commonly used technique for the immobilisation of enzymes and antibodies.

1.5.10   Microbial Biosensors for Environmental Applications

Table 1.5 Microbial Biosensors for Environmental Applications

Analysis	Microorganism	Transducer/ immobilization	Detection limit	Reference
BOD	*Trichosperum cutaneum*	Miniature oxygen electrode (UV cross-linking resin (ENT – 3400)	0.2 – 18 mg/*l*	Yang et.al (1996)
BOD	*T. cuteneum*	Miniature oxygen electrode array (photo cross-linkable resin)	<32 mg/*l*	Yang et.al (1997)
BOD	*T.cutaneum*	Oxygen electrode (entrapment)	10-70 mg/*l*	Marty et. al (1997)
BOD	*P.putidex*	Oxygen electrode (adsorption on porous nitro cellulose membrane)	> 0.5 mg/*l*	Chee et. al (1999)
BOD	Activated sludge (mixed microbial consortium)	Oxygen electrode/flow injection system (entrapped in dialysis membrane)	> 3.5 mg/*l*	Lin et. al (2000)
BOD	Salt tolerant mycelia yeast A. adeinvarans 1.53	Oxygen electrode (PVA)	2.61-524 mg/*l*	Tag et. al (2000)
Bioavailable organic carbon in oxic sediments	Yeast cells	Oxygen electrode (PVA)	Microscale	Neudoerfer and Meyer (1997)

Table 1.5 *contd…*

Analysis	Microorganism	Transducer/ immobilization	Detection limit	Reference
Aniomic surfactants (linear alky benzene sulfonates (LAS)	LAS degrading bacteria isolated from activated sludge	Oxygen electrode, (reactor type sensor, ca-alginate)	< 6 mg/l	Nomura et. al (1994)
Acrylamide acrylic acid	*Broxibacterium.s p*	Oxygen electrode (free celis)	0.01-0.075 and 0.01-0.1 g/l	Ignatov et. al. (1997)
Phenotic compounds	*Ps. parido*	Oxygen electrode (reactor with cells adsorbed on PEI glass)	100 uM	Nandakumar and Mattiason (1999 a)
Nitrite	*Nurobacter vulgaris* DSM 10236 *S.cerevisine*	Oxygen electrode (adsorption on Whatman paper)	> 10 μm	Reshetilov et. al (2000)
Cyanide	*S.cerevisiae*	Oxygen electrode (PVA)	0.15-15 nM	Tkebukaro et. al (1996)
Chlorophenol s	*Rhodococcus sp., Trichosporon beigelli Ps. Putida*	Oxygen electrode (PVA)	0.004-0.04 and 0.002-0.04 mM	Riedel et. al (1993, 1995)
3-Chloro-benzoate	*Ps. putida*	Oxygen electrode (PVA)	40-200 μN	Riedel et. al (1991)
Chlorinated and brominated hydrocarbons (I-chlorobutane and ethylenebromide)	*Rhodococcus sp.* DSM 6344	Ion selective electrodes (alginate)	0.22 and 0.04 mg/l	Peter et. al (1996)
Polycyclic aromatic hydrocarbons (Naphthalene)	*Sphingomonus yanolkuvate* B1 or *Ps. Fluorescens* WW 4	Oxygen electrode	0.01-3.0 mg/l	Keenig et al. (1996, 1997a)

Table 1.5 *contd…*

Analysis	Microorganism	Transducer/ immobilization	Detection limit	Reference
Organophosp hate nerve agents (paraxon, methyl parathion, diazinon)	GEM[b] *E.coli* (organophosphor ous hydrolase)	Potentiometric (adsorption on electrode surface)	0.055-1.8, 0.06-0.91 and 0.46-8.5 μM	Mulchandani et. al. (1998a)
Organophosp hate nerve agents (paraxon, parathion, coumaphos)	GEM[b] *E.coli* (organophosphor ous hydrolase)	Fiber-optic (agarose)	0.0-0.6, 0.0-0.03 and 0.0-0.075 μM	Mulchandani et.al. (1998b)
Pollutants such as diuron and mercuric chloride	*Synechacaccus sp.* PCC 7942	Photoelectro chemical (photo cross linkable PVA bearing styrylpyridium group)	0.2 and 0.06 μM	Rouillon et al (1999)
Herbicides (diuron and atrazine)	Chloroplast/thyla koid membranes	Pt-electrode in microelectrochemi cal cell (photo cross linkable PVA bearing styrylpyridium group	2×10^{-5} and 2×10^{-4} μM	Rouition et al (1995)
Mono and polyphenols (atrazine)	Potato (S. tuberosum) slices (polyphenol oxidase inhibition)	Oxygen electrode (tissue slice sandwitched between membranes)	20-130 μM	Mazzel et. al (1993)

Table 1.6 Applications of Bioluminescence-based Biosensors

Application	Microorganism	Reference
Monitoring toxicity of compounds to eukaryoles	*S. cerevislae* was genetically modified to express firefly luciferase	Hollis et. al. (2000)
On-line monitoring of microbial growth	*E.coli* engineered for constitutive bioluminescence	Marincs (2000)
Toxicity of Zn, Cu and Cd, alone or in combination	*E.coli* HB101 and Ps. Fluorescens 10586 genetically modified with luxCDABE	Presion et. al (2000)
Polycyclic aromatic hydrocarbons	Ps. Fluorescens HK44 genetically modified with luxCDABE	Webb et.al. (1997), Sayler et al. (1999), Ripp et. al. (2000)
Exotoxicity assessment of organotins and their initial breakdown products (tributyltin, dibutyltin, triphenyltin and diphenyltin)	Microtox and hexCDABE modified *Ps. Fluorescens*	Bundy et. al. (1997)
Ethanol as a model toxicant	*E.coli TV* 1061, *harboring* the plasmid pGrpELux5	Gu et. al. (1996), Rupani et al. (1996)
Monitoring of biocides	Bioluminescent strain of E.coli produced by recombinant DNA technology.	Fabricant et. al. (1995)
Metals, solvents, crop protection chemicals etc	*E.coli* heat shock promoters, dnak and grpE were fused with lux genes of V,fischeri	Van Dyk et. al (1994)
Identifying constraints to bioremediation of BTEX contaminated sites	luxCDABE modified Ps. Fluorescens	Sousa et. al. (1998)
Assessment of the toxicity of metals in soils amended with sewage sludge	luxCDABE modified Ps. Fluorescens	McGrath et. al. (1999)

1.6   Protein Engineering

Protein Engineering is a term that refers to the study of proteins. The design of novel enzymes or proteins with new or desirable functionalities is known as protein engineering. It is based on the modification of amino acid sequences using recombinant DNA technology. Within the broader area of genetic engineering, protein engineering might be regarded a sub-discipline. Protein engineering is distinguished by the end product, which is a protein with a modified amino acid sequence rather than a new (or modified) live organism. Many of the concerns raised in the broader field of genetic engineering (e.g., the current debate over genetically modified species) do not apply to protein engineering because proteins do not reproduce. In this way, designed proteins are more akin to new chemical compounds derived from non-biological sources, which raise safety and toxicity issues but are biodegradable by their very nature.

1.6.1 The following are the Steps in Protein Engineering

(i)   **Identification:** Protein engineering begins with the discovery of a protein with a specific function that can be altered to meet a specific purpose.

(ii) **Protein Isolation and Characterization:** Identified proteins are isolated and biochemically characterised. After that, the 3D structure and function of the protein, as well as the link between structure and function, are discovered.

(iii) **Protein Modification:** Based on the foregoing facts and established principles of protein conformation, protein modification may be suggested as a means of achieving desired results.

(iv) **Change Incorporation:** Changes are incorporated into the protein using side-directed mutagenesis, biochemical, or molecular methods. A new protein's activity must be evaluated. Protein design begins with an understanding of protein structural fundamentals.

A sequence of amino acids is created using these principles with the goal of causing the protein to take up a specific 3D structure and perform the required function. DNA is produced according to the amino acid of choice. Then, using recombinant DNA technology, it is cloned into an expression vector system. Tests and the next stage of the design process will be performed on the expressed protein.

1.6.2   Methods of Protein Engineering

There are two main approaches for protein engineering, rational design and directed evolution (irrational design).

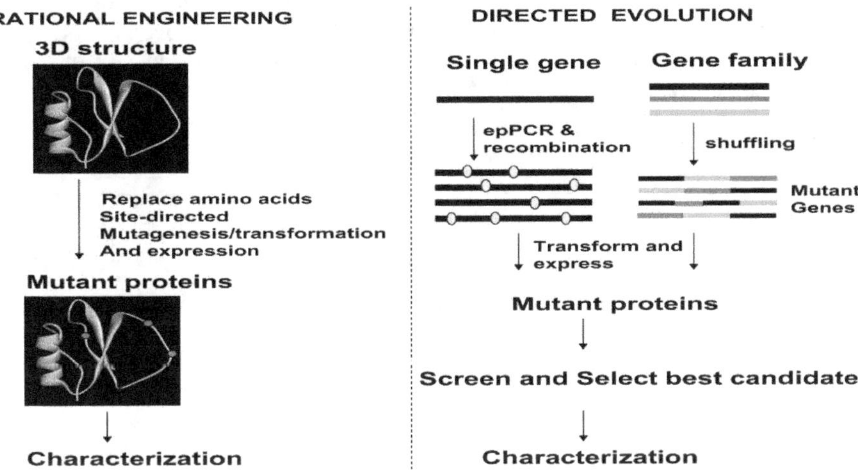

Fig. 1.16 Schematic Diagram of Protein Engineering

In the case of rational design, the protein's structure and function are taken into account, and a reasonable gene mutation is designed. This is usually accomplished by making rationally designed alterations to the gene of the protein cloned in a heterologous translation expression vector. Site directed or site-specific mutagenesis of protein genes alters the synthesis of protein molecules. However, in other circumstances, protein structure is unavailable, necessitating the use of a directed evolution approach. Random changes (mutation) are made to the protein in this process, and a mutant version with desired features is chosen.

1. **Rational design:** The so-called "rational design" approach, which incorporates "site-directed mutagenesis" of proteins, is the most well-known method in protein engineering. Site-directed mutagenesis allows specific amino acids to be introduced into a target gene. The "overlap extension" method and the "whole plasmid single round PCR" method are two common methods for site-directed mutagenesis.

(i) **The "overlap extension" approach:** This method employs two primer pairs, one of which carries the mutant codon with the mismatched sequence. These four primers are used in the first polymerase chain reaction (PCR), which involves two PCRs and the production of two double-stranded DNA products. Two heteroduplexes are generated during denaturation and annealing, and each strand of the heteroduplex contains the desired mutagenesis codon. The non-mutated primer set is then used to amplify the mutagenic Protein Engineering DNA, and DNA polymerase is employed to fill in the overlapping 3' and 5' ends of each heteroduplex.

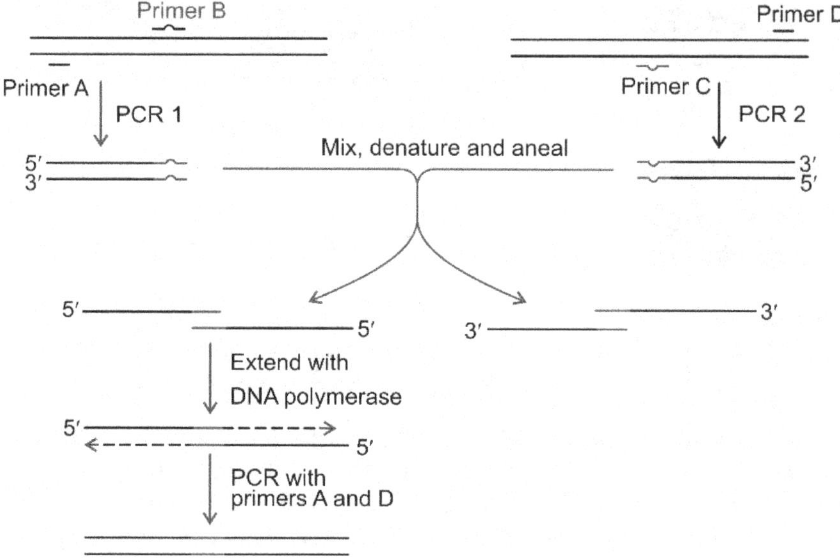

Fig. 1.17 Schematic Diagram of Rational design Protein Engineering

(ii) The complete plasmid single round PCR: Stratagene's commercial "Quick-change Site-Directed Mutagenesis Kit" is based on this technology. It requires two oligonucleotide primers that are complementary to the opposite strands of a double-stranded DNA plasmid template and contain the desired mutation(s). PCR is performed with DNA polymerase, and both strands of the template are reproduced without displacing the primers, yielding a modified plasmid with non-overlapping breaks. After that, DpnI methylase is employed to selectively digest the vector to generate a circular, nicked vector containing the mutant gene. The nick in the DNA is repaired when the nicked vector is transformed into competent cells, yielding a circular, altered plasmid.

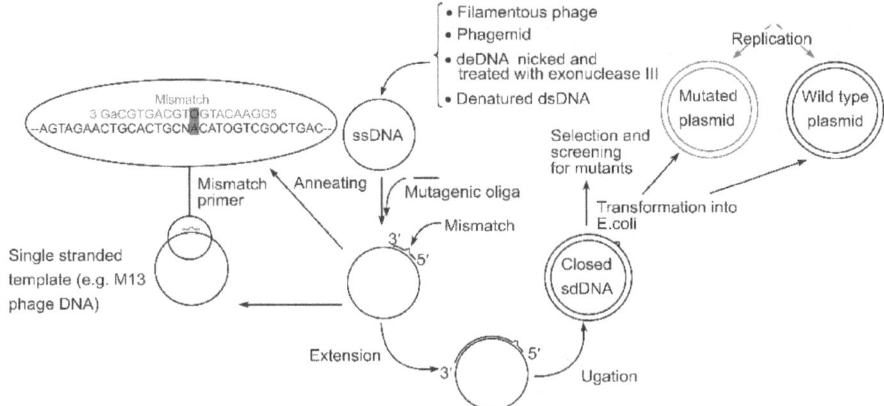

Fig. 1.18 Schematic Diagram plasmid single round PCR

When the structure and mechanism of the protein of interest are well known, rational design is a viable option. However, in many cases of protein engineering, there is a scarcity of information about the structure and processes of the protein in question. As an alternative, the use of "evolutionary approaches" such as "random mutagenesis and selection" for the desired protein qualities was introduced. Random mutagenesis could be a useful tool, especially when there is little knowledge about the structure and mechanism of a protein. The sole stipulation is that a sufficient selection technique that favours the desired protein characteristics be available. "Saturation mutagenesis" is a simple and widespread approach for random mutagenesis.

Saturation mutagenesis

Saturation mutagenesis is when a single amino acid in a protein is replaced with each of the natural amino acids, resulting in all conceivable variants at that point. Another strategy that combines rational and random techniques to protein engineering is "localised or region-specific random mutagenesis." It entails replacing a few amino acid residues in a specific location at the same time to produce proteins with new specificities. As with site-directed mutagenesis, this approach makes use of overlap extension and whole-plasmid, single-round PCR mutagenesis. However, the codons for the selected amino acids are randomised, resulting in the employment of a variety of 64 distinct forward and reverse primers, depending on a statistical mixture of four bases and three nucleotides in a randomised codon.

Random Mutagenesis (PCR based) with degenerated primers (Saturation mutagenesis)

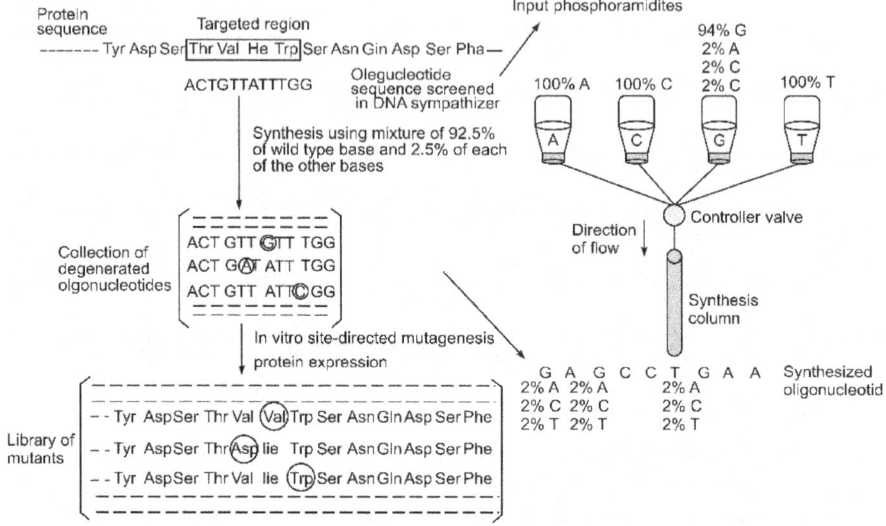

Fig. 1.19 Schematic Diagram of Saturation mutagenesis

2. **Irrational design (directed evolution):** "In vitro protein evolution systems" are based on the notion of gene hierarchy evolution. Modern genes are thought to have evolved from tiny genetic units through hierarchical and combinatorial processes. MolCraft, an in silico developed microgene, is an example.

DNA shuffling method

A set of genes with double-stranded DNA and similar sequences is collected from various organisms or created by error-prone PCR in the DNA shuffling method. These genes are digested with DNase I, which results in randomly cleaved tiny pieces that are purified and re-joined using an error-prone and thermostable DNA polymerase. The fragments are employed as PCR primers, aligning and cross-priming one another. As a result, a hybrid DNA with portions from many parent genes is created.

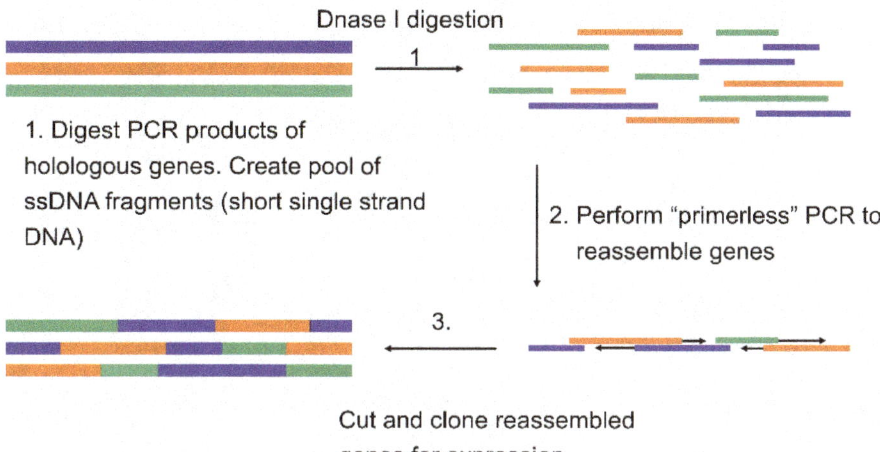

Fig. 1.20 DNA Shuffling

1.6.3   Protein Engineering's Applications

Protein engineering is being used to:

(a)   Create superior enzymes with the ability to catalyse the production of high-value specific chemicals;

(b)   Produce enzymes for large-scale use in the chemical industry; and

(c)   Produce biological compounds that are superior to natural ones, such as synthetic peptides, storage proteins, and specific drugs.

Protein engineering technology has been used to change a long variety of proteins. A mutation of isoleucine to cystine in 'T4 Lysozyme' results in the creation of a disulphide bridge, resulting in thermal stability and a 200-fold increase in enzyme activity at 670°C. The stability of the human beta interferon enzyme was improved by removing one of the three cysteine residues. It's possible that the enzyme 'Trypsin' might be modified to have a different substrate selectivity. By substituting the active site methionine with alanine, the substrate selectivity of lactic protease (in E. coli) was drastically altered.

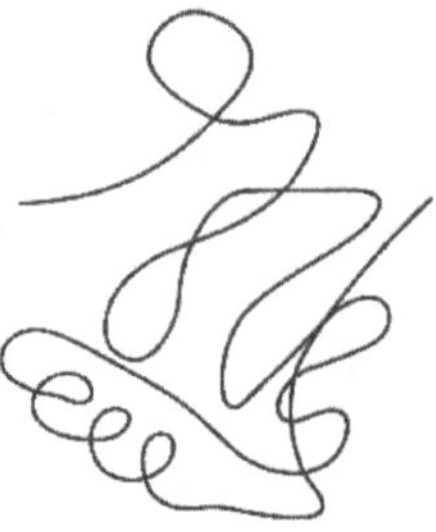

Native protein

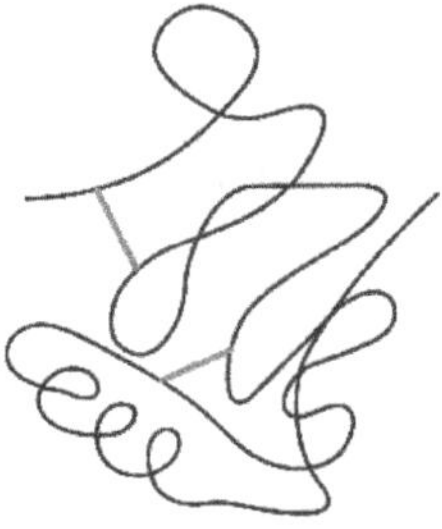

Engineered protein

Fig. 1.21 Structure of Protein

- Immunotoxins, which are conjugates of cell-binding antibodies or antigens covalently attached to a plant or bacterial toxin, are another application of protein engineering. These immunotoxins are made through the fusion of genes with sequences coding for antibodies and hazardous peptides. When a patient is given immunotoxins, the antibody or antigen aids in the recognition of the cells that need to be killed, and the toxin component aids in the destruction of those cells. So immunotoxins are made up of two parts: a) a toxin polypeptide or a portion of it with toxin activity, called A chain, and b) a cell binding recognition polypeptide or antibody, called B chain, or a portion of it with binding site. For example, the plant toxin ricin was utilised as an immunotoxin in a study of its effect on mice tumour cells.

- Another emerging field in biotechnology is drug design. Drug design can be altered by inhibiting enzyme activity, depending on the mode of action used by the medications. Trimethoprim (TMP), for example, is a therapeutically relevant antibacterial medication that works by inhibiting the enzyme dihydrofolate reductase (dHFR) in bacteria, and is used to treat urinary tract infections. However, at high doses, it begins to damage human dHFR, making it toxic. TMP has been synthesised, and it will have a rigid three-dimensional structure in connection with the bacterial enzyme dHFR, preventing it from attacking human dHFR.

- Renin is another example of an enzyme. Modelling of inhibitors of the enzyme 'renin' is also underway. The enzyme catalyses the first step in a chain of events that results in high blood pressure. Nonpeptide inhibitors that imitate the intermediate products in the reaction of renin with its substrate and thereby halt renin's function are being developed. These inhibitors will aid in the treatment of high blood pressure.

1.6.4   Production of Enzyme

Microbial enzymes have been used for ages without being fully understood. Taka-diastase (a fungus amylase) was the first enzyme produced commercially in the United States in 1896. It was used to treat digestive problems as a medicinal agent.

Before tanning, softening the hides with the faeces of dogs and pigeons was a century-old technique in Europe. In 1905, a German scientist (Otto Rohm) demonstrated that extracts from animal organs (pig and cow pancreases) may be utilised as a source of enzymes (proteases) for leather softening.

In 1915, enzymes (mostly proteases) were first used for washing applications. However, due to allergic reactions to contaminants in enzymes, it was not maintained. Special procedures for the manufacturing and application of enzymes in washing powders are now available (without allergic reactions). Enzymes for commercial use can be made from a variety of biological sources. At the moment, microbial sources account for the vast bulk (80%).

The following are the many organisms and their proportionate contributions to the creation of commercial enzymes:

Fungi – 60%

Bacteria – 24%

Yeast – 4%

Streptomyces – 2%

Higher animals – 6%

Higher plants – 4%

Enzymes derived from microorganisms: Commercial enzymes are derived from microorganisms, which are the most important and convenient sources. They can be induced to produce large amounts of enzymes under the right conditions. Microorganisms can be cultured on low-cost media, and manufacturing can be completed quickly.

Furthermore, using genetic engineering techniques, it is simple to control microbes to boost the production of desired enzymes. Microbial enzymes are easier to recover, isolate, and purify than enzymes derived from animals or plants.

In reality, microorganisms have effectively manufactured the majority of industrial enzymes. This is accomplished using a variety of fungi, bacteria, and yeasts.

Table 1.7 List of Industrially Produced Enzymes

Enzyme	Source(s)	Application(s)
α-Amylase	Asperigilus cryzae Aspergillus niger Bacilus subilus Bacillus icenforms	Production of bear and alcohol Preparation of glucose syrups As a digestive aid Removal of starch sizes
Amyloglucosidase	Aspergilus niger Rhizopus niveus	Starch hydrolysis
Cellulase	Aspergillus niger Tricoderma koningi	Alcohol and glucose production
Glucoamylase	Aspergillus niger	Production of beer and alcohol Starch hydrolysis
Glucoamylase	Aspergillus niger Bacillus amyloliquefaciens	Production of beer and alcohol Starch hydrolysis
Glucose Isomerase	Arthrobacter sp Bacillus sp	Manufacture of high fructose syrups
Glucose oxidase	Aspergillus niger	Antioxidant in prepared foods
Invertase	Saccharomyces cerevisiae	Sucrose inversion Preparation of artificial honey confectionaries

Table 1.7 *contd...*

Enzyme	Source(s)	Application(s)
Keratinase	Streptomyces fradiae	Removal of hair from hides
Lactase	Kluyveromyus sp Saccaromyces fragilis	Lactose hydrolysis Removal of lactose from whey
Lactase	Kluyveromyus sp Saccharomyces fragilis	Lactose hydrolysis Removal of lactose from whey
Lipase	Candida lipolytica Asperigilus niger	Preparation of cheese Flavour production
Pectinase	Aspergilus sp Sclerotina libertine	Clarification of fruit juices and wines Alcohol production, coffee concentration
Penicillin acylase	Escherichia coli	Production of 6-aminopenicillanic acid
Penicillanase	Bacillus subtilis	Removal of penicillin
Protease, acid	Aspergillus niger	Digestive aid Substitute for calf rennet
Protease, neutral	Bacillus amyloliquefaciens	Fish and meat tenderizer
Protease, alkaline	Aspergilus oryzae Streptomyces griseus Bacillus sp	Meat tenderize Detergent additive Beer stabilizer
Pollulanase	Klebsiella aerogens	Hydrolysis of starch
Takadiastase	Aspergillus oryzae	Supplement to bread Digestive aid

Niger (a fungus) is unique among microorganisms in that it is capable of producing a vast variety of enzymes in high amounts. A. Niger is capable of producing well over 40 commercial enzymes. A-amylase, cellulase, protease, lipase, pectinase, phytase, catalase, and insulinase are examples of these enzymes.

General consideration in the Production of Enzymes

The salient features for production of enzymes are as follows:

1. Selection of organisms
2. Formulation of medium
3. Production process
4. Recovery and purification of enzymes.

An outline of the flow chart for enzyme production by microorganisms

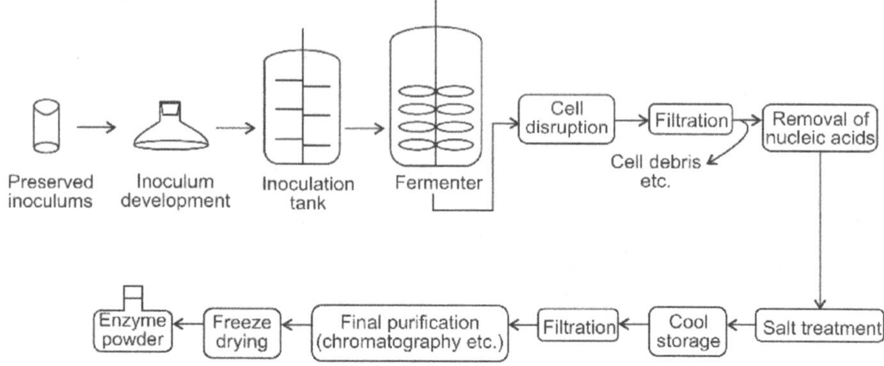

Fig. 1.22 Schematic outline of the flow chart for enzyme production by microorganisms

Selection of Organism

The most significant factors for choosing a microbe are that it should produce the largest amount of the required enzyme in the shortest amount of time while producing the least number of other metabolites. After the organism has been chosen, strain improvement can be done using appropriate methods to optimise enzyme production (mutagens, UV rays). Inoculum can be made in a liquid media from the organism chosen.

Formulation of medium

The culture medium used should contain all of the nutrients necessary to enable optimal microbe development, which will eventually result in large amounts of enzyme synthesis. The medium's elements should be easily accessible at a minimal cost and nutritionally sound. Starch hydrolysate, molasses, maize steep liquor, yeast extract, whey, and soy bean meal are some of the most often utilised substrates for the medium. There have also been some grains (wheat) and pulses (peanut) used. For optimal microbial growth and enzyme synthesis, the pH of the medium should be kept at 7.0.

Production process

Enzyme production in industry is generally done under submerged liquid conditions, with some solid-substrate fermentation thrown in for good measure. The yields are higher and the chances of infection are lower when using the submerged culture approach. As a result, this is the favoured method. Solid substrate fermentation, on the other hand, has a long history and is still used to produce fungal enzymes such as amylases, cellulases, proteases, and pectinases.

Batch or continuous sterilisation techniques can be used to sanitise the medium. Inoculating the medium kicks off the fermentation process. The appropriate growth circumstances (pH, temperature, O2 supply, and nutrition input) are maintained. Antifoam substances can be used to reduce the production of froth.

Batch fermentation and, to a lesser extent, continuous fermentation are the most common methods for producing enzymes. Throughout the fermentation process, the bioreactor system must be kept sterile. Fermentation lasts anywhere from 2 to 7 days in most manufacturing processes. Several additional metabolites are created in addition to the intended enzyme(s). It is necessary to recover and purify the enzyme(s).

Enzyme recovery and purification

The desired enzyme generated may be expelled into the culture media (extracellular enzymes) or present within the cells (intracellular enzymes) (intracellular enzymes). The commercial enzyme can be crude or highly refined, depending on the use. It could also take the shape of a solid or a liquid. The downstream processing processes, such as recovery and purification, will be determined by the nature of the enzyme and the degree of purity desired.

Recovery of an extracellular enzyme present in the broth is generally easier than recovery of an intracellular enzyme. Special cell disruption techniques are required for the release of intracellular enzymes. Physical measures can be used to break down microbial cells (sonication, high pressure, glass beads). The enzyme lysozyme can lyse the cell walls of bacteria. The enzyme glucanase is employed in yeasts. Enzymatic approaches, on the other hand, are costly.

Once the cells are disturbed and intracellular enzymes are liberated, the recovery and purification stages will be the same for both intracellular and extracellular enzymes. The most crucial factor is to keep the amount of desired enzyme activity as low as possible.

Removal of cell debris

Cell debris removal can be accomplished using filtration or centrifugation.

Removal of nucleic acids

Nucleic acids must be removed because they obstruct the recovery and purification of enzymes. Poly-cations such as polyamines, streptomycin, and polyethyleneimine can be used to precipitate and remove them.

Enzyme precipitation

Precipitation of enzymes: Salts (ammonium sulphate) and organic solvents can be used to precipitate enzymes (isopropanol, ethanol, and acetone). Precipitation is useful because the enzyme can be dissolved in a small amount of water to concentrate it.

Liquid-liquid partition

Using polyethylene glycol or polyamines, liquid-liquid extraction can be used to increase the concentration of desired enzymes.

Separation by chromatography

Separation and purification of enzymes can be accomplished using a variety of chromatographic techniques. Ion exchange, size exclusion, affinity, hydrophobic interaction, and dye ligand chromatography are some of these techniques. Ion-exchange chromatography is the most widely used method for enzyme purification among these.

Drying and Packing

Drying produces a concentrated version of the enzyme. Film evaporators or freeze dryers can help with this (lyophilizers). The dried enzyme is ready to be packaged and sold. Stability can be achieved for some enzymes by storing them in ammonium sulphate suspensions.

All enzymes used in foods or medicinal treatments must be of high purity and meet regulatory criteria. These enzymes must be completely devoid of poisonous chemicals, dangerous bacteria, and allergic reactions.

General Considerations on Microbial Enzyme Production Regulation

By optimising the fermentation conditions, the maximum production of microbial enzymes can be attained (nutrients, pH, O2, temperature etc.). This necessitates a thorough grasp of the genetic regulation of enzyme synthesis. Some of the general aspects of microbial enzyme control are briefly explained.

Induction

Several enzymes are inducible, meaning they can only be generated in the presence of inducers. The inducer could be a substrate, a product, or an intermediary (sucrose, starch, galactosides) (fatty acid, phenyl acetate, xylobiose).

A list of inducible enzymes and their corresponding inducers.

Table 1.8 list of inducible enzymes

Enzyme	Inducer
Invertase	Sucrose
Amylase	Starch
Lipase	Fatty acids
β-Galactosidasc	Galactosidcs
Penicillin G amidase	Phenylacetate
Xylanase	Xylobiose

Inducible Enzymes

Inducible enzymes are expensive and difficult to handle (sterilisation, adding at a specified time). In recent years, researchers have attempted to create microorganism mutants that are not dependent on inducers.

Feedback repression

The final product (typically a tiny molecule) regulates the enzyme synthesis in a major way. This happens when a huge quantity of the end product accumulates. The manufacture of feedback-regulated enzymes on a large scale is problematic. To circumvent this challenge, mutants lacking feedback repression have been produced.

Nutrient repression

The native metabolism of microorganisms is designed in such a way that no superfluous enzymes are produced. In other words, microbes do not produce enzymes that they do not require because it is a waste of time. Nutrient repression is used to stop the development of undesirable enzymes. In the growing media, the nutrients could be carbon, nitrogen, phosphate, or sulphate sources. Nutrient suppression must be overcome in order to produce enzymes on a big scale.

Repression of glucose is a classic example of nutritional (or, more accurately, catabolite) repression. That is, the enzymes required for the metabolism of the other chemicals are not produced in the presence of glucose. Glucose repression can be circumvented by providing carbohydrate to the fermentation medium at a pace that keeps the glucose concentration near zero at all times. Attempts have been made in recent years to select mutants that are resistant to glucose-induced catabolite suppression. Other carbon sources, such as pyruvate, lactate, citrate, and succinate, operate as catabolite repressors for some microbes.

In microorganisms, nitrogen source suppression is also found. Ammonium ions or amino acids could be to blame. As a nitrogen source, ammonium salts are most typically utilised. Ammonium salt repression can be circumvented by creating mutants resistant to this nitrogen source.

Microbial Enzyme Production by Genetic Engineering

Enzymes are the functional products of genes. As a result, enzymes are theoretically ideal candidates for genetic engineering-assisted manufacturing. Advances in recombinant DNA technology have undoubtedly aided in expanding microbial production of commercial enzymes over the last 15 years. The desired enzyme genes can now be transferred from one organism to another. The required gene can be cloned and introduced into a suitable production host once an enzyme with potential industrial use has been found.

Cloning strategies

Cloning procedures entail creating a cDNA library for the mRNA and designing oligonucleotide probes for the targeted enzyme. The specific cDNA clones can be identified by hybridization with oligonucleotide probes.

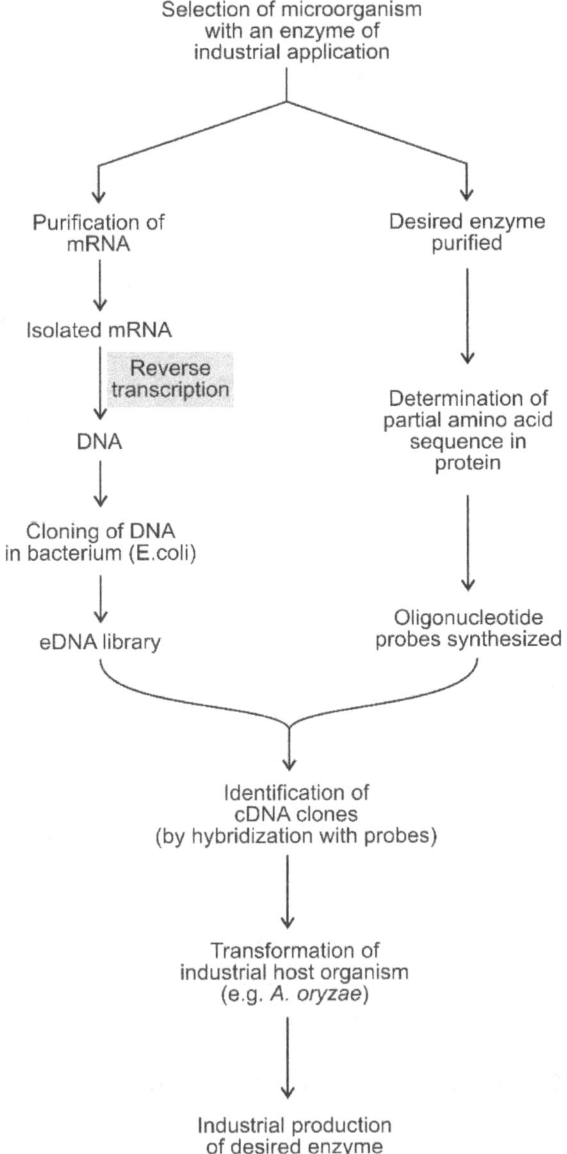

Fig. 1.23 Schematic diagram of Cloning strategies

Cloning Strategy for Industrial Production

The next stage is to turn an industrially relevant host organism (such as Aspergillus oryzae) into the enzyme of choice. It is possible to produce high-quality industrial enzymes using this method. The following are some of the enzymes that have been created through cloning techniques:

Lipolase, an enzyme found in the fungus Humicola lanuginose, is particularly good at removing fat stains from fabrics. However, due to a relatively low degree of synthesis, industrial manufacturing of lipolase by this organism is not conceivable. The lipolase gene was extracted, cloned, and introduced into the Aspergillus oryzae fungus.

As a result, large-scale production of this enzyme has been realised. Lipolase is extremely stable and resistant to proteases, which are typically found in detergents. All of these characteristics make lipolase an excellent candidate for fabric washing.

Rennet (chymosin) is a widely utilised enzyme in the production of cheese. The stomachs of new born calves are the most common source. As a result, there is a scarcity in its supply. The gene for chymosin synthesis has been cloned, allowing for large-scale manufacture.

Protein engineering for industrial enzyme modification

Protein engineering and site-directed mutagenesis have now made it possible to change the structure of a protein/enzyme. Increased enzyme stability and catalytic performance, resistance to oxidation, modified substrate preference, and increased tolerance to alkali and organic solvents are all goals of the alterations to the enzymes.

Select amino acids at specified places (in an enzyme) can be modified using site-directed mutagenesis to make an enzyme with desired features. Protein engineering has been used to structurally change phospholipase A2 such that it can withstand high acid concentrations. As a food emulsifier, the modified enzyme performs better. Genetic engineering has had a huge impact on the cost-effective industrial manufacture of enzymes with desired characteristics.

1.7   Genetic Engineering Principles

Genetic engineering entails the direct and pre-determined alteration of genetic material to achieve a certain goal. Recombinant DNA technology or gene cloning are other terms for the same thing.

Basic Procedure

Gene cloning is the process of inserting a specific piece of 'desired DNA' into a host cell in such a way that the inserted DNA is duplicated and passed down to daughter cells during cell division.

The following are the most important factors in gene cloning

- Isolation of the gene to be cloned.

- Insertion of the gene into another piece of DNA called vector which will allow it to be taken by bacteria and replicated within them as the cells grow and divide.

- Transfer of the recombinant vector into bacterial cells, either by transformation or by infection using viruses.

- Selection of those cells which contain the desired recombinant vectors.

- Growth of the bacteria, that can be continued indefinitely, to give as much cloned DNA as needed.

- Expression of the gene to obtain the desired product.

Isolation of DNA Fragments

There are four techniques for isolating desired DNA fragments.

• Restriction endonuclease digestion

This method cleaves the desired area of DNA using restriction enzymes. They are a class of enzymes that detect nucleotide sequences in DNA, usually 4 or 6 base pairs long, and cut both strands of DNA within the recognition site. They are unique to each location.

These enzymes can do two sorts of cuts:

Blunt ends - If it cleaves both DNA strands at exactly opposite locations on both strands, it results in blunt end fragments that are difficult to ligate or attach to the vector in the next step.

Cohesive ends - In some situations, the two DNA strands are not severed at the same time, but rather staggered, resulting in cohesive ends (sticky ends). Sticky ends are ideal for cloning because the staggered ends make it easier to attach another bit of DNA.

• Mechanical shearing

Sonication (using sound waves to shear the DNA) or pushing the DNA molecule with a syringe are two methods for mechanical shearing.

• Duplex cDNA synthesis

Synthesis of a complementary DNA (cDNA) strand to the intended DNA: It is sometimes possible to synthesise a complementary DNA (cDNA) strand to the desired DNA.

There are two ways to do it:

Classical method: In this method, oligonucleotide dT primers, klenow fragment of T4 DNA polymerase and S1nuclease is used to synthesize cDNA.

New method: In this method, terminal transferase and dCTP primer is used. After removing any contaminating mRNA by sucrose gradient, oligo dGTP primer is added to synthesize the second DNA strand.

Direct chemical synthesis

The desired DNA fragment can be synthesized if the sequence of the desired DNA is known.

Vector Installation of the Desired Gene

After obtaining the necessary DNA fragment, it must be transmitted to the host cell. Small plasmids, phage, or (animal virus DNA molecules) are utilised as cloning vehicles to transport a DNA fragment into a live cell. Vehicles for cloning are also known as vectors. They must possess the following characteristics:

- Replication origin to allow for independent replication.
- The presence of restriction enzyme recognition sites for insertion of the DNA fragment.
- After transfer, the bacteria must be able to multiply in the host cell.
- The presence of many selection/screening markers.

Different approaches can be used to insert or ligate the desired gene into the vector

- **Homopolymer tailing:** Homopolymer tailing entails adding the identical bases to the terminal end of the polymer, for example, 8 mol of poly G tail is added using terminal transferase. As a result, the complementary strand produces a poly C tail. As a result, the entering DNA does not need to be chopped.

- **Linker molecule:** A brief sequence containing a site for a specific restriction enzyme is inserted and ligated to the DNA by the enzyme DNA ligase in the absence of restriction enzyme sites. Linkers and adaptors are utilised to create non-complementary single strands. Adaptors aim to complement each other.

- **Blunt end ligation:** When the DNA and the vector have blunt ends, a high concentration of both the plasmid and insert DNA is required, and DNA ligase is utilised to ligate them. Low concentrations of self-ligation have been discovered.

- **Ligation of cohesive terminals:** is is more effective and occurs naturally.

The Host Cell: An Introduction

After the vector and desired DNA molecule have been ligated, the vector must be transferred to a host cell, where it will replicate and produce copies of the desired gene, as well as its products. The following approaches can be used to accomplish this transfer.

Transfection with recombinant phage DNA: If the vector is a phage, it can infect the host cell, allowing the gene to be transferred.

Recombinant plasmid transformation: If the vector is a plasmid, it can be transferred to the host by recombination.

Screening or Selection

After being delivered to the host via the vector, the recombinant DNA is integrated into the host cell DNA and begins reproducing alongside the host or independently with the phage within the host. In both circumstances, the host cells become factories for replicating and expressing the target gene. Following that, the host cells are screened to see if the target gene has been successfully integrated and replicated, as well as the expression of its products. The following strategies are used to do this:

Genetic Method

This entails the expression of specific characteristics. These qualities are usually encoded via the vector or, if a direct selection mechanism is available, by the desired cloned sequence. Antibiotics are one of the easiest strategies for selecting for the presence of vector molecules. For example, the Ampr and Tcr genes in pBR322 provide resistance to Ampicillin and Tetracycline, respectively.

Nucleic Acid Hybridization Screening

This is a very powerful method of screening clone banks and one of the most important approaches in gene manipulation. It employs a nucleic acid probe that detects the presence of a certain gene sequence. The power of nucleic acid hybridization comes from the fact that complementary sequences will attach to each other with extreme fidelity.

cDNA, genomic DNA, and oligonucleotides are the three basic types of probes employed.

Immunological Screening

An immunological approach is used to identify the protein product of a cloned gene. A particular antibody is utilised instead of a nucleic acid probe. The method of detection can be radioactive or non-radioactive.

Analysis of Cloned Genes: This method entails determining the protein product using two methods based on in vitro mRNA translation. Hybrid release translation (HRT) and hybrid arrest translation (HAT) are the terms for these techniques (HART). The preferred method is HRT.

Techniques for Blotting

The samples are first processed through a gel electrophoresis, after which the separated fragments are transferred to a nitrocellulose or nylon membrane using a blotting procedure. The capillary technique is used in the original procedure. A radioactive probe can then be hybridised with the filter. The filter is rinsed after hybridization, then exposed to X-ray film and an autoradiogram is created, which offers information on the clone's structure.

Southern Blotting: It's used to test DNA samples. E.D Southern was the first to develop it, hence the name. An agarose gel is utilised in this experiment.

Northern Blotting: Here RNA samples are been made to run. Here also agarose gel is used.

Western Blotting: It used to find the proteins. Here SDS PAGE method is followed. Membrane is then probed with an antibody to detect the protein.

Questions

1. Define the term "biotechnology." Explain branches, applications in detail.

2. Create an essay on enzyme biotechnology.

3. Explain the concept of enzyme immobilization and how it can be used.

4. Describe how biosensors works and its applications.

5. Have a conversation about protein engineering.

6. Describe genetic engineering and its applications in detail

CARRIER, VECTORS, RESERVOIRS

2.0 Carrier, Vectors, Reservoirs

Carrier

The commonest source of infection for humans is humans themselves. The parasite may originate from a patient or a carrier. A carrier is a person who harbours the pathogenic microorganism without suffering from only ill effect because of it.

Definitions of Some Important Carriers

Healthy carrier is one who harbours the pathogens but who displays no symptoms of the disease and capable of transmitting the pathogens, while Convalescent carrier is one who has recovered the pathogen in his body but still capable of transmitting the pathogens to others.

Temporary carrier state lasts less than six months. Chronic carrier may last for several years and sometimes even for the rest of one's life. Paradoxical carrier refers to a carrier who acquires the pathogen from another carrier.

Reservoirs

Many pathogens are able to infect both human beings and animals. Animals may, therefore act as sources of human infection. Such animals serve to maintain the parasite in nature and act as the reservoirs of human infections. They are therefore called reservior hosts. Infectious diseases transmitted from animals to human beings are called zoonoses.

Zoonotic diseases may be bacterial (plague from rats), viral (Rabies from dogs) proto zoal (toxo plasmosis from cats), helminthic (hydatid disease from dogs) and fungi (zoophilic dermatophytes from cats and dogs).

Vectors

Blood sucking insects transmit pathogens to human beings. The diseases so caused are called arthropod borne disease. Insects such as mosquitoes, ticks, mites, flies, fleas and lice that transmit infections are called "vectors". Such vectors are called mechanical vectors in other instances; the pathogen multiplies in the body of the vector, often undergoing part of its development at cycle in it. Such vectors are termed biological vectors. The interval between the times of entry of pathogen into the vector in the vector becoming infective is called the extrinsic incubation period.

Besides acting as vectors, some insects may also act as reservoir hosts. Infection is maintained in such insects by transovarial (certain arthropod vectors they transmit disease-causing bacteria from parent arthropod to offspring arthropod) or transstadial passage (passage of a microbial parasite, such as a virus or rickettsia, from one developmental stage (stadium) of the host to its subsequent stage or stages, particularly as seen in mites).

Arthropod Vectors

Some disease producing organisms are transmitted by insects (*e.g.*, Flies and Mosquitoes) and other arthropods (*e.g.*, Flex's and Ticks).

In certain cases the vectors simply act as accidental carriers of the organisms from filth to food or to the human host. In this way, plague and typhoid fever are transferred by fleas and house-flies respectively. In other cases, the micro-organisms are transmitted by blood-sucking arthropods and spend part of their life cycle in the vector.

E.g.,   Transmission of malaria by Anopheles mosquito

Transmission of yellow fever by *Aedes albopictus* mosquito,

Sleeping sickness by the tsetse fly and

Murine typhus by rat fly

2.1 Cloning Vector

A cloning vector is a small piece of DNA that can be kept stable in the body and into which a foreign DNA fragment can be put for cloning. A virus's DNA, a higher organism's cell, or a bacterium's plasmid can all be used as cloning vectors. The inclusion of restriction sites, for example, allows for the easy insertion or removal of a DNA segment into the vector. A restriction enzyme can be used to cleave the vector and foreign DNA, resulting in DNA pieces with blunt or sticky ends. After that, molecular ligation can be used to link foreign DNA with compatible ends. After cloning a DNA fragment into a cloning vector, it can be subcloned into a more specific vector.

Cloning vectors come in a variety of shapes and sizes, but genetically modified plasmids are the most frequent. Plasmids, bacteriophages (such as phage), cosmids, and bacterial artificial chromosomes are all used as cloning vectors in E. coli (BACs). However, some DNA pieces, such as very large DNA fragments, cannot be kept stable in E. coli and must be transferred to another cell, such as yeast. Yeast artificial chromosomes are one type of cloning vector (YACs).

Cloning Vectors Attributes

A good cloning site and a selectable marker are required elements of all regularly used cloning vectors in molecular biology. Others may include characteristics that are unique to their application. Cloning is commonly done with E. coli because it is simple and convenient. As a result, many cloning vectors include features required for propagation and maintenance in E. coli, such as a functional replication origin (ori). Several plasmids have the ColE1 replication origin. Shuttle vectors are vectors that have components that allow them to be maintained in organisms other than E. coli.

Every cloning vector has features that make it easy to insert or remove a gene. It's possible that this is a multiple cloning site (MCS) or polylinker, which has a lot of different restriction sites. The restriction sites in the MCS are first cleaved by restriction enzymes, and then a PCR-amplified target gene, which has also been digested with the same enzymes, is ligated into the vectors with DNA ligase. If you like, you can insert the target DNA sequence into the vector in a precise direction. If necessary, the restriction sites can be employed to subclone the vector into another vector.

Other cloning vectors may substitute topoisomerase for ligase, allowing for faster cloning without the need to restriction digest the vector or insert. A linearized vector is activated by attaching topoisomerase I to its ends in this TOPO cloning procedure, and this "TOPO-activated" vector may then accept a PCR product by ligating both of the PCR product's 5' ends, releasing the topoisomerase and producing a circular vector in the process. DNA recombination, as employed in the Gateway cloning system, is another method of cloning without the usage of DNA digest and ligase. Once cloned into the cloning vector (referred to as the entry clone in this procedure), the gene can be easily introduced into a number of expression vectors.

Selectable Marker

The vector contains a selectable marker that allows positively transformed cells to be selected. Antibiotic resistance is frequently employed as a marker, with the beta-lactamase gene, which imparts resistance to the penicillin group of beta-lactam antibiotics, such as ampicillin, being one example. Some vectors have two selectable markers, such as the ampicillin and kanamycin resistance genes in plasmid pACYC177. Although some selectable markers, such as zeocin and hygromycin B resistance, are effective in diverse cell types, a shuttle vector that is supposed to be maintained in two different organisms may also require two selected markers. Auxotrophic selection markers may also be utilised to allow an auxotrophic organism to grow in a minimal growth media.

Positive selection of plasmid with cloned gene is possible using another type of selectable marker. Barnase, Ccda, and the parD/parE toxins are examples of genes that kill host cells. This usually works by interrupting or deleting the fatal gene during the cloning process, and because failing clones with the lethal gene intact would kill the host cells, only successful clones are chosen.

Types of Cloning Vectors

There are several cloning vectors to choose from, and the vector you use may be determined by a variety of parameters like the size of the insert, the number of copies, and the cloning process. Large inserts, especially those with a high copy number, may not be stably maintained in a general cloning vector, hence cloning large fragments may need the use of a more specialised cloning vector shown in Fig. 2.1.

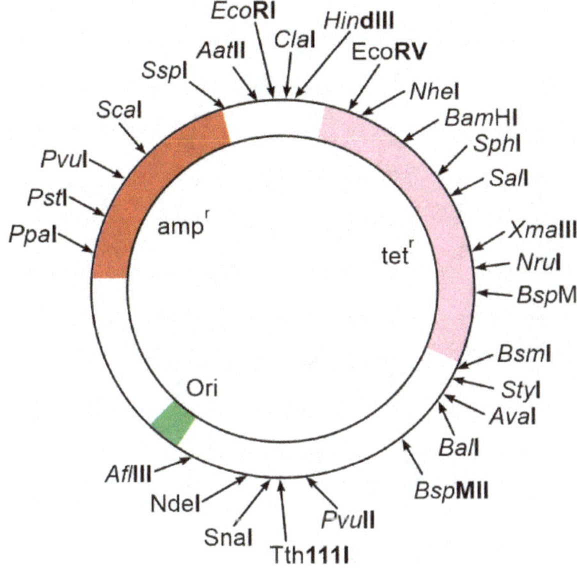

Fig. 2.1 Structure of Cloning Vector

Plasmid Vector

Plasmids replicate circular extrachromosomal DNA on their own. They are the most often used and standard cloning vectors. Cloning DNA inserts up to 15 kb in size is possible with most generic plasmids. The pBR322 plasmid was one of the first widely used cloning vectors. Other cloning vectors include the pUC series of plasmids, as well as a wide range of cloning plasmid vectors. Many plasmids have a high copy number, such as pUC19, which has 500-700 copies per cell, and a high copy number is advantageous since it results in a higher yield of recombinant plasmid for manipulation. Low-copy-number plasmids, on the other hand, may be preferable in some situations.

Some plasmids have an M13 bacteriophage replication origin that can be utilised to make single-stranded DNA. The pBluescript series of cloning vectors is an example of what would be known as phagemid shown in Fig. 2.2.

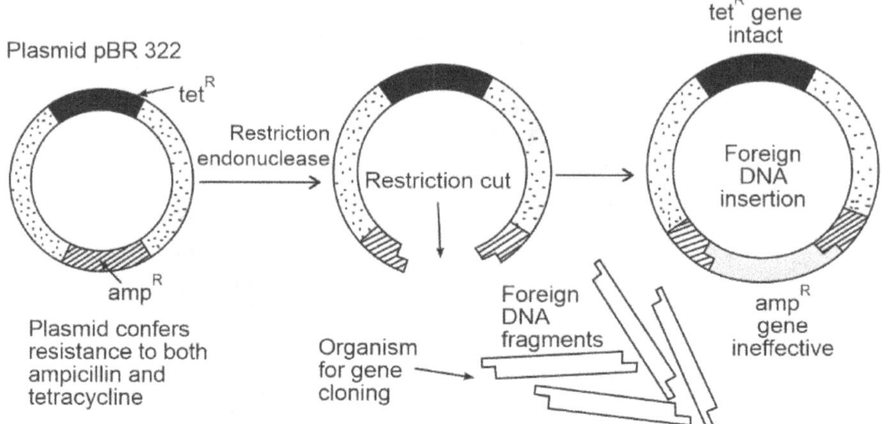

Fig. 2.2 Diagrammatic representation of Plasmid Vector

Bacteriophage Vector

The phage and M13 bacteriophages were employed in the cloning process. Because the quantity of DNA that can be packed into a phage is limited (up to 53 kb), phage cloning vectors may need to have some non-essential genes removed, such as lysogeny genes, as phage cloning vectors are only used for the lytic cycle. Insertion vectors and replacement vectors are the two types of phage vectors available. Foreign DNA with a size of 5-11 kb can be introduced into insertion vectors thanks to a specific cleavage site.

In addition, the size of DNA that can be packed into a phage has a limit, and vector DNA that is too small will not fit inside the phage effectively. This attribute can be utilised for selection - a vector without an insert may be too small for propagation, so only vectors containing an insert can be chosen.

Cosmid Vector

Cosmids are plasmids that contain a region of bacteriophage λDNA called the cohesive end site (cos), which contains the ingredients needed to package DNA into λ particles. It's usually utilised to clone big DNA segments that are between 28 and 45 kb in size.

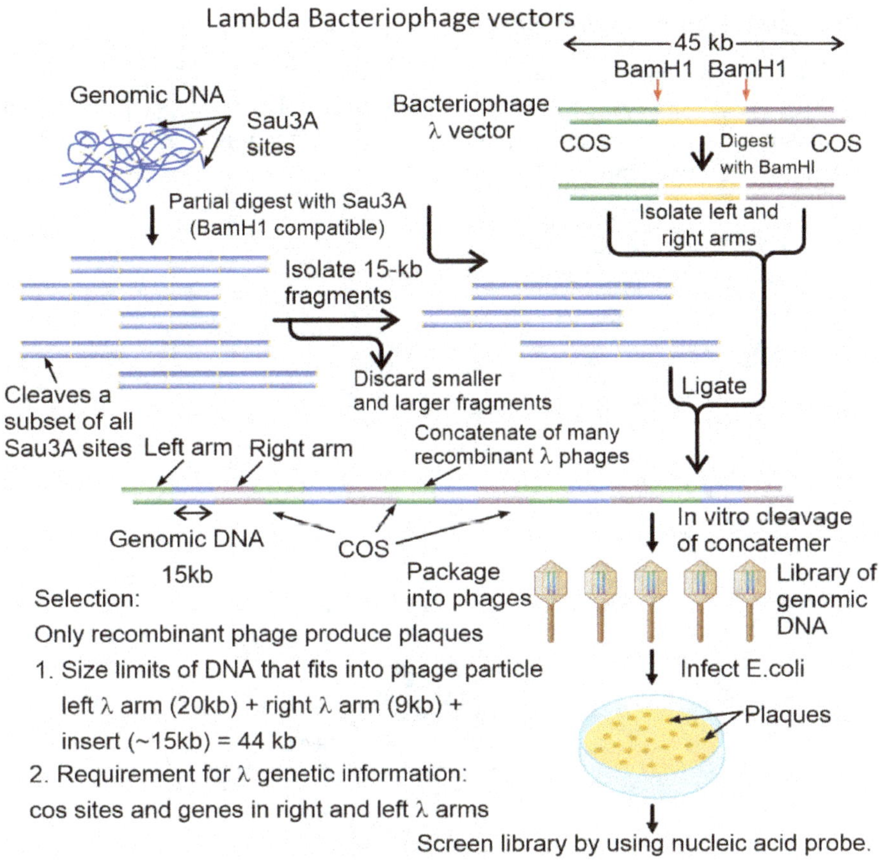

Lambda Bacteriophage vectors
45 kb
BamH1 BamH1
Genomic DNA
Sau3A
sites
Bacteriophage
λ vector
COS
Digest
with BamHI
COS
Partial digest with Sau3A
(BamH1 compatible)
Isolate left and
right arms
Isolate 15-kb
fragments
Discard smaller
and larger fragments
Ligate
Cleaves a
subset of all
Sau3A sites
Left arm
Right arm
Concatenate of many
recombinant λ phages
Genomic DNA
15kb
COS
In vitro cleavage
of concatemer
Package
into phages
Library of
genomic
DNA
Selection:
Only recombinant phage produce plaques
1. Size limits of DNA that fits into phage particle
left λ arm (20kb) + right λ arm (9kb) +
insert (~15kb) = 44 kb
2. Requirement for λ genetic information:
cos sites and genes in right and left λ arms
Infect E.coli
Plaques
Screen library by using nucleic acid probe.

Fig. 2.3 Diagrammatic representation of Bacteriophage Vector

Polylinker
Cosmid vector
Ampicillin
resistance
gene
Cos site
CoiE1
Ori

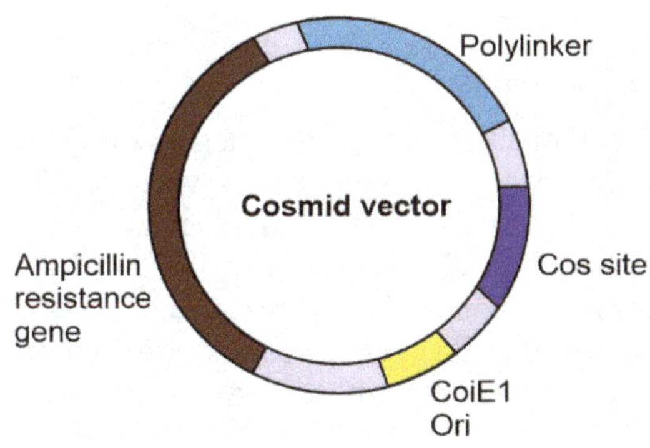

Fig. 2.4 Structure of Cosmid Vector

Bacterial Artificial Chromosome

In bacterial artificial chromosomes, inserts up to 350 kb can be cloned (BAC). In E. coli, BACs are maintained with only one copy per cell. The F plasmid is used in BACs, while the P1 phage is used in the PAC artificial chromosome.

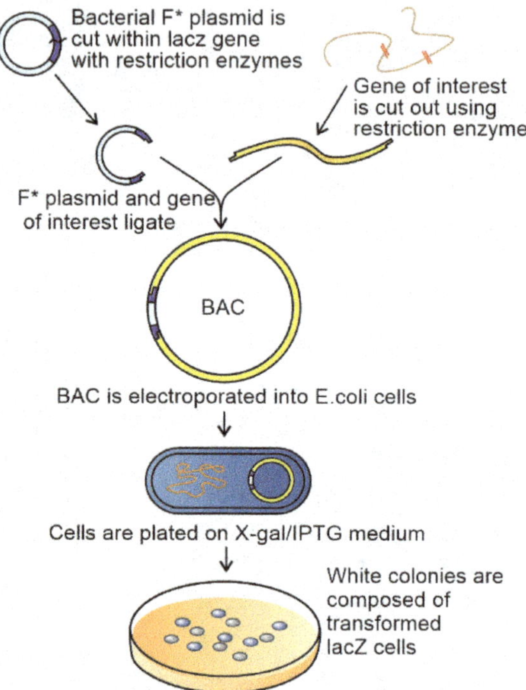

Fig. 2.5 Diagrammatic representation of Bacterial artificial chromosome

Yeast Artificial Chromosome

To clone DNA fragments larger than 1 mega base (1Mb=1000kb), yeast artificial chromosomes are employed as vectors. They're helpful for copying bigger DNA pieces, which are needed for genome mapping projects like the Human Genome Project. It has a telomeric sequence, which replicates itself independently (features required to replicate linear chromosomes in yeast cells). These vectors also have restriction sites for cloning foreign DNA and selectable marker genes.

Human Artificial Chromosome

Human artificial chromosomes could be used as gene delivery vectors, as well as a tool for expression research and evaluating human chromosomal function. It can carry very large DNA fragments (for practical purposes, there is no upper limit), so it overcomes the problem of other vectors' limited cloning capacity, as well as the risk of insertional mutagenesis produced by viral vector integration into host chromosomes.

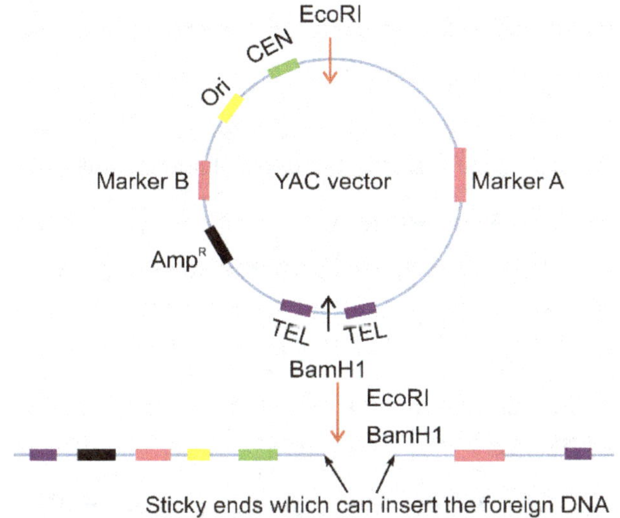

Fig. 2.6 Diagrammatic representation of Yeast artificial chromosome

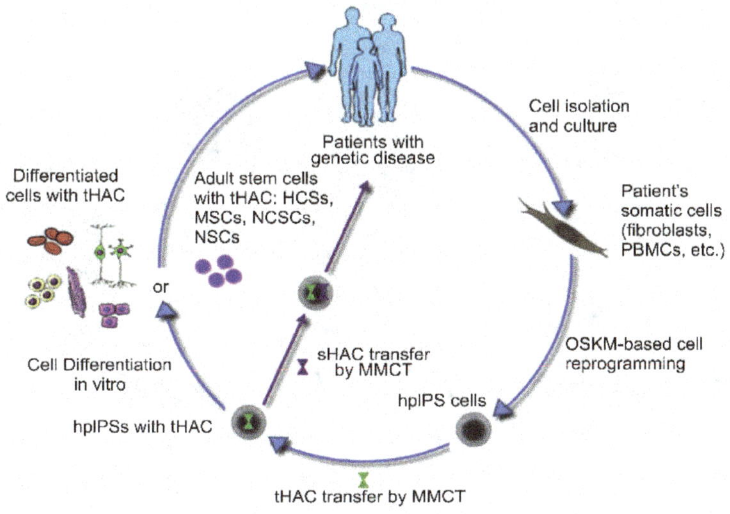

(a)

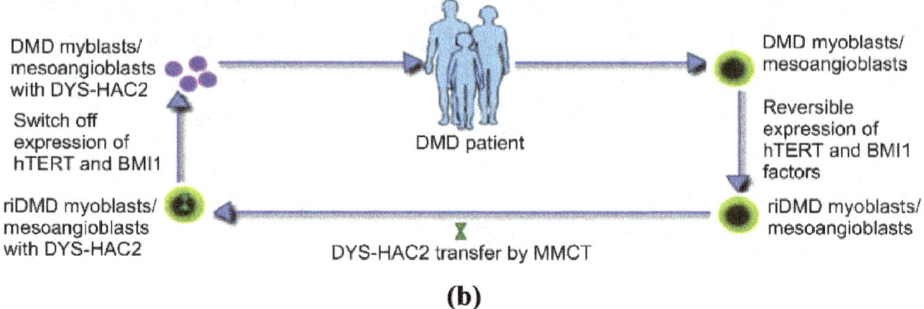

Fig. 2.7 Diagrammatic representation of Human artificial chromosome

Animal and Plant Viral Vectors

Foreign genes have been introduced into plant and animal cells using viruses that infect plant and animal cells. Viruses are suitable vehicles for transferring foreign DNA into eukaryotic cells in culture because of their innate capacity to adsorb to cells, introduce their DNA, and multiply. In the first mammalian cell cloning experiment, a vector based on Simian virus 40 (SV40) was utilised. To clone genes in mammals, a multitude of vectors based on various types of viruses, such as Adenoviruses and Papillomaviruses, have been utilised. Retroviral vectors are widely used to clone genes in mammalian cells at the moment. Cauliflower mosaic virus, Tobacco mosaic virus, and Gemini viruses have all been employed with limited success on plants.

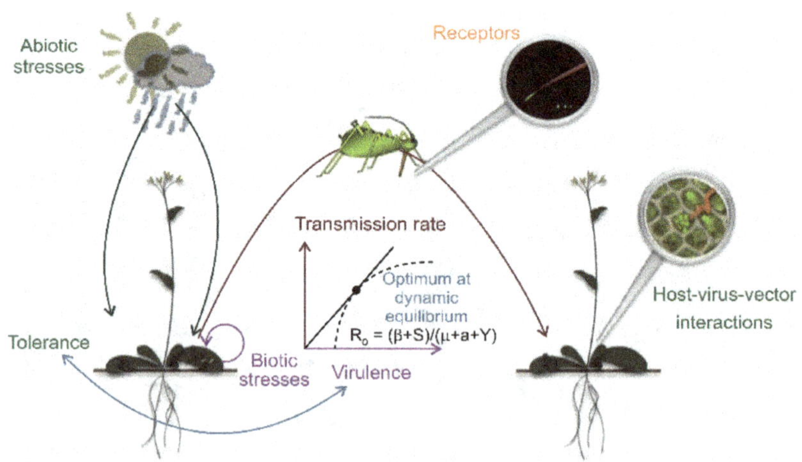

Fig. 2.8 Plant Viral Vectors

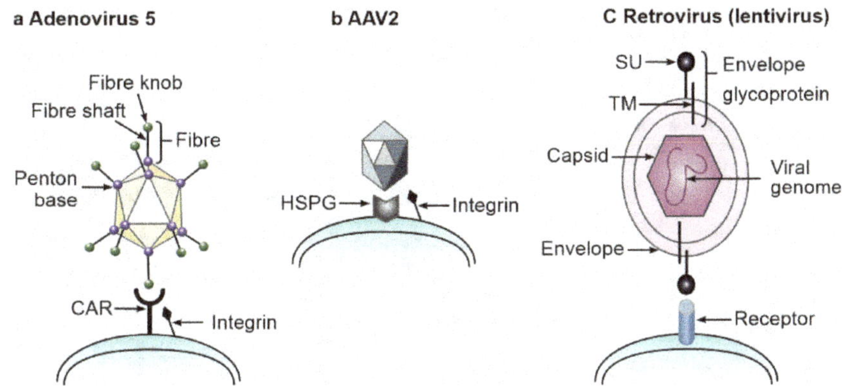

Fig. 2.9 Animal Viral Vectors

2.2   Recombinant DNA Technology

Recombinant DNA (rDNA) molecules are DNA molecules created in the laboratory using genetic recombination (such as molecular cloning) to combine genetic material from numerous sources, resulting in sequences not seen in biological organisms. Because DNA molecules from all creatures have the same chemical structure, recombinant DNA is feasible. The only difference is the sequence of nucleotides inside that identical overall structure. As a result, when foreign DNA is connected to host sequences capable of driving DNA replication and then introduced into a host organism, the foreign DNA replicates alongside the host DNA.

Biology relies heavily on recombinant DNA technology for study. It enables researchers to modify DNA fragments in the lab for research purposes. It entails implanting a fragment of DNA into a bacterial or yeast cell using a number of laboratory methods. Once inside, the bacteria or yeast will duplicate the DNA as well as their own. Important proteins required in the therapy of human ailments, such as insulin and growth hormone, have been effectively made using recombinant DNA technology.

Enzymes and other laboratory procedures are used to alter and isolate DNA segments of interest in recombinant DNA technology. This approach can be used to mix (or splice) DNA from various species, as well as to create new genes with new functions. Recombinant DNA refers to the copies that result from the process. The recombinant DNA is usually propagated in a bacterial or yeast cell, which uses its cellular machinery to copy the modified DNA alongside its native DNA.

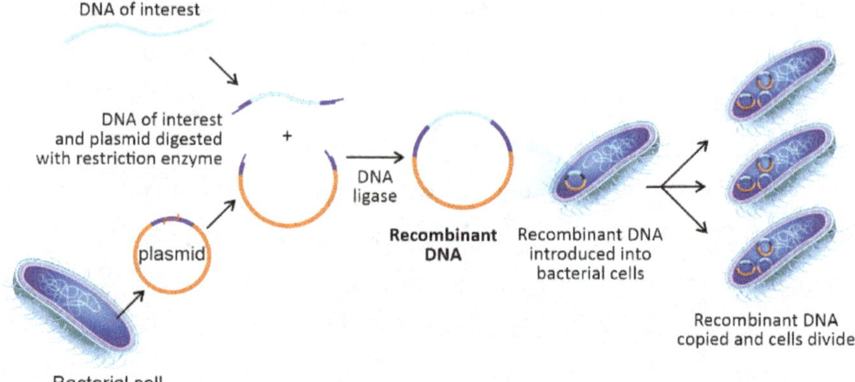

Fig. 2.10 Structure of rDNA

The following are the steps involved in rDNA technology

1. Isolation of the Genetic Material (DNA)
2. Cutting of DNA at Specific Locations
3. Isolation of Desired DNA Fragment
4. Amplification of Gene of Interest using PCR
5. Ligation of DNA Fragment into a Vector
6. Insertion of Recombinant DNA into the Host Cell/Organisms
7. Obtaining or Culturing the Foreign Gene Product.

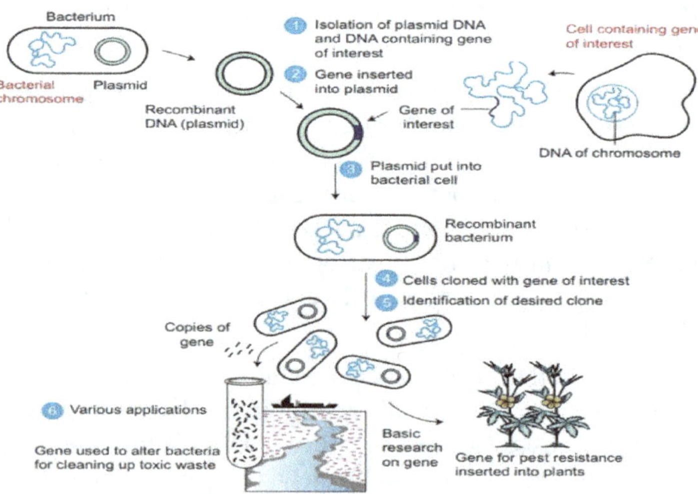

Fig. 2.11 The steps involved in rDNA technology are
diagrammatically illustrated

1. **Isolation of the Genetic Material (DNA):** Nucleic acid is the genetic material found in all living creatures. This is found in the majority of organisms in the form of deoxyribonucleic acid (DNA). In order for restrictor enzymes to cut DNA, it must be in pure form, that is, free of other macromolecules (such as proteins, RNA, enzymes, and so on).

   Isolation of genetic material (DNA) is carried out in the following steps:

   (a) Although DNA is encased in membranes, bacterial cells/plants/animal tissues are treated with the enzymes lysozyme (bacteria), cellulose (plant cells), and chitinase (fungus) to liberate DNA along with other macromolecules such as proteins, polysaccharides, and lipids.

   (b) Ribonuclease can be used to remove RNA, whereas protease can be used to remove proteins.

   (c) After adding cold ethanol, other molecules can be eliminated with proper procedures, and purified DNA will precipitate out. In the suspension, this can be viewed as a collection of fine Threads.

2. **Cutting of DNA at Specific Locations:** Restriction enzyme digestions are performed by incubating purified DNA molecules with the restriction enzyme. This is done at the optimal conditions for that specific enzyme.

3. **Isolation of Desired DNA Fragment:** The activity of restriction enzymes can be determined using agarose gel electrophoresis. Because DNA is negatively charged, it gravitates towards the positive electrode or anode, causing DNA to separate. The desired DNA fragment is then rinsed out.

4. **Amplification of Gene of Interest using PCR:** The DNA replication in vitro is best described by Polymerase Chain Reaction (PCR). Kary Mullis invented this approach in 1985 and was awarded the Nobel Prize in Chemistry in 1993 for it. Using two sets of primers, PCR is used to amplify a gene of interest.

The basic requirements of a PCR reaction are the following

(a) **DNA Template:** The double-stranded DNA that needed to be amplified.

(b) **Primers:** These are chemically synthesised oligonucleotides (short segment of DNA) that are complementary to a region of DNA template.

(c) **Enzymes:** Two enzymes are commonly used.

i. Taq Polymerase: It was isolated from Thermus aquaticus, a thermophilic bacteria. It possesses the ability to remain active in the presence of high temperatures that cause denaturation of double-stranded DNA.

ii. It also aids in the amplification of a DNA segment to around a billion times, i.e., I billion copies are created when the DNA replication process is repeated several times.

iii. Polymerase Vent (isolated from Thermococcus litoralis).

Three main steps involved in PCR technique are

a) **Denaturation:** The double-stranded DNA is denatured for 15 seconds at a high temperature of 95°C. Each single-strand that has been split now serves as a template for DNA synthesis.

b) **Annealing:** To anneal, two sets of oligonucleotide primers are used (hybridise). Depending on the length and sequence of the primers, this step is performed at a somewhat lower temperature (40-60°C) with Mg2+ and dNTPs (deoxynucleoside triphosphates).

c) **Extension:** In this reaction, the thermostable enzyme Taq DNA polymerase is utilised, which can withstand the high temperature of 72 °C the primer extension reaction by adding nucleotides complementary to the template.

Note: The thermostable DNA polymerase, such as Taq polymerase, requires Mg2+ as a cofactor. These steps are repeated many times in order to obtain several copies of desired DNA.

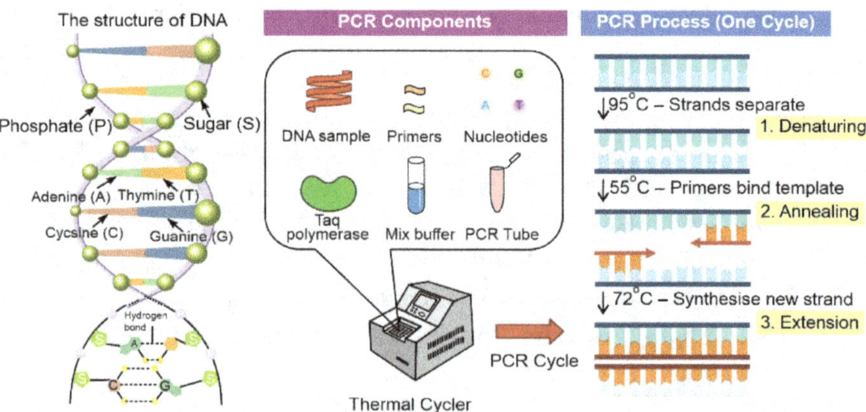

Fig. 2.12 The steps involved in PCR

5. **Ligation of DNA Fragment into a Vector:** This process requires a vector DNA and a source DNA. In order to obtain sticky ends, both of these should cut with the same endonuclease. After which both are ligated by mixing vector DNA, gene of interest and enzyme DNA ligase to form the recombinant DNA/hybrid DNA.

6. **Insertion of Recombinant DNA into the Host Cell/Organisms:** This can occur by several methods, before which the recipient cells are made competent to receive the DNA. If a recombinant DNA bearing gene for resistance to an antibiotic (e.g., ampicillin) is transferred into E. coli cells, the host cells become transformed into ampicillin resistant cells.

   The ampicillin resistance gene in this case is called a selectable marker. When transformed cells are grown on agar plates containing ampicillin, only transformants will grow and others will die.

7. **Obtaining or Culturing the Foreign Gene Product:** When you insert a piece of alien DNA into a cloning vector and transfer it into a bacterial cell, the alien DNA gets multiplied

2.3   Applications of Recombinant DNA Technology in Medicine

By replacing damaged and defective genes in the body with new genes, recombinant DNA technology has made it feasible to treat a wide range of ailments. It has ushered in dramatic developments in the world of medicine, introducing previously unimaginable techniques of treating ailments and delivering pharmaceuticals.

❖ **Human Insulin:** Insulin produced by humans Insulin is a protein-based hormone that regulates blood sugar levels. This hormone is produced by cells in the pancreas known as the 'Islets Of Langerhans.' Because a low level of insulin can lead to diabetes, this hormone plays a crucial role in managing glucose levels in the body.By employing bacteria as a host cell, scientists were able to generate human insulin using recombinant DNA technology. There are several different types of recombinant insulin formulations on the market. Inserting the human insulin gene into E. coli, which then generates insulin for human usage, yields recombinant insulin. This is said to be a safer alternative to conventionally prepared medications.

❖ **Human Growth Hormones:** A polypeptide hormone, human growth hormone is a hormone that is made up of several different amino acids. In both humans and animals, it is responsible for cell reproduction, growth, and regeneration. It is produced in the pituitary glands by somatotroph cells. HGH for therapeutic purposes was previously derived from cadavers' pituitary glands before recombinant HGH became accessible. Some patients developed Creutzfeldt-Jakob disease as a result of this risky technique. This problem was solved by using recombinant HGH, which is presently utilised as a treatment. Athletes and others have also utilised it as a performance enhancer. Many growth hormones have recently been produced thanks to biotechnology. This hormone has been found to be effective in treating dwarfism.

❖ **Vaccines:** A vaccine is a biological material made from a suspension of disease-causing cells that are either weak or dead. It is injected into the body in order to boost antibody production against a specific antigen. By cloning the gene for protective antigen protein using recombinant DNA technology, scientists have made it easier to develop vaccinations. Virus vaccines, such as those for herpes, influenza, hepatitis, and foot-and-mouth disease, are usually created using this method.

❖ **Monoclonal Antibodies:** When a foreign substance enters the body, the immune system generates an antibody, which is a type of protein. Monoclonal antibodies can now be created using the hybridoma process. Lymphocytes or B cells are fused with myeloma cells in this procedure, resulting in a Hybridoma material. In culture, this hybridoma generates an endless supply of antibodies. Monoclonal antibodies are the antibodies that are created. Vaccines against several viral illnesses are made using these antibodies.

❖ **Interferon:** Interferons are glycoproteins that have the ability to prevent viruses from multiplying or dividing in cells or surrounding cells. Hairy cell leukaemia is one type of malignancy that can be treated with it. E.coli is used to manufacture this protein utilising recombinant DNA technology. Lymphoma and myelogenous leukaemia are treated with interferon alpha.

❖ **Antibiotics:** Antibiotics are a class of drugs that are used to treat bacterial infections. They can be created both in the lab and by microbes. They have the power to kill bacteria in the body that cause infections. In 1928, Alexander Fleming used recombinant DNA technology to find Penicillin. Antibiotics are also made using other biotechnological processes.

❖ **Diagnosis of infection with HIV:** Recombinant DNA was utilised to generate each of the three widely used procedures for diagnosing HIV infection. A recombinant HIV protein is used in the antibody test (ELISA or western blot) to check for the presence of antibodies produced by the body in response to HIV infection. Using reverse transcriptase polymerase chain reaction, the DNA test looks for HIV genetic material (RT-PCR). The molecular cloning and sequence analysis of HIV genomes enabled the development of the RT-PCR test.

2.4   Interferon

Interferons (IFNs) are proteins that host cells produce and release in response to pathogens such as viruses, bacteria, parasites, or tumour cells. They allow cells to communicate in order to activate the immune system's defensive defences, which eliminate infections or malignancies. The term "interferon" comes from the fact that this molecule interferes with virus reproduction. It was first found by Alick Isaacs and Jean Lindemann in 1957 and was thought to be a single compound.

IFNs are members of the cytokine family of glycoproteins. The ability of interferons to "interfere" with viral replication within host cells gives them their name. Other activities of IFNs include activating immune cells like natural killer cells and macrophages, increasing recognition of infection or tumour cells by up-regulating antigen presentation to T lymphocytes, and improving the ability of uninfected host cells to resist fresh virus infection. Aching muscles and fever are two symptoms linked to the production of IFNs during infection.

In animals, there are about 10 different IFNs; seven of them have been described for humans. Type I IFN, Type II IFN, and Type III IFN are the three IFN classes most commonly used. IFNs from all IFN classes are critical in the fight against viral infections.

Interferon type I (IFN-I) binds to a specific cell surface receptor complex called the

IFN-receptor (IFNAR), which is made up of two chains: IFNAR1 and IFNAR2.

IFN-α, IFN-β and IFN-ω are the three types of type I interferons found in humans.

Interferons' mechanism of action is as follows

When mammalian cells are infected with viruses, they create interferons. The virus induces the host DNA to create interferons by releasing its nucleic acid into the cellular cytoplasm. Interferons are proteins released by cells that attach to cells nearby. They do this by inducing a sequence of antiviral enzymes in the cellular DNA. The proteins that are generated in this way prevent viral replication and protect the cells. The protective (enzymes) proteins are thought to bind to virus mRNA and prevent protein synthesis. Interferons appear to have a species-specific activity. Human interferons work in humans in this way. Interferons from other animals (dogs, mice) are useless in humans.

Recombinant interferon production

The complementary DNA (cDNA) was made from a specific interferon's mRNA. This is placed into a vector (for example, a plasmid) that is then introduced into E. coli or other cells. Intracellularly, the recombinant product forms inclusion bodies. It is possible to separate the interferon from the culture media. The basic mechanism for manufacturing recombinant interferons is as follows.

An early fermentation stage is required for large-scale production. The E. coli cells are homogenised after harvesting, and the inclusion bodies are retrieved by centrifugation. The interferon is purified to homogeneity using a mixture of chromatographic processes after solubilization and refolding. In the presence of a phosphate buffer and sodium chloride, the final product is created. It comes in glass vials with a 30 mg/ml solution and has a shelf life of 24 months when stored at 2–8°C'.

Interferon production is lower in bacterial hosts, despite the fact that E. coli was the first to be employed. This is due to the fact that most interferons are glycoproteins in nature, and bacteria lack the machinery needed to glycosylate proteins.

The manufacture of Betaferon

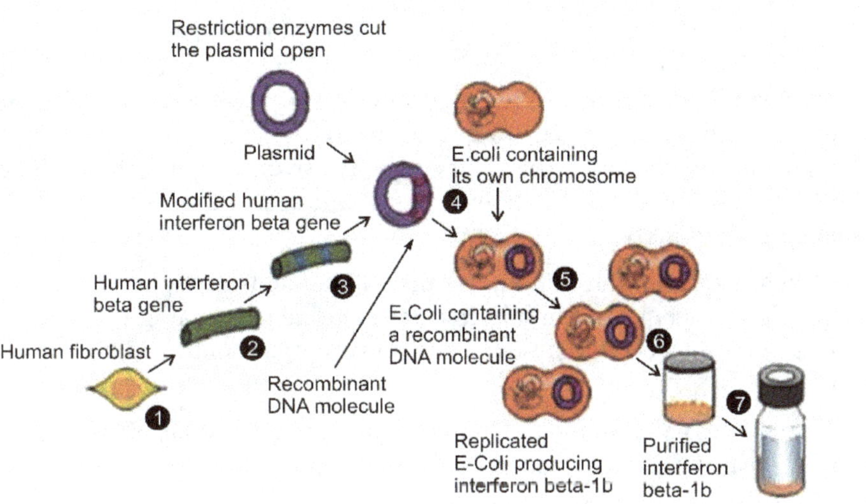

Fig. 2.13 Recombinant interferon production

2.4.1   Vaccine

A vaccination is a biological preparation that boosts your immune system against a certain disease. A vaccination usually contains an agent that looks like a disease-causing germ and is manufactured from weakened or destroyed microbes, their toxins, or one of their surface proteins. The agent induces the immune system to recognise the agent as foreign, destroy it, and "remember" it so that the immune system can recognise and eliminate any of these germs it encounters in the future.

Vaccines can be either preventive (to avoid or mitigate the symptoms of a future infection by any natural or "wild" disease) or therapeutic (to treat an existing infection) (e.g., vaccines against cancer are also being investigated; see cancer vaccine).

Recombinant Vaccines

The biotechnology industry has also contributed to the development of vaccinations against specific diseases. Recombinant vaccines are vaccines that make use of recombinant DNA technology. Subunit vaccines are another name for it.

Vaccine against Hepatitis B

Hepatitis is a viral infection that causes liver damage. Hepatitis is derived from the terms "hepato" and "itis," which mean "liver" and "inflammation." It is one of the most devastating viral diseases, affecting almost 7 million individuals each year. It can infect and harm the liver in both acute and chronic forms. Damage to the liver, which is the centre of all body reactions and metabolism, results in death. It's a serious illness that spreads quickly.

Hepatitis B immunisation, on the other hand, can prevent it. The hepatitis B vaccine is administered intramuscularly. It is given in three doses, with the second and third doses given one month and six months apart.

Hepatitis B vaccine was originally produced using hepatitis virus. It wasn't clear whether the vaccine was live or attenuated.

Hepatitis B Vaccine Production

A live vaccine is one that uses a live hepatitis virus. However, attenuation reduces the pathogenicity of the virus. When a weak virus is injected into the body, they can no longer be pathogenic. However, due to virulence issues in immune-compromised patients, these vaccinations are dangerous and unreliable. There is also a downward tendency in human immunity. As a result, once given, vaccinations can become virulent and cause infection. Hepatitis-B subunit vaccinations are used to avoid this and provide effective prophylaxis.

The steps required in making Hepatitis B Vaccine

1. Isolation of the hepatitis B virus's whole genome:
2. Plasmid-mediated genome cloning and multiplication
3. Publication of the HBs antigen sequence.
4. Ligate using a yeast expression vector.
5. Transform in saccharomyces and wait for the vaccine to develop.

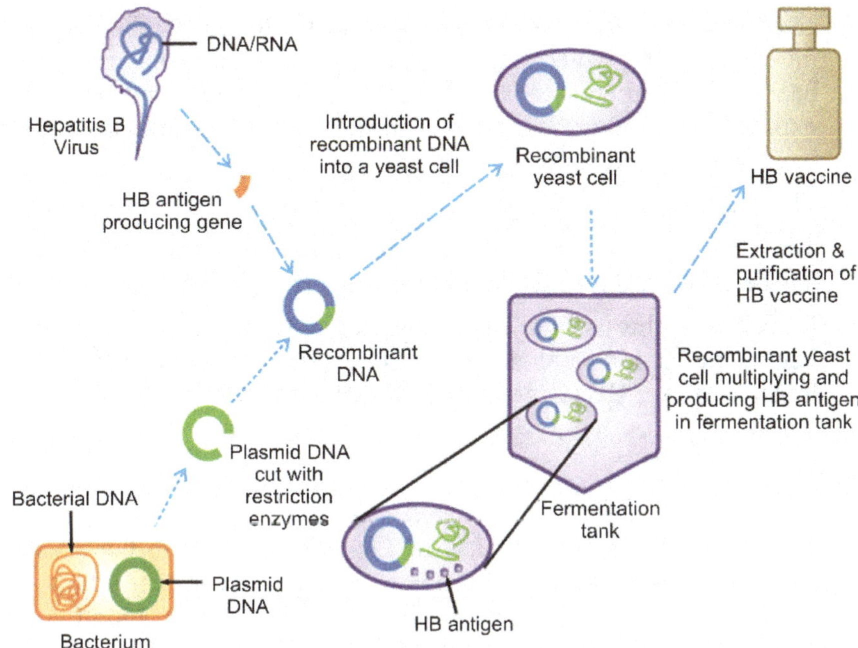

Fig. 2.14 Production of Hepatitis B Vaccine

Procedure

- The first step is to isolate the genome from the virus. The whole 2kb genome that codes for HB ag on the viral body has been isolated. However, the number may be low, and the virus is not easily multiplied in laboratories. As a result of the plasmid, the gene is multiplied. Plasmids have a natural proclivity for multiplying. This genome-encoded plasmid is given to bacteria for replication and multiplication. Many plasmids containing the gene are created.

- Using restriction endonucleases, the necessary gene coding for HBs is cleaved from these adequate genomes.

- These are the enzymes that precisely cleave DNA molecules.

- Once the appropriate gene has been created, it is extracted and cloned using a different vector, the yeast expression vector.

- Alcohol dehydrogenase-1 (a strong promoter gene) is flanked by alcohol dehydrogenase-1 (a strong promoter gene) in this yeast expression vector. Leucin 2 is also used as a marker.

- The enzyme DNA ligase is employed to ligate (clone) the gene with the yeast vector, which is then turned into the saccharomyces cervatia bacteria. The altered cells are allowed to proliferate and boost gene expression in culture conditions. In the body of a bacterial cell, the vaccine is made and present.

- The solution is centrifuged after the bacterial cells have been lysed.

- The HBs gene is acquired in the supernatant this way. This vaccine has been isolated and allowed to form silver aggregates.

- Rather than the usual rDNA technology steps, we use two vectors here. One is for viral gene multiplication, while the other is for transferring the HBs gene into bacteria, where it is expressed.

2.4.2   Insulin

The J-cells of the pancreas' islets of Langerhans produce the hormone insulin. Insulin is made up of 51 amino acids that are organised into two polypeptide chains. There are 21 amino acids in chain A and 30 amino acids in chain B. Disulphide bonds hold both of them together.

Recombinant Insulin Production

In the late 1970s, attempts were made to synthesise insulin using recombinant DNA technology. The basic procedure was putting the human insulin gene and the lac operon promoter gene on E. coli plasmids. This approach was used to create human insulin. In July 1980, at Guy's Hospital in London, seventeen human volunteers were given recombinant insulin for the first time to treat diabetes. Insulin was the first recombinant DNA-based medicinal product to be delivered to people. Human insulin was approved for marketing by Eli Lilly Company in 1986 under the trade name Humulin.

The initial method of insulin production in E. coli has undergone various modifications to improve yield, such as the insertion of a signal peptide, independent synthesis of the A and B chains, and so on. Both genes are expressed via the lac operon system (inducer gene, promoter gene, operator gene, and structural gene Z for -galactosidase). Lactose in the culture medium causes the synthesis of both the A and B chains of insulin in separate cultures. The isolated, purified, and linked insulin chains can be used to make full-fledged human insulin.

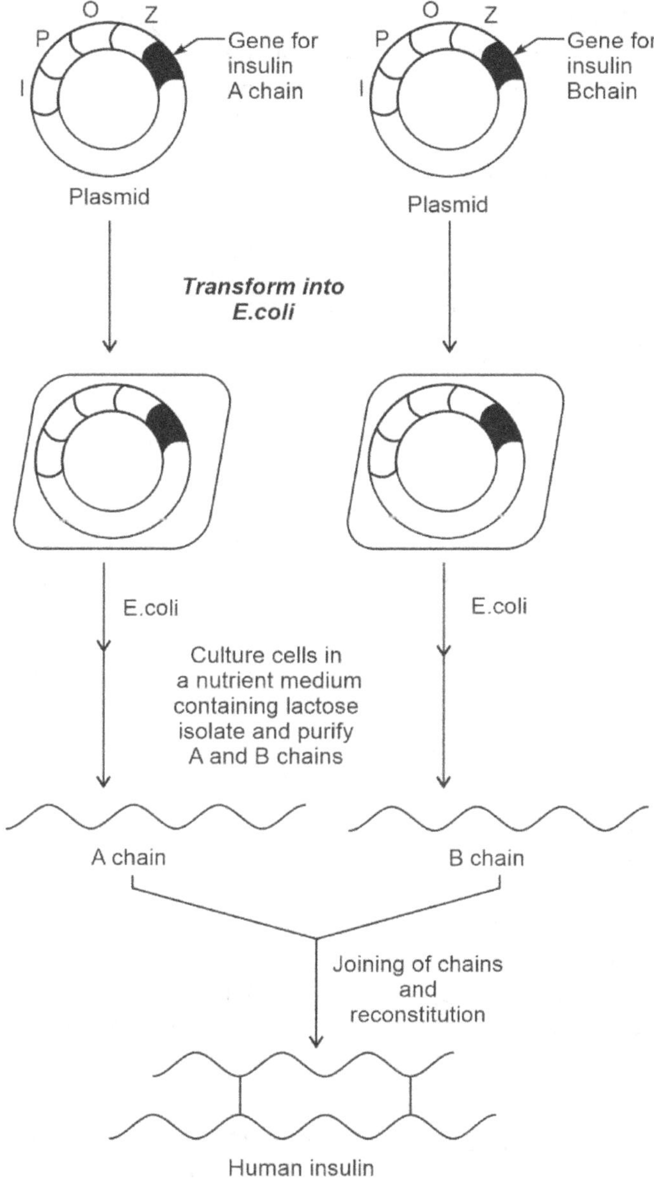

Fig. 2.15 Production of Recombinant Insulin in E.coli

Recombinant Insulins of the Second Generation

The insulin concentration in the blood progressively rises after injection. As a result, insulin injections must be given at least 15 minutes prior to a meal. Furthermore, the drop in insulin levels is gradual, putting patients at risk of hyperinsulinemia. This is owing to the fact that therapeutic insulin exists as a hexamer (six molecules linked together) that slowly dissociates into the physiologically active dimer or monomer.

In recent years, site-directed mutagenesis and protein engineering have been used to try to make second-generation insulin. Muteins are the second generation of recombinant proteins. The goal of developing a high number of insulin muteins was to speed up the dissociation of hexamers into biologically active forms. Insulin lispro, which has changed amino acid residues in the B-chain of insulin, is one of them. Insulin lispro can be injected right before a meal because it quickly reaches pharmacologically effective levels.

2.5   Polymerase Chain Reaction

Polymerase chain reaction (PCR) is a method widely used to rapidly make millions to billions of copies (complete or partial) of a specific DNA sample, allowing scientists to take a very small sample of DNA and amplify it (or a part of it) to a large enough amount to study in detail. PCR was invented in 1983 by the American biochemist Kary Mullis at Cetus Corporation; Mullis and biochemist Michael Smith, who had developed other essential ways of manipulating DNA, were jointly awarded the Nobel Prize in Chemistry in 1993.

PCR is fundamental to many of the procedures used in genetic testing and research, including analysis of ancient samples of DNA and identification of infectious agents. Using PCR, copies of very small amounts of DNA sequences are exponentially amplified in a series of cycles of temperature changes. PCR is now a common and often indispensable technique used in medical laboratory research for a broad variety of applications including biomedical research and criminal forensics.

The majority of PCR methods rely on thermal cycling. Thermal cycling exposes reactants to repeated cycles of heating and cooling to permit different temperature-dependent reactions specifically, DNA melting and enzyme-driven DNA replication. PCR employs two main reagents primers (which are short single strand DNA fragments known as oligonucleotides that are a complementary sequence to the target DNA region) and a DNA polymerase. In the first step of PCR, the two strands of the DNA double helix are physically separated at a high temperature in a process called nucleic acid denaturation. In the second step, the temperature is lowered and the primers bind to the complementary sequences of DNA. The two DNA strands then become templates for DNA polymerase to enzymatically assemble a new DNA strand from free nucleotides, the building blocks of DNA. As PCR progresses, the DNA generated is itself used as a template for replication, setting in motion a chain reaction in which the original DNA template is exponentially amplified.

Principle

A precise section of a DNA strand is amplified using the PCR method (the DNA target). Although certain techniques allow for amplification of segments up to 40 kbp, most PCR methods amplify DNA fragments between 0.1 and 10 kbp. The available substrates in the reaction, which become limiting as the reaction develops, dictate the amount of amplified product.

A basic PCR set-up requires several components and reagents, including:

- A DNA template containing the amplificable DNA target region

- A DNA polymerase, which polymerizes new DNA strands;

- Two DNA primers complementary to the 3' (three prime) ends of each of the sense and anti-sense strands of the DNA target (DNA polymerase can only bind to and elongate from a double-stranded region of DNA; without primers, there is no double-stranded initiation site at which the polymerase can bind);*deoxynucleoside triphosphates*, or dNTPs (sometimes called "deoxynucleotide triphosphates"; nucleotides containing triphosphate groups), the building blocks from which the DNA polymerase synthesizes a new DNA strand

- A buffer solution that provides a chemical environment conducive to the DNA polymerase's optimal activity and stability

- Bivalent cations, such as magnesium (Mg) or manganese (Mn) ions; Mg2+ is the most frequent, although Mn2+ can be utilised for PCR-mediated DNA mutagenesis since a higher Mn2+ concentration increases the error rate during DNA synthesis; and monovalent cations, such as potassium (K) ions;

In a thermal cycler, the reaction is usually carried out in small reaction tubes (0.2–0.5 mL volumes) with a volume of 10–200 L. The reaction tubes are heated and cooled by the thermal cycler to achieve the temperatures required at each phase of the process.

Many modern thermal cyclers make use of the Peltier effect, which allows the block carrying the PCR tubes to be heated and cooled by merely reversing the electric current. Thermal conductivity is improved by thin-walled reaction tubes, allowing for rapid thermal equilibrium. To prevent condensation at the top of the reaction tube, most thermal cyclers feature heated covers. A layer of oil on top of the reaction mixture or a ball of wax inside the tube is required in older thermal cyclers without a heated cover. Process involved in PCR

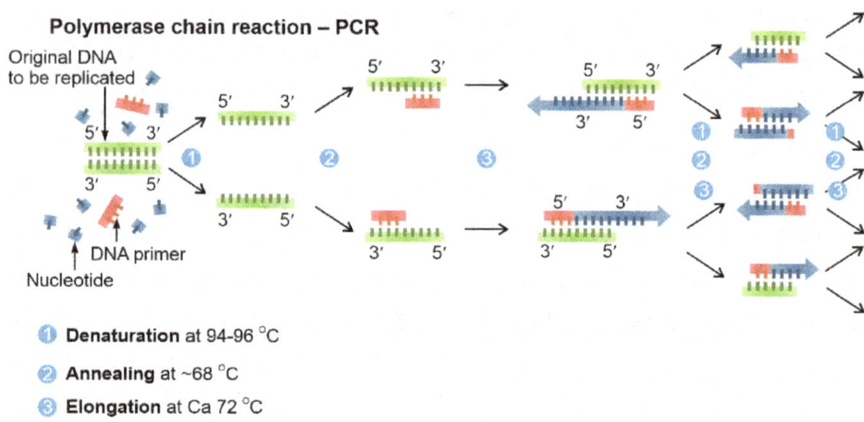

Fig. 2.16 Diagrammatic representation of Polymerase chain reaction

1. **Denaturation:** The DNA template is heated to a temperature of 94° C. This causes the weak hydrogen bonds that link DNA strands together in a helix to dissolve, allowing single-stranded DNA to form.

2. **Annealing:** The mixture is chilled to between 50 and 70 °C. This permits the primers to attach (anneal) to the template DNA's complementary sequence.

3. **Extension:** Thereafter, the process is heated to 72 °C, which is the ideal temperature for DNA polymerase to function. Using the target DNA as a template, DNA polymerase expands the primers by sequentially adding nucleotides to the primers.

A single double-stranded DNA template segment is amplified into two autonomous pieces of double-stranded DNA in one cycle. In the next cycle, these two pieces will be accessible for amplification. As the cycles are repeated, additional copies of the template are created, and the number of copies of the template grows exponentially.

Types of PCR

1. Reverse transcriptase PCR (RT-PCR)
2. Nested PCR
3. Real- Time PCR (Quantitative PCR-qPCR)
4. Inverse PCR
5. LATE (Linear-After-The-Exponential) PCR
6. Fast cycling PCR
7. Variable Number of Tandem Repeats (VNTR) PCR
8. Thermal Asymmetric interlaced PCR (TAIL-PCR)
9. Suicide PCR
10. Touch Down PCR
11. Ligation-mediated PCR
12. Long-Range PCR
13. Methylation-specific PCR
14. Reverse Transcriptase Real-Time PCR
15. RNase H-dependent PCR
16. Single Specific Primer-PCR
17. Solid-phase PCR
18. Miniprimer PCR
19. Multiplex PCR
20. Nanoparticle Assisted PCR (Nano PCR)
21. Amplified Fragment length polymorphism (AFLP) PCR
22. Inter Sequence-Specific PCR
23. Allele-specific PCR
24. Arthrobacter luteus (Alu) PCR
25. Hot start PCR
26. Asymmetric PCR
27. COLD-PCR
28. In-Situ PCR
29. Colony PCR
30. Digital PCR (dPCR)
31. High- Resolution Melt (HRM) PCR

1. **Reverse transcriptase PCR (RT-PCR):** Reverse transcription PCR (RT-PCR) is a variant of traditional PCR in which RNA molecules are transformed into complementary DNA (cDNA) molecules before being amplified by PCR.

   - In RT-PCR, reverse transcriptase is used to convert the RNA template into complementary DNA (cDNA). The cDNA is subsequently used as a template for PCR-based exponential amplification.

   - RT-PCR can be performed in a single tube or in two phases in separate tubes. With less chances of contamination and variation assimilation, the one-step technique is more effective.

   - Research methodologies, gene insertion, genetic illness diagnostics, and cancer detection all require RT-PCR.

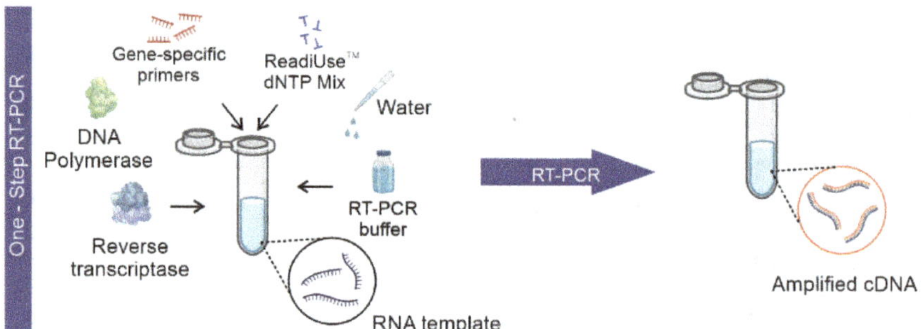

Fig. 2.17 Reverse transcription PCR

2. **Nested PCR**
   - Nested PCR is a beneficial modification of PCR technology that improves the reaction's specificity by preventing non-specific binding using two sets of primers.

   - The first pair of primers binds to the outside of our target DNA and amplifies a bigger fragment, whereas the second set of primers binds to the target spot specifically.

   - The second set of primers amplifies only the target DNA in the second round of amplification.

   - Nested PCR is an effective approach for phylogenetic analysis and pathogen detection.

   - Since the technology is more sensitive, even if the sample contains less DNA, it can be amplified, which is not possible with traditional PCR.

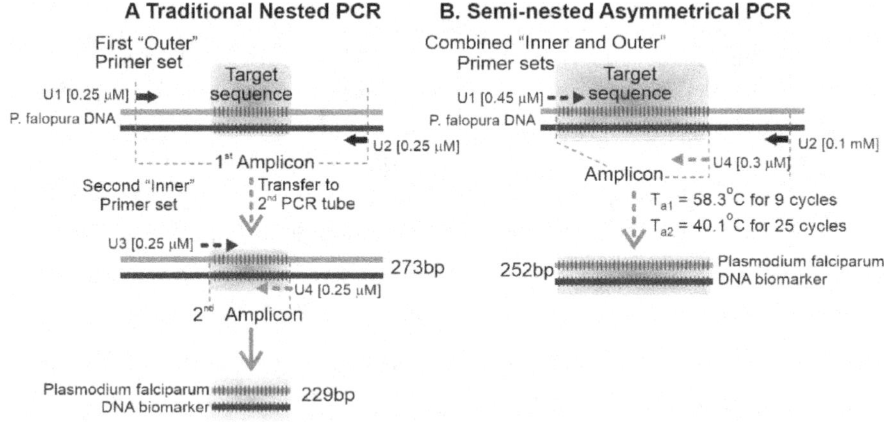

Fig. 2.18 Nested PCR

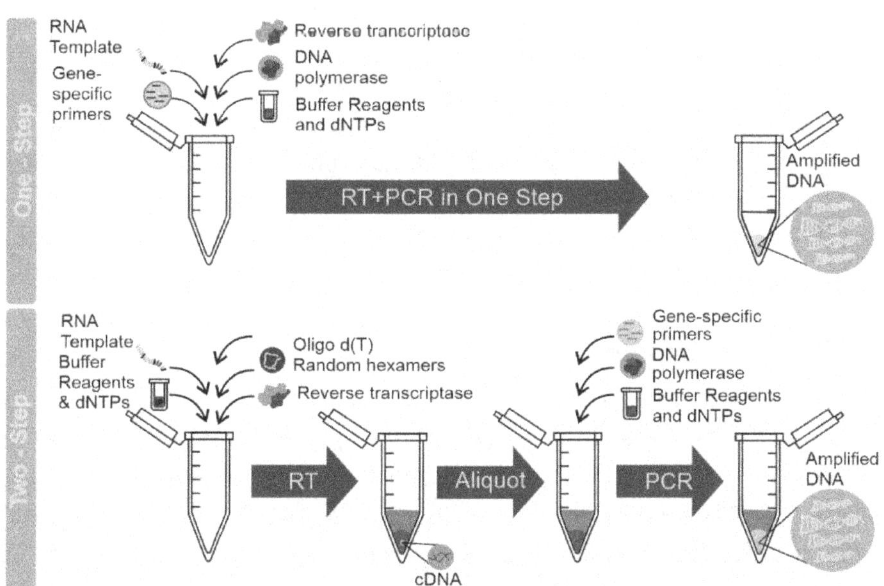

Fig. 2.19 Real- Time PCR (Quantitative PCR-qPCR)

3. Real- Time PCR (Quantitative PCR-qPCR)

- Quantitative PCR (qPCR), also known as real-time PCR or quantitative real-time PCR, is a PCR-based technology that combines the amplification of a target DNA sequence with the quantification of that DNA species' concentration in a reaction.

- Traditional PCR is a time-consuming procedure that involves analysing PCR results using gel electrophoresis. qPCR simplifies the analysis by detecting products in real time during the exponential phase.
- The use of fluorescent dye is required for real-time PCR to work.
- Pathogen genotyping and quantification, microRNA analysis, cancer detection, microbial load assessment, and GMO detection are all applications of q-PCR.

4. **Inverse PCR**

- Inverse polymerase chain reaction (Inverse PCR) is a polymerase chain reaction variant that is used to amplify DNA when only one sequence is known.

- Unlike traditional PCR, which requires primers that are complementary to both terminals of the target DNA, Inverse PCR allows for amplification even if only one sequence is available from which to create primers.

- Inverse PCR uses restriction digestion followed by ligation to create a looping segment that may then be primed for PCR using a single section of known sequence.

- The temperature-sensitive DNA polymerase then amplifies the DNA, similar to other polymerase chain reaction procedures.

- Inverse PCR is particularly beneficial for determining the position of transposons' inserts.

5. **LATE (Linear-After-The-Exponential) PCR**

- LATE (Linear-After-The-Exponential) PCR is a variant of Asymmetric PCR that employs a limiting primer with a higher melting temperature than the surplus primer to preserve reaction

- efficiency while the limiting primer concentration drops in the middle of the reaction.

- LATE-PCR starts with an exponential phase with amplification efficiency comparable to traditional PCR. The reaction quickly shifts to linear amplification once the limiting primer is

- depleted, and the single-stranded product is sustained for several more heat cycles.

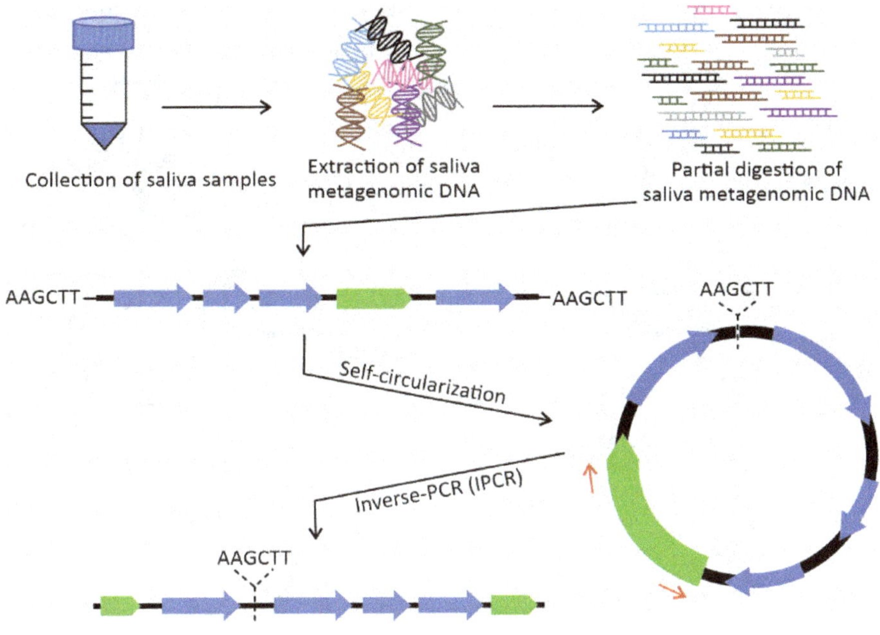

Fig. 2.20 Inverse PCR

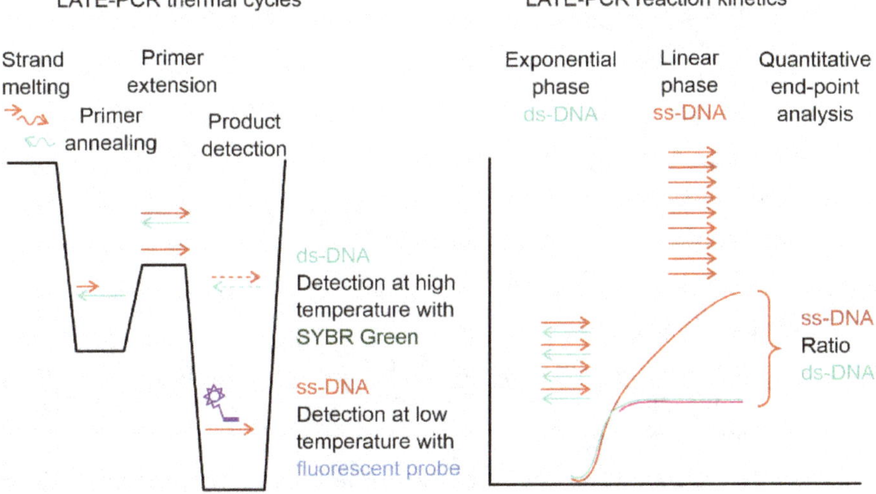

Fig. 2.21 LATE (Linear-After-The-Exponential) PCR

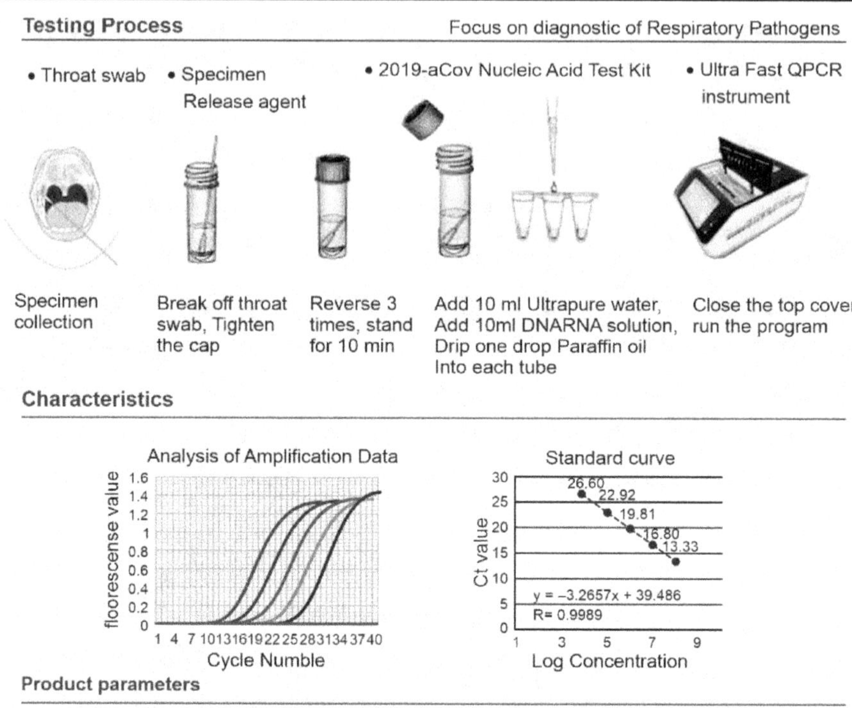

Ultrafast real-time qPCR system	
Sample flux	8
Reaction volume	10-25ul
Maximum beating up-rate	8°C/sec
Temperature range	30-100 °C (tube) ; modular-150°C
Temperature accuracy	40.3°C
Temperature uniformity	0.3°C-0.5°C
Fluorescence channels	4
Weight	3.2 kg (Including power adapter 3.8kg)
Dimension	25cm "19cm" 12 cm

Fig. 2.22 Fast cycling PCR

6. Fast cycling PCR

- Fast cycling PCR is a PCR-based technology that allows amplification of specific PCR products with significantly reduced cycling time.

- The principle in this process is the same as conventional PCR, the only difference being the time of amplification.

- The buffer used in this PCR increases the affinity of Taq DNA polymerases for short single-stranded DNA fragments, reducing the time required for successful primer annealing to just 5 seconds.

- Fast cycling PCR is essential for processes requiring quick cycles and also helps in the rapid diagnosis of diseases and mutations.

7. Variable Number of Tandem Repeats (VNTR) PCR

- In VNTR PCR, fragments that exhibited little variation within a species but did indicate differences across species are amplified, making them significant markers for individualization in forensic research.

- It can successfully amplify genomic deoxyribonucleic acid (DNA) from a very little amount of DNA using the polymerase chain reaction (PCR).

- PCR-based variable-number tandem repeat (VNTR) analysis was a promising method for typing M. tuberculosis among the genotyping tools.

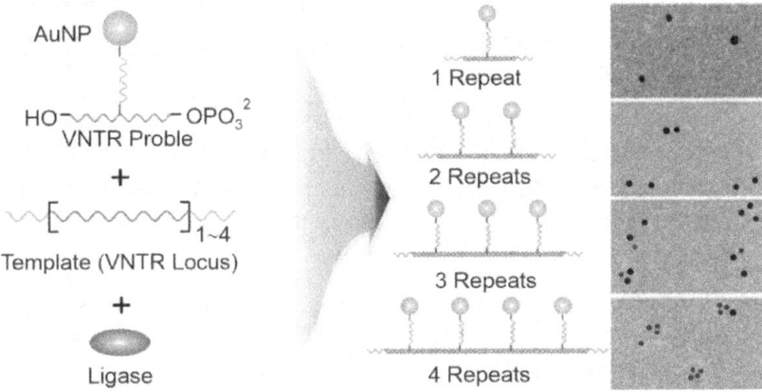

Fig 2.23 Variable Number of Tandem Repeats (VNTR) PCR

8. Thermal Asymmetric interlaced PCR (TAIL-PCR)

- TAIL PCR is an effective method for recovering DNA fragments that are close to known sequences.

- TAIL –PCR employs three nested primers in consecutive reactions, as well as an arbitrary degenerate primer with a low melting temperature, to control the relative amplification frequencies of specific and non-specific products.

- This method is highly accurate, allowing unpurified TAIL-PCR products to be directly sequenced, as well as the cloning of full-length functional genes.

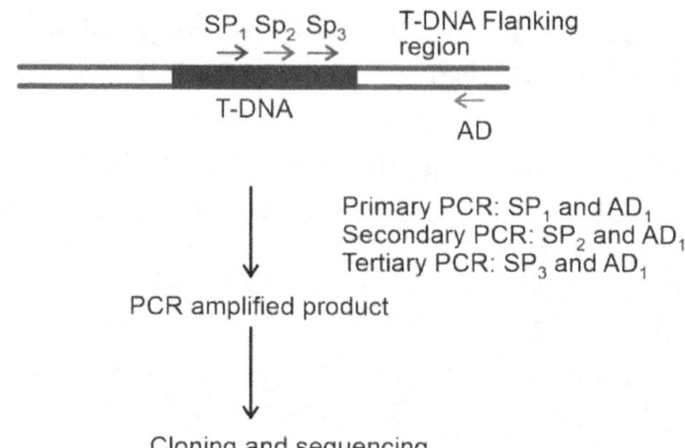

Fig. 2.24 Thermal Asymmetric interlaced PCR

9. Suicide PCR

- Suicide PCR is a widely utilised technique in research where eliminating false positives and verifying the specificity of the amplified fragment are critical.

- These primers must always target a genomic region that has never been amplified before using this primer or any other set of primers. • This arrangement ensures that no contaminating DNA from previous PCR reactions is present in the lab, which could otherwise generate false positives.

- Suicide PCR is employed in paleogenetics research, which examines conserved genetic material from ancient species remnants.

10. Touch Down PCR

- Touch Down PCR is a type of PCR in which the starting annealing temperature is greater than the primers' optimal Tm and is gradually reduced over successive cycles until the Tm temperature, or "touchdown temperature," is reached.

- Touchdown PCR improves reaction specificity at higher temperatures while also increasing efficiency by lowering the annealing temperature near the end.

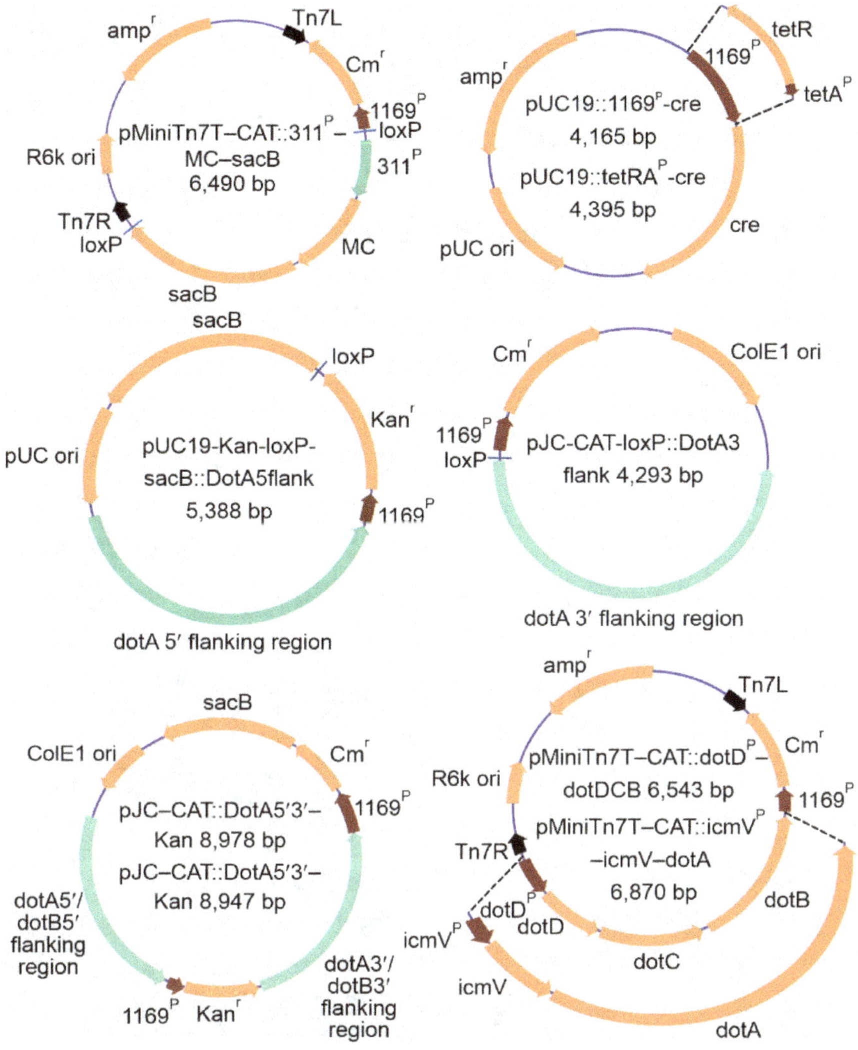

Fig. 2.25 Suicidal Plasmids

11. Ligation-mediated PCR

- Ligation-mediated PCR is a modified form of conventional PCR in which only one end is known at first and the second end is added later by ligation of a unique DNA linker.

- Ligation-mediated PCR employs tiny DNA fragments known as 'linkers' (or adaptors) that are first ligated to target DNA fragments.

- The target fragments are then amplified using PCR primers that bind to the linker sequences.

- This method is used for genome walking, DNA foot printing, and DNA sequencing.

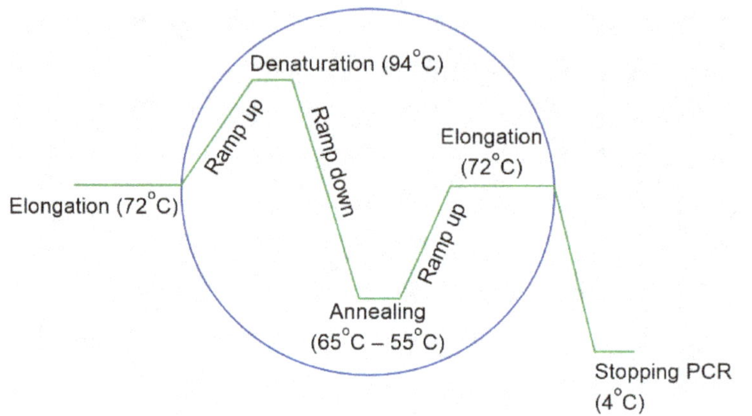

Fig. 2.26 Touch Down PCR

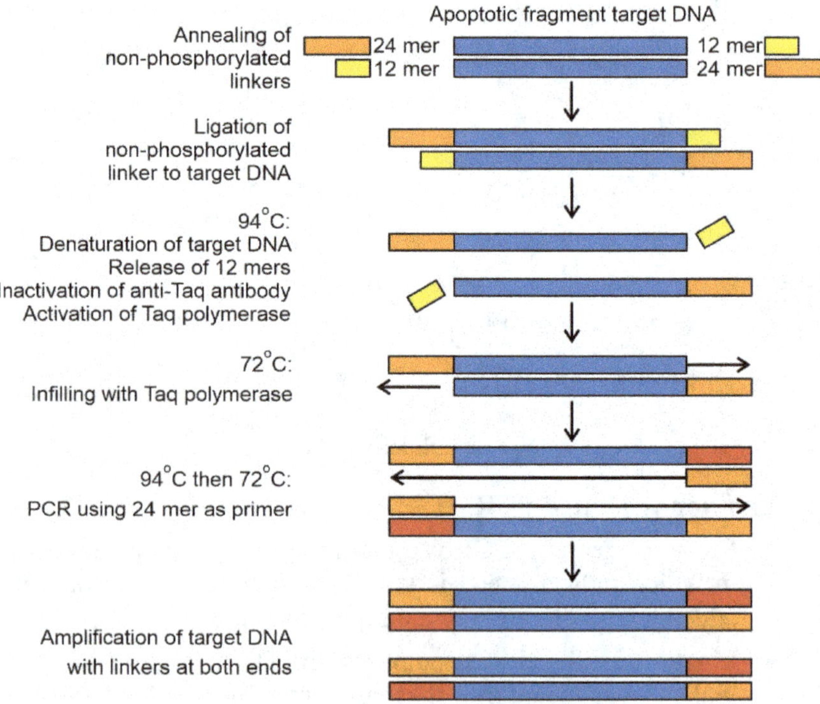

Fig. 2.27 Ligation-mediated PCR

12. Long-Range PCR

- Long-Range PCR is a technique for amplification of longer DNA sequences that can't be amplified using standard PCR reagents.

- Lengthy-range PCR can be done by utilising modified high-efficiency polymerases with increased DNA binding, resulting in highly processive and accurate amplification of long fragments.

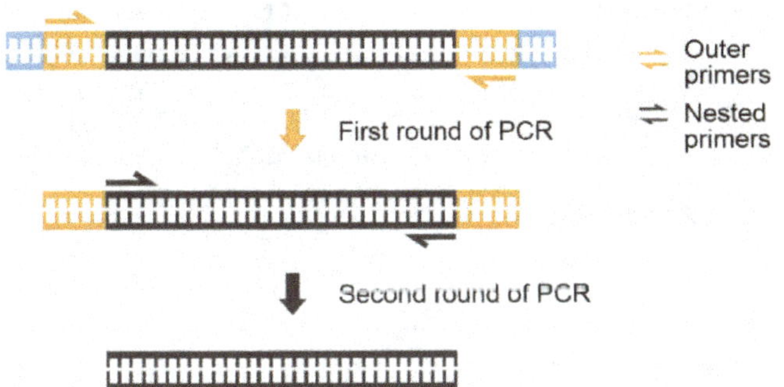

Fig. 2.28 Long-Range PCR

13. Methylation-specific PCR

- Methylation-specific PCR (MSP) is a technique for detecting and analysing CpG island DNA methylation patterns.

- To perform MSP, DNA is changed and PCR is performed using two primer pairs, one for detectable methylated DNA and the other for unmethylated DNA.

- The DNA is bisulfite-treated to convert cytosine to uracil, and then the methylated regions are amplified selectively with primers specific for them.

- Methylation patterns must be detected because excessive methylation of CpG dinucleotides in the promoter suppresses gene expression.

14. Reverse Transcriptase Real-Time PCR (RT-qPCR)

- RT-PCR is commonly associated with q-PCR forming Reverse Transcriptase Real-Time PCR (RT-qPCR).

- This allows quantification of DNA in real-time after the amplification.

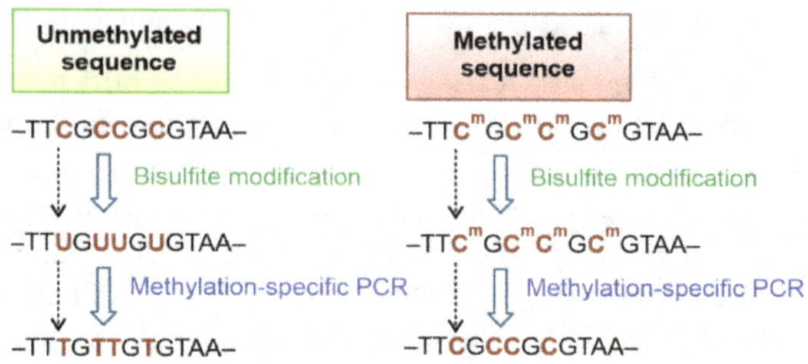

Fig. 2.29 Methylation-specific PCR

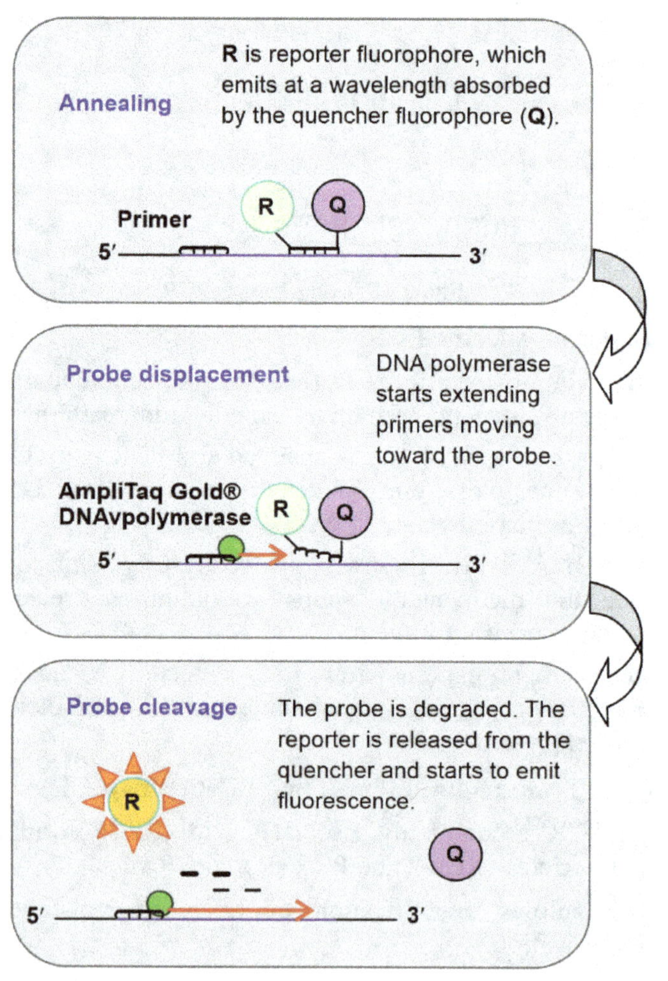

Fig. 2.30 Reverse Transcriptase Real-Time PCR (RT-qPCR)

15. RNase H-dependent PCR

- The blocked primer can only perform amplification depending on the cleavage activity of an RNase Henzyme during hybridization to the complementary target sequence in RNase H-dependent PCR.

- The blocked primer can only perform amplification depending on the cleavage activity of an RNase Henzyme during hybridization to the complementary target sequence in RNase H-dependent PCR.

- Non-specific binding and primer dimer production are minimised when the RNase H enzyme is active, allowing efficient hybridization.

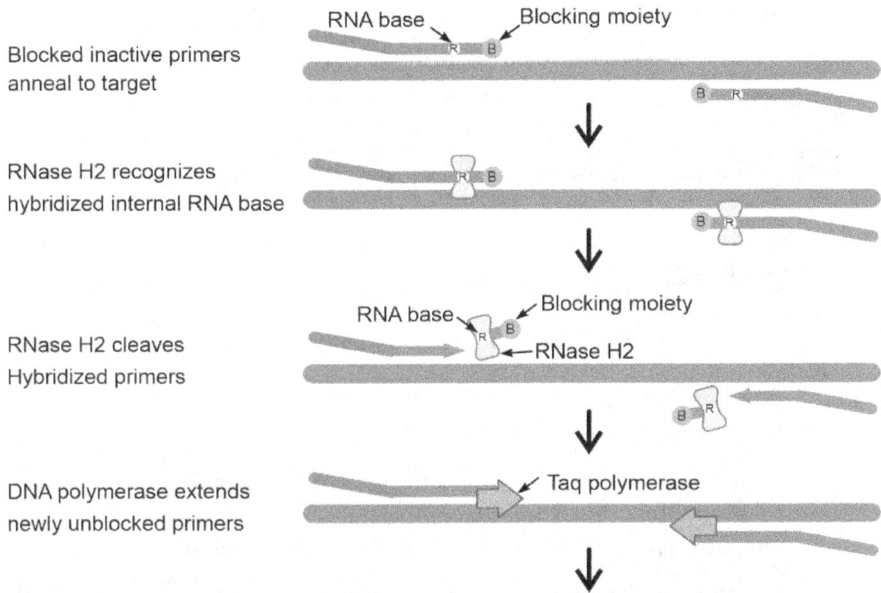

Fig. 2.31 RNase H-dependent PCR

16. Single Specific Primer-PCR

- SSP-PCR (single specific primer-PCR) is a PCR-based method that allows for the amplification of genes for which only a partial sequence is available.

- It permits unidirectional genome walking from known to unknown portions of the chromosome, allowing double-stranded DNA amplification even when sequence information is only available at one end.

- The single specific primer-PCR (SSP-PCR) method allows for the amplification of genes for which only a partial sequence is available, as well as unidirectional genome wandering from known to unknown chromosome regions.

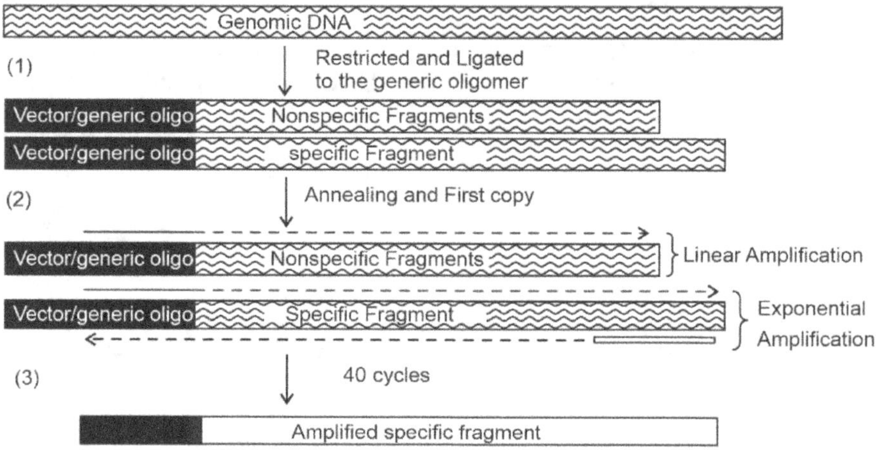

Fig. 2.32   Single Specific Primer-PCR

17. Solid-phase PCR

- Solid-phase PCR (SP-PCR) is a PCR technique that allows for target nucleic acid amplification on a solid support with one or both primers bound on the surface.

- The spatial separation of the primers reduces unfavourable primer interactions, preventing primer-dimers from forming and allowing for better multiplexing amplification.

- Instead of letting the primers freely diffuse in a bulk solution, this innovative approach attaches the 5'-end of the primers to a surface.

- The polymerase can capture a freely diffusing DNA target on the surface and then copy it.

- After the annealing stage, the copy remains attached to the surface, whilst the original DNA molecule returns to the solution.

- The free end of the attached copy hybridizes to the primer (attached to the surface) complementary to its sequence, and the amplification process can start.

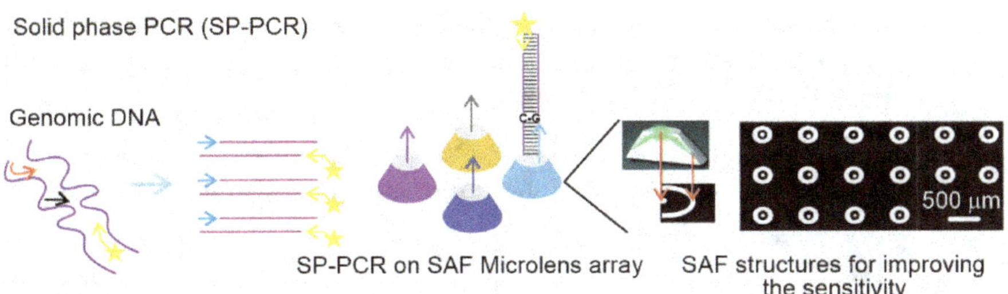

Fig. 2.33 Solid-phase PCR

18. Miniprimer PCR

- Miniprimer PCR is a novel PCR technology that uses a modified polymerase and 10-nucleotide "miniprimers."

- This approach has been discovered to reveal unique 16S rRNA gene sequences that would have been missed using regular primers.

- A thermostable polymerase enzyme is used in miniprimer PCR, which can extend from short primers (9 or 10 nucleotides).

- This approach allows PCR to target smaller primer binding areas, which is useful for amplification of highly conserved DNA sequences like the 16S (or eukaryotic 18S) rRNA Gene.

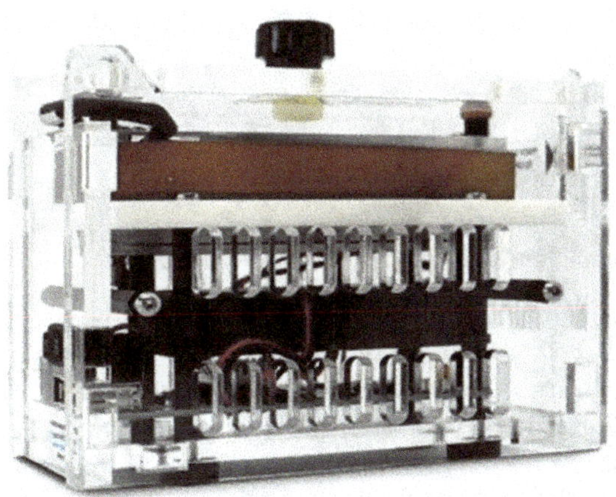

Fig. 2.34 Miniprimer PCR

19. Multiplex PCR

- Multiplex PCR is a common molecular biology technique used for the amplification of multiple targets in a single PCR test run.

- In Multiplex PCR, multiple primers and a temperature-mediated DNA polymerase are used for the amplification of DNA in a thermal cycler.

- All the primers pairs designed for Multiplex PCR have to be optimized so that the same annealing temperature is optimal for all the pairs during PCR.

- When multiple sequences are targeted at once, additional information can be generated from a single test run which otherwise would require a larger amount of the reagents and extensive time and effort to perform.

- This technology has been applied in many areas such as genotyping, mutation and polymorphism analysis, microsatellite STR analysis, detection of pathogens or genetically modified organisms, etc.

- In diagnostic laboratories, multiplex PCR is useful to detect different microorganisms that cause the same types of diseases.

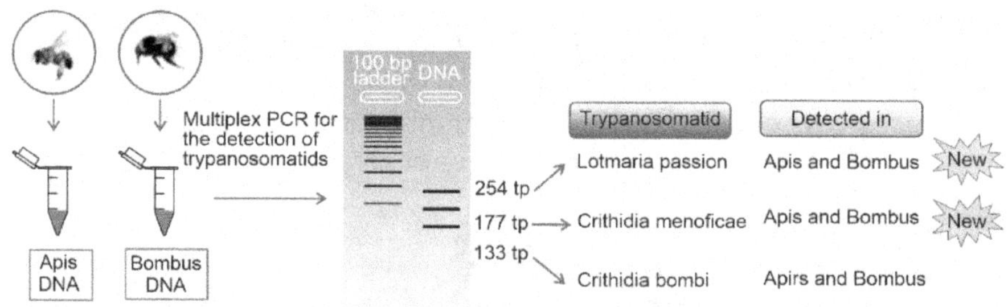

Fig. 2.35 Multiplex PCR

20. Nanoparticle Assisted PCR (Nano PCR)

- In a nanoparticle assisted PCR, tiny molecular compounds with specific physical properties that improve the reaction are used. According to one theory employing gold nanoparticles, these particles adsorb some of the polymerase and regulate the amount of polymerase left in the system, which may be crucial for improving the reaction's specificity.

- Another theory claims that nanoparticles adsorb primer pairs and lower the melting temperature at duplex formation between perfectly paired and mispaired primers, increasing the reaction's specificity.

- Nanoparticle assisted PCR has high sensitivity, specificity, and selectivity, and is widely used in virus detection and gene sequencing.

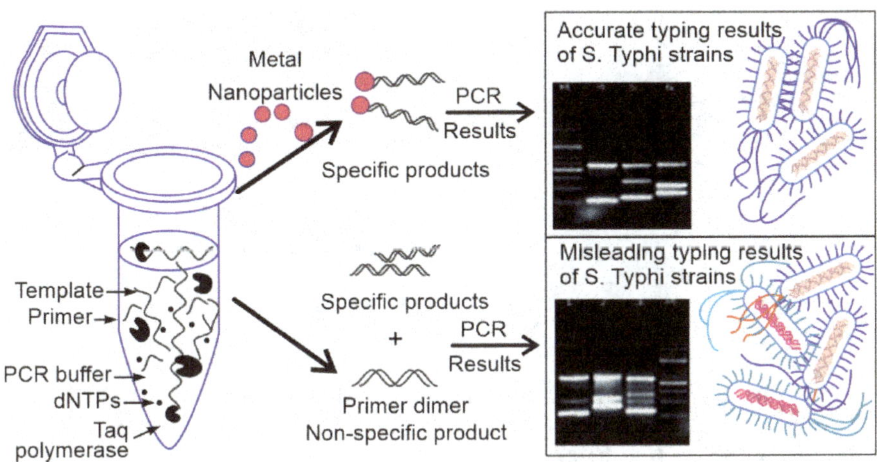

Fig. 2.36 Nanoparticle Assisted PCR (Nano PCR)

21. Amplified Fragment length polymorphism (AFLP) PCR

- It's a PCR-based approach that generates unique fingerprints for genomes of interest by selectively amplification of a segment of digested DNA fragments.

- Without knowing the genome sequence, this approach may swiftly synthesise vast numbers of marker fragments for any organism.

- AFLP PCR digests genomic DNA with restriction enzymes, allowing adaptors to be attached to the sticky ends of the fragments.

- Primers that are complementary to the adaptor sequence are used to amplify a portion of the restriction fragments.

- The amplified sequences are separated and seen on agarose gel electrophoresis after denaturing. AFLP PCR is employed for a varicty of applications, as to assess genetic diversity within species or among closely related species, to infer population-level phylogenies and biogeographic patterns, to generate genetic maps and to determine relatedness among cultivars.

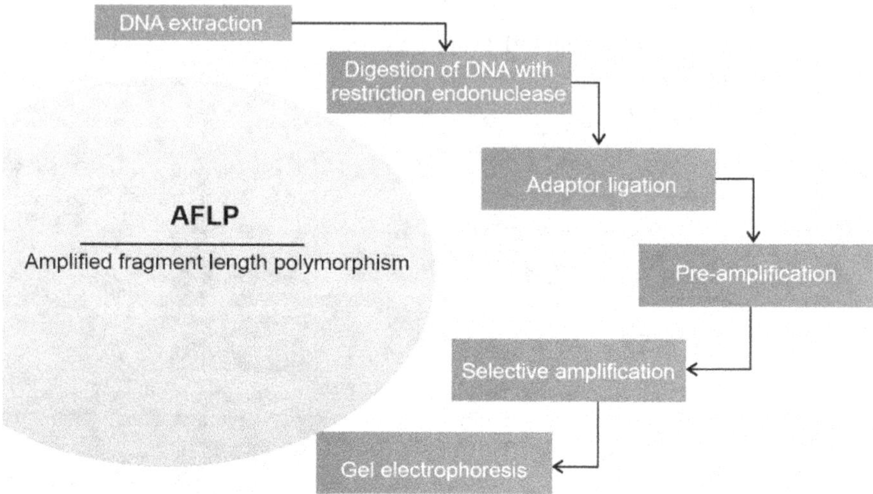

Fig. 2.37 Amplified Fragment length polymorphism (AFLP) PCR

22. InterSequence-Specific PCR

- InterSequence-Specific PCR (or ISSR-PCR) is a method for DNA fingerprinting that uses primers selected from specific segments repeated throughout a genome to produce a unique fingerprint.

- The technique uses microsatellites as primers in a single primer PCR reaction targeting multiple genomic loci to amplify primarily the inter-SSR sequences of various sizes. •Genomic fingerprinting, genetic diversity and phylogenetic research, genome mapping, and gene tagging can all benefit from ISSR PCR.

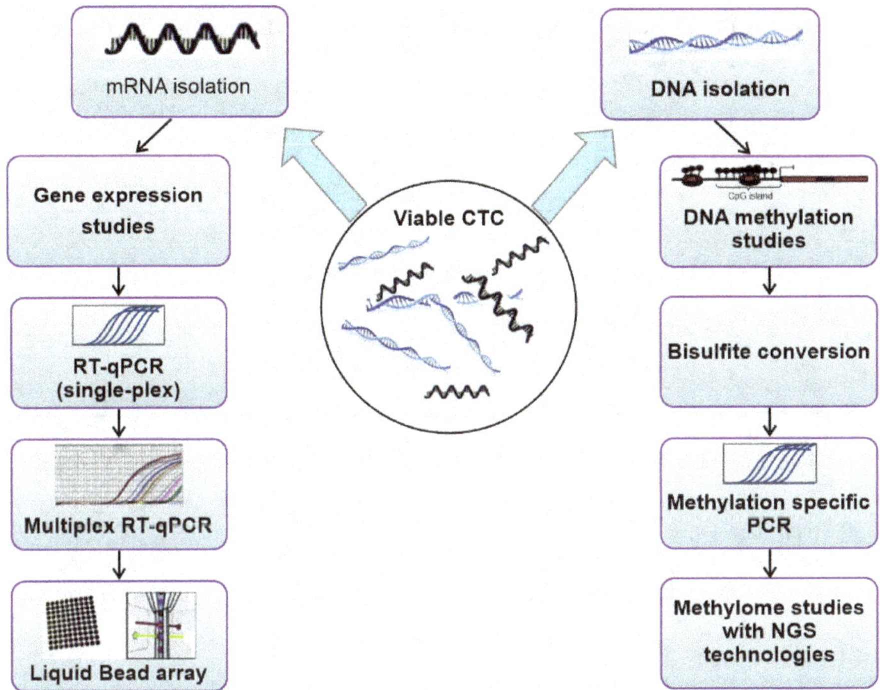

Fig. 2.38 InterSequence-Specific PCR

23. Allele-specific PCR

- Allele-specific polymerase chain reaction (AS-PCR) is a technique based on allele-specific primers, which can be used to analyze single nucleotide polymorphism.

- The *allele-specific PCR* is also called the (amplification refractory mutation system) ARMS-PCR corresponding to the use of two different primers for two different alleles.

- One is the mutant set of primers which are refractory (resistant) to the normal PCR, and the other is the normal set of primers, which are refractory to the mutant PCR reaction.

- The 3' ends of these primers are modified such that one set of the primer can amplify the normal allele while others amplify the mutant allele.

- This mismatch allows the primer to amplify a single allele.

- It is widely applied in the single gene point mutation detection such as sickle cell anemia and thalassemia.

- It is also used for the direct determination of ABO blood group genotypes.

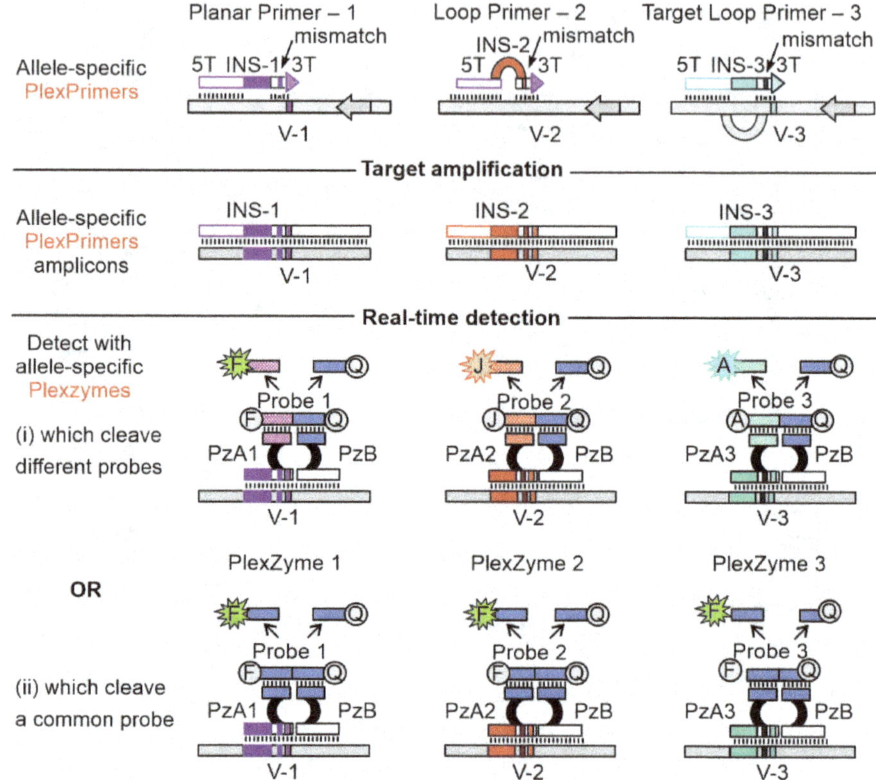

Fig. 2.39 Allele-specific PCR

24. Arthrobacter luteus (Alu) PCR

- Alu PCR is a rapid and easy DNA fingerprinting technique based on the simultaneous analysis of many genomic loci surrounded by Alu repetitive elements.

- Alu elements are short stretches of DNA initially characterized by the action of the *Arthrobacter luteus* (Alu) restriction endonuclease.

- Alu elements are one of the most abundant transposable elements and found throughout the human genome, and they play a role in the evolution and have been used as genetic markers

- In Alu PCR, two fluorochrome-labelled primers complementary to those sequences are used to perform the PCR, and the PCR products are then analysed by

- Alu insertions have been used in several genetically inherited human diseases and various forms of cancer. Thus, this PCR plays an essential role in the detection of these diseases and mutations.

Assembly PCR

- Assembly PCR is a method for the assembly of large DNA oligonucleotides from multiple shorter fragments.

- In PCR, the size of oligonuleotides used is 18 base pairs, while in assembly PCR lengths of up to 50bp are used to ensure correct hybridization.

- During the PCR cycles, the oligonucleotides bind to complementary fragments and then are filled in by polymerase enzyme.

- Each cycle of this PCR thus increases the length of various fragments randomly depending on which oligonucleotides find each other.

- Assembly PCR is used to improve the yield of the desired protein and can also be used to produce large amounts of RNA for structural or biochemical studies.

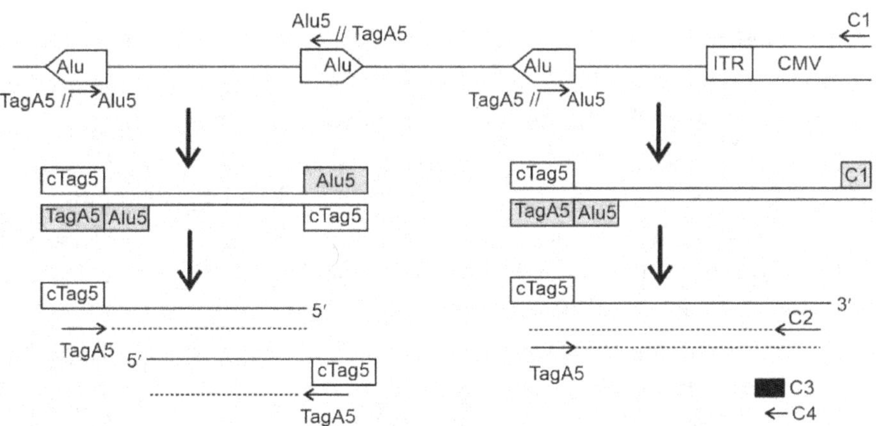

Fig. 2.40 Arthrobacter luteus (Alu) PCR

25. Hot start PCR

- Hot start PCR is a newer version of polymerase chain reaction (PCR) that decreases the creation of primer-dimers and unwanted products caused by non-specific DNA amplification at room temperature.

- Hot start PCR decreases non-specific binding, the production of primer-dimers, and often boosts product yields by separating one or more reagents from the reaction mix until the mixture reaches the denaturation temperature following heating. It also takes less time and effort, and it lowers the chance of contamination.

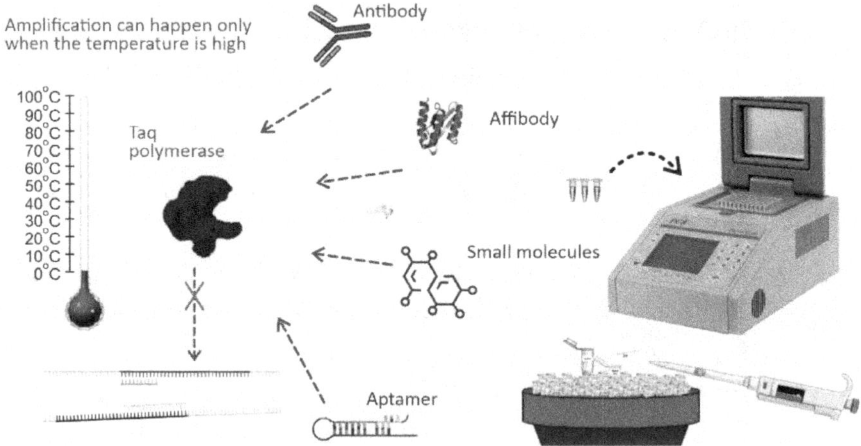

Fig. 2.41 Hot start PCR

26. Asymmetric PCR

- Asymmetric PCR is a type of PCR in which one strand of the original DNA is amplified more than the other.

- Asymmetric PCR is distinguished from conventional PCR by the use of an excessive number of primers for a single strand.

- The lower concentration limiting primer is quantitatively integrated into newly produced double-stranded DNA and used up as the asymmetric PCR advances.

- It's advantageous when only one of the two complementary strands needs to be amplified, such as in sequencing and hybridization probing, because it results in linear synthesis of the desired single DNA strand from the excess primer when the limiting primer is depleted.

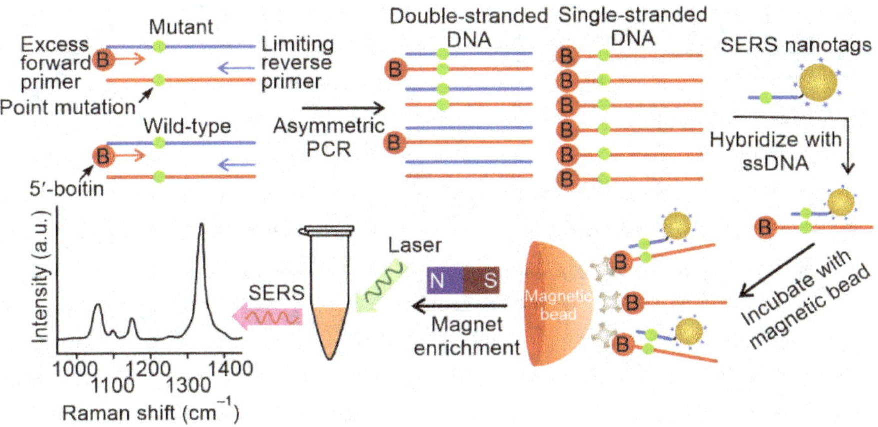

Fig. 2.42 Asymmetric PCR

27. COLD-PCR

- COLD-PCR (co-amplification at lower denaturation temperature-based polymerase chain reaction) is a new type of PCR that selectively amplifies low-abundance DNA variants from mixtures of wild-type and mutant-containing (or variant-containing) sequences, regardless of mutation type or position on the amplicon.

- This approach is based on changing the critical temperature at which mutation-containing DNA melts faster than wild type DNA.

- After denaturation, there is an intermediate annealing process that permits wild-type and mutant alleles to hybridise.

- These heteroduplexes will melt and be employed as a template because of the mismatch in the melting temperature of the ds DNA. As a result, a higher percentage of minor variation DNA will be amplified and available for following

- PCR rounds. PCR plays a vital role in the detection of mutations in oncology specimens, especially in heterogeneous tumours as well as bodily fluids.

- This PCR also assists in the assessment of residual disease after surgery or chemotherapy and disease staging and molecular profiling for prognosis or tailoring therapy to individual patients.

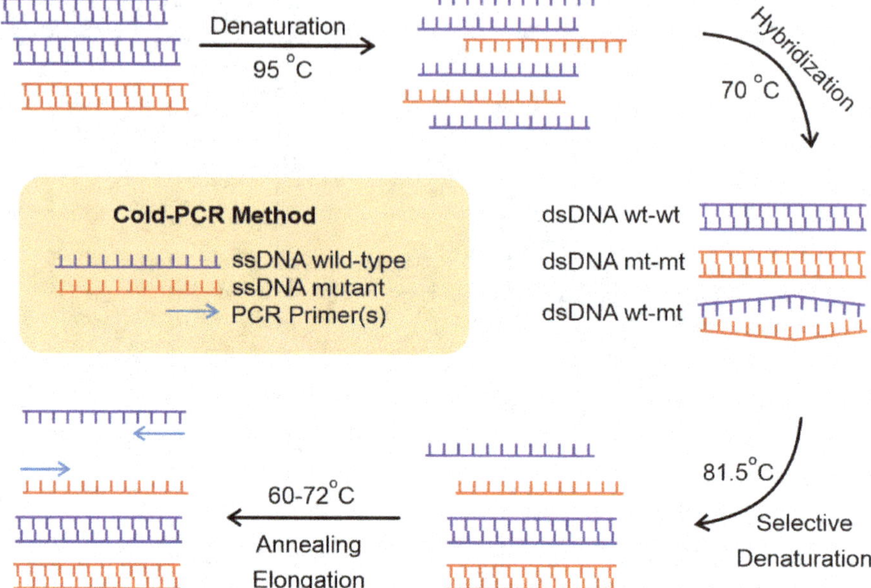

Fig. 2.43 COLD-PCR

28. *In-Situ* PCR

- *In-Situ* Polymerase Chain Reaction (In-situ PCR) is an effective method for detecting minute quantities of rare nucleic acid sequences in frozen or paraffin-embedded cells or tissue sections for compartmentalization of those sequences within the cells.

- This method involves tissue fixing, which preserves cell morphology, followed by treatment with proteolytic enzymes to provide an entry point for the PCR reagents to act on the target DNA. The reagents amplify the target sequences, which are subsequently identified using normal immunocytochemical techniques.

- *In-situ* PCR is widely used in the study of organogenesis and embryogenesis and can be used to diagnose infectious illnesses, quantify DNA, and detect even small amounts of DNA.

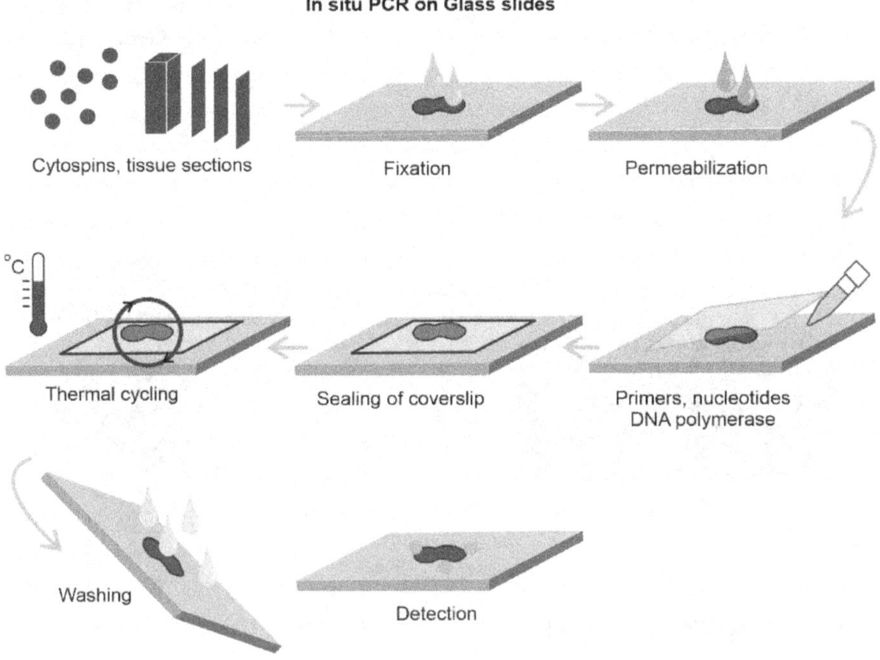

Fig.2.44 *In-Situ* PCR

29. Colony PCR

- Colony PCR is a method for identifying DNA of interest that has been inserted into a plasmid by developing inserted DNA specific primers.

- Using two sets of primers, the plasmid-containing bacterial colony can be amplified directly.

- The first set contains insert-specific primers that amplify the insertion sequence, while the second set contains vector-specific flanking primers that amplify plasmid DNA other than the inserted DNA.

- A bacterial colony is taken and mixed with all of the other PCR reagents in the master mix.

- The most common use of colony PCR is for determining proper ligation and incorporation of inserted DNA into bacteria and yeast plasmids.

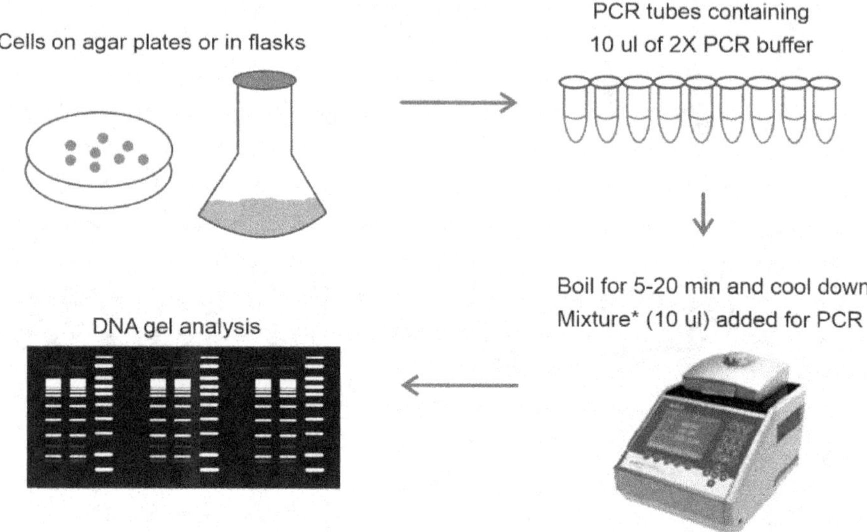

Fig.2.45 Colony PCR

30. Digital PCR (dPCR)

- Digital PCR (dPCR) is a quantitative PCR technology that provides a sensitive and efficient way for the measurement of the amount of DNA or RNA present in a sample.

- For dPCR, the initial sample mix is divided into a large number of individual wells prior to the amplification step, resulting in either target sequence being present in each well or not.

- Based on the presence or absence of fluorescence in the amplified reaction wells calculation of the absolute number of targets present in the original sample is done.

- Wells with a fluorescent signal are considered positives and scored as "1" while wells with no such signal are negatives and scored as "0".

- The concentration of the target sequence present in the initial sample is then determined through Poisson statistical analysis.

- dPCR is used to determine the total numbers of DNA and RNA viruses, bacteria, and parasites in a variety of clinical specimens, mainly when a well-calibrated standard is not available.

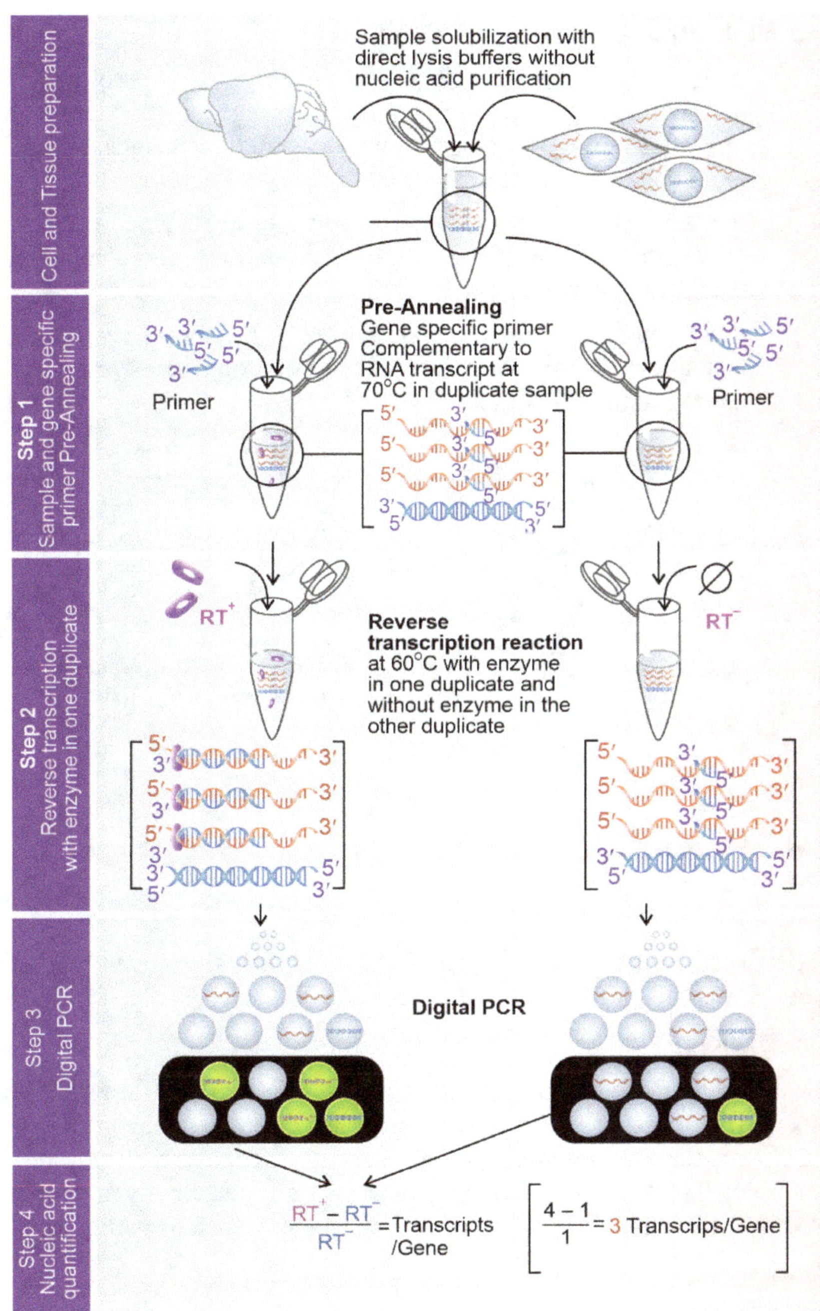

$$\frac{RT^{+} - RT^{-}}{RT^{-}} = \text{Transcripts/Gene} \qquad \left[\frac{4-1}{1} = 3 \text{ Transcrips/Gene}\right]$$

Fig. 2.46 Digital PCR

31. High- Resolution Melt (HRM) PCR

- It is far less expensive than other genotyping technologies such as sequencing and Taqman SNP typing for the detection of mutations, polymorphisms, and epigenetic changes in double-stranded DNA samples.

- It's perfect for large-scale genotyping projects since it's fast and powerful, allowing it to accurately genotype large numbers of samples in a short amount of time.

- Non-geneticists in any laboratory with access to an HRM capable real-time PCR system can do strong genotyping using a good quality HRM test.

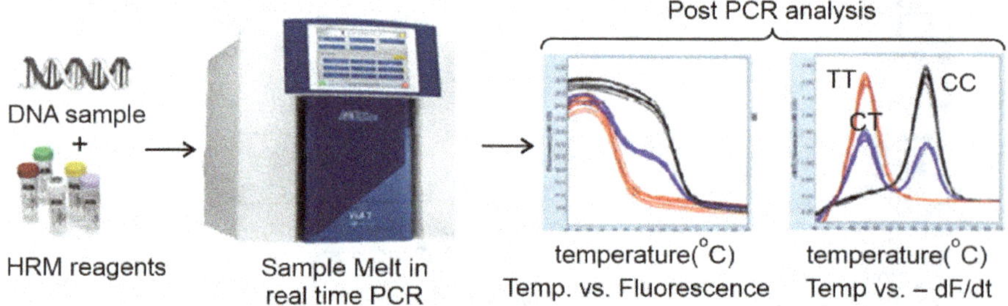

Fig.2.47 High- Resolution Melt (HRM) PCR

2.6   Applications of PCR

Diagnostic

The assessment of quantitative HIV viral load is a significant marker for illness outcome and is used to diagnose the disease.

Bio-Marker

As a bio-marker for diseases processes Bio-markers are the genes specially induced or down regulated during diseases. They are called as gene sigmatures which identifies a number of neoplastic disease process Example: Cytokines-chemokines- receptors are selectively induced and used to detect infectious diseases without the presence of pathogens.

Medicine

Clinical microbiology is a branch of molecular biology that deals with microorganisms that are difficult to identify and cultivate in the medical field. The application of PCR technology solves a number of problems, including culturing and identifying problems. The application of the PCR technology in blood banks has resulted in the selection and assurance of good blood samples. PCR technique, which provides patients with speed and sensitivity, is used to characterise many viruses, including influenza. Thus, molecular biology can be used to identify mutations and carriers of diseases such as diabetes, obesity, neurological disorders, cardiac, metabolic, and congenital diseases.

Forensic Science

In the field of forensic science, Molecular approaches can be used to explore the genetic foundation of disorders that cause sudden death. Forensic molecular pathology is the use of molecular biology in medical research to investigate the genetic basis of disease pathophysiology. Alleles discovered in different areas of DNA indicated by the genetic marker STR have a genetic profile.

Plant Research

In Plant Research In plant research it can be used in the following methods, they are

a. Insert analysis

b. Phyto-pathology

c. Molecular system and evolution

Insert Analysis The screening and analysis of clones in the complementary DNA group is a standard method in molecular biology. It also entails bacterial cultivation, followed by the isolation of vectors and DNA inserts for purification.

Phyto-pathology It aids in the detection and monitoring of plant infection caused by viruses, bacteria, and fungi. Only a few plant pathogens, such as pseudomonas, xanthomonas, and mycoplasmas, have nucleotide sequences. RAPD is also used to identify and distinguish plant diseases, as well as to generate a set of unique DNA fragments.

Molecular Systematics

Systematic evolution at the molecular level Morphological features can be based on phytogenetic correlations, and molecular approaches for plant gene analysis have become increasingly prominent in recent decades.

Molecular Systematic can be used in the following ways:

1. Analysis-comparisons of allozymes
2. Isolation-sequencing of proteins
3. Analysis of RAPD fingerprints
4. Analysis of restriction patterns
5. Sequence comparisons of marker genes.

Agricultural Sciences

In Agricultural Sciences Identification of multiple infectious diseases is the most useful application of PCR technique.

The following are the milestone achievements in agricultural fields.

a. Identification of a mutated gene EDA with ectodermal dysplasia in Holstein cattle
b. Identification of polymorphism in ABCB1 gene in phenobarbitol responsive-resistant idiopathic epileptica.
c. Deletion of Meq gene (which decreases immune suppresion in chickens).
d. MTM/ mutated gene with X-linked Myotubular myopathy in dog species.
e. Insertion mutation in ABCD4 with gall bladder mucocele formation in dogs
f. Agricultural techniques can also be used for the identification and characterization of specific pathogens of animals.
g. Bursal diseases virus-Avian samples
h. Bovine respiratory syncytial virus
i. Actinobacillus pleurop neumoniae-pgs samples
j. Canine parvo-virus type-2-faecal samples of dogs
k. Feline immunodeficiency virus
l. Feline leukemia virus (FeLV).

Virology PCR

The PCR technique is used in virology to evaluate antiviral medication in HIV-1, HBV, HSV-1, and HSV-2. The real-time polymerase chain reaction (RT-PCR) is a technique used in the investigation of infectious illnesses. Due to the expensive expense of lab work and the low sensitivity of the data, diagnosis was a major issue. The use of PCR technology aided and enhanced the detection and diagnosis of a variety of genes.

Microbiology Conventional PCR

The most often used technology in microbiology is conventional PCR. Bacillus anthracis, Variola major, and Anthrax species are among the species for which standard PCR procedures have been established. It has a high sensitivity, is simple to use, and takes minimal time. Conventional PCR can identify and classify 50-75 percent of anaerobic bacteria. Lactobacillus, Gadnarella vaginalis, Mycoplasmas horminis, and Fusobacterium species can all be detected with it. For diverse species such as M TB, M avium complex, C trochomatis, and N gonorrhoea, commercial assays are available. As a result, molecular detection is a faster and less time-consuming invasion method.

Dentistry

In Dentistry They can be useful in the following conditions such as

1. Periodontal diseases
2. Dental caries
3. Oral cancer
4. Endodontic infections

Periodontal Diseases

Periodontal Diseases are a group of diseases that affect the gums and PCR techniques can detect the following viruses in periodontal diseases: HCMV, EBV, HSV, and HPV. In the oral cavity, QRT-PCR was employed to evaluate gene expression in vivo. For the detection and quantification of peridontopathogenic bacteria such as A. actinomycete, M comitans, P. gingivalis, T. dentioola, T. socranskci, and others, many investigators have compared traditional PCR with RT-PCR.

Dental Caries

S. cricettus, S. ratti, S. mutans, S. sobrinus, S. downei, S. ferus, and S. macacae are dental health-destroying bacteria, and mutant genes of S. mutans/ S. sobrinus may be easily recovered from the human oral cavity. This PCR procedure provided speedy and accurate results, as well as a quick reaction completion.

Endodontic Infections

T. denticola, D. pseudomosintes, F. alocis, T. forsythia, T. malthopilum, T. socranskii, and P. tannearae are all important endodontic infections. These strains can be easily found and identified using PCR methods. The use of PCR techniques has propelled the discipline of medical microbiology to new heights.

Oral Cancer

S. anginosus can be easily discovered, diagnosed, and treated using RT-PCR. The RT-PCR technique can be used to determine the prognosis of oral malignancies. The PCR technique is used to detect EBV virus in nasopharyngeal cancer and squamous cell carcinoma in lymph nodes in head and neck cancer. Breast cancer, follicular lymphoma, stomach cancer, prostate cancer, and Ewling's sarcoma can all be detected with the PCR approach.

Mycology- Parasitology

In the field of mycology and parasitology, Fluroscent PCR uses marked primers/probes to detect fungi in environmental samples, whereas conventional PCR is a qualitative approach. In HIV-positive patients, Pneumocystis jiroveci produces severe pneumonia, which can be detected using an immune-fluroscence technique. Immunofluorescent techniques can also be used to detect Aspergillus species. Plasmodium and histopathiological species are among the other species that can be found.

Infectious Diseases

Hepatitis C virus causes liver inflammation, which leads to cirrhosis and cancer, according to the area of infectious diseases. PCR is a method for detecting HCV infection.

HIV-AIDS Quantitative PCR

Quantitative PCR is used to detect HIV in HIV-AIDS patients. Three drug combinations are used to treat HIV, and PCR can be used to monitor the levels of these three drugs in the body on a regular basis.

Cancer-Therapy

Cancer-Therapy is a term that refers to the treatment of cancer. In order to detect pathogenic strains, both qualitative and quantitative PCR approaches can be used. The p53 gene aids in the monitoring of cellular divisions, which may be discovered using the PCR technique, regardless of whether it is out of control and leads to the development of malignant cells. A procedure known as Promoter Methylation is employed in the PCR technique to control cancer illnesses. Although cellular divisions cannot be modified, they can be turned off. The cell attaches tiny molecules (-CH3 groups) to the DNA building blocks in the DNA region. As a result, polymerases that typically read genes and generate working copies can no longer encapsulate and begin in another location. As a result, the cell remains silent and no new cells are created.

Questions

1. Describe rDNA technology and its consequences in detail.

2. Elaborate Cloning vectors. Add a note on types of plasmids.

3. Discuss the role of interferon's in the body.

4. Describe how Hepatitis is produced.

5. Describe Insulin's manufacturing process.

6. Demonstrate the process of PCR and its applications

3 IMMUNOGENICITY

3.1 Immunogenicity

Recognition of Foreignness

- antibodies produced in the cells of the B-lymphocyte (B cell).

- Secreted antibodies bind to antigens on the surfaces of invading microbes (such as viruses or bacteria).

- Humoral immunity is so named because it involves substances found in the humus, or body fluids.

- Humoral immunity participates in the pathogenesis of immediate (types 1, 2 and 3) hypersensitivity and certain autoimmune diseases.

3.1.1 Chemical Nature of Antibodies

- *Antibodies*: They are proteins found in the blood serum and related fluids produced in response to antigens.

- The antibody will react specifically with the inducing antigen but its presence may or may not be related to the immune status of the host.

- Antibodies may be separated from other serum proteins by specific methods involving reaction with the antigen responsible for their induction, or by non-specific methods based on the physical and chemical properties of the antibody molecule.

- Each protein is composed of different amino acids, the total net charge on the proteins would be different and this would determine their rate of migration in an electric field.

The four major plasma protein groups include:

1. The fast-moving albumin and
2. The three globulins groups include respectively.

The globulins which showed antibody activity were found to be primarily in the gamma fraction and secondarily in the slow-moving globulins.

The primary importance was the realization of the basic unit of all antibody molecules which is a four polypeptide chain arrays.

3.1.2   Structure of Antibody

Ab molecules are inverted-γ-shaped structures, made up of two identical heavy and two identical light polypeptide chains held together by disulphide (S-S) bonds. The longer chains are called 'heavy' (H) and the shorter one's 'light' (L) chains.

Each L chain is attached to the H chain by a disulphide bond. The two symmetrical chains are held together by one to five s-s (disulphide) bonds, depending on the types of Ig.

The Ab chains are structurally and antigenically distinct and contain constant and variable regions based on the structure of constant region of heavy chains, gamma, Mu, alpha, delta and epsilon, Igs are classified into IgG, IgM, IgD and IgE respectively (Fig. 3.1).

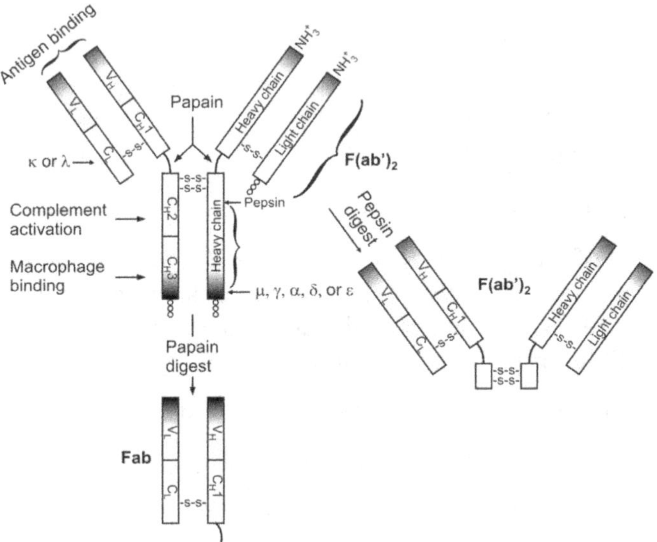

Fig. 3.1 Schematic representation of an Antibody Molecule

The L chains exists, its two forms Kappa and lambda. Each immunoglobulin molecule shows either two kappa's or two combinations. The light chains are named kappa and lambda after Korngold them. The kappa chains are preponderant in most of the immunoglobulins. and chains are present in a ratio of about 2:1 in any one individual.

♦ Antibodies Table 3.1 (Immunoglobulins, Ig) are proteins derived from the 'immunoglobulin supergene'.

Table 3.1 An overview of Antibody Molecules Classes and Subclasses

Antibody	Human and Mouse					
	Light Chain	**Subtype**	**Heavy Chain**			
IgA	κ or λ	IgA_1	α_1			
	κ or λ	$IgA2$	α_2			
IgE	κ or λ	None	ε			
IgD	κ or λ	None	δ			
IgM	κ or λ	None	μ			
IgG	κ or λ	IgG_1	γ_1	κ or λ	IgG_1	γ_1
	κ or λ	IgG_2	γ_2	κ or λ	IgG_{2a}	γ_{2a}
	κ or λ	IgG_3	γ_3	κ or λ	IgG_{2b}	γ_{2b}
	κ or λ	IgG_4	γ_4	κ or λ	IgG_3	γ_3

♦ One end of the Ig binds to antigens (the F_{ab} portion, so called because it is the fragment of the molecule which is antigen binding), and the other end which is crystallizable, and therefore called F_c, is responsible for effectors functions.

♦ Each immunoglobulin contains 4 polypeptide chains.

♦ Shorter ones are called light chains (made up of 107 amino acids)

♦ Big ones are called heavy chains (made up of 214 amino acids)

♦ Light chains and heavy chains are joined by one inter disulphide bond.

- Light chains exist in two classes, λ (lambda) and κ (kappa). Each antibody molecule has either λ(lambda) or κ (kappa) light chains, not both.

- The light chain (L) has a molecular weight of approximately 25,000 Daltons.

- The heavy chain has a molecular weight of 50,000 D.

- IgA exists in monomeric and dimeric form.

- IgM exists in pentameric form; molecular weight is 900,000 k D.

- The links between monomers are made by a J chain.

- The heavy and light chains consist of amino acid sequences. In the regions concerned with antigen binding, these regions are extremely variable, whereas in the other regions of the molecule, they are relatively constant. Thus, each heavy and each light chain possesses a variable and constant region.

- Light chains and heavy chains are polypeptide chains. They show polarity.

- Heavy chains have 1-13 inter disulphide bonds only to show flexibility called as Hinge region or neck region.

- Trace amount of carbohydrates like fructose and mannose found in the hinge region.

- If papain and pepsin are used immunoglobulin breaks into two parts.

  One half – F_c (fragment crystallisable)

  Another half – F_{AB} (fragment antigen binding)

- The region of antibody reacting with antigen called prototype/antibody determinant region.

3.1.3   Production of Antibodies

The production of antibodies consists of three steps:

1. The entry of the antigen, its distribution and fate in the tissues and its contact with appropriate immunocompetent cells. (The afferent limb).

2. The processing of antigen by cells and the control of the antibody forming process (central functions)

3. The secretion of antibody, its distribution in tissues and body fluids and the manifestations of its effects (efferent limb)

Antibody production follows a characteristic pattern consisting of:

(a) A lag phase, the immediate stage following antigenic stimulus during which no antibody is detectable in circulation.

(b) A log phase in which there is a steady rise in the titer of antibodies.

(c) A plateau of steady state when there is equilibrium between antibody synthesis and catabolism.

(d) The phase of decline during which the catabolism exceeds the production and the titer falls.

Antibodies are globulin proteins (proteins that have a compact, globular form) – therefore, we have come to use the term immunoglobulins (Ig) for Abs.

Abs are made in response to an antigen and can recognize and bind to the Ag. Bacterium or virus may have several epitopes that cause the production of different Abs.

Each antibody has at least two identical sites that bind to the epitope. These sites are known as antigen binding sites. The number of Antigen-binding sites on an Ab is called the valence of that Ab.

e.g., As most humans have two binding sites; they are bivalent.

3.1.4   Primary and Secondary Responses

Primary responses: The term primary response refers to the antibody response to an initial antigenic stimulus.

♦ The primary response is slow, sluggish and short-lived, with a long lag phase and low titer of antibodies that does not persist for long.

♦ The antibody formed in the primary responses is predominantly IgM.

Secondary response: It is the response to subsequent stimuli with the same antigen.

♦ The secondary response is prompt, powerful and prolonged, with a short or negligible lag phase and a much higher level of antibodies.

♦ The antibody formed in the secondary response is IgG.

◆ A single injection of an antigen helps more in sensitizing or priming the immune competent cells producing the particular antibody than in the actual elaboration of high levels of antibody.

◆ Effective levels of antibody are usually induced only by subsequent injections of the antigens. It is for this reason non-living vaccines are given multiple doses of active immunization.

◆ The first injection is known as the priming dose and subsequent injections as booster doses.

◆ When an antigen was injected into an animal already carrying the specific antibody in circulation, a temporary fall in the level of circulating antibody occurs due to the combination of the antigen with the antibody. This has been called the negative phase.

3.2   Immunoglobulin Classes

The simplest and most abundant Igs are monomers, but they can also assume some differences in size and arrangement.

The five classes of Igs are designated IgG, IgA, IgM, IgD and IgE, each class has a different role in the immune response. Molecules of IgA and IgM are aggregated to two or five monomers respectively that are joined together. Thus, each of these isotypes occupies a particular site in the body and has a particular role in defending the body against extracellular pathogens and their toxic products. Antibodies can accomplish this by direct interactions with pathogens or their products, for example by binding to active sites of toxins and neutralizing them or by blocking their ability to bind to host cells through specific receptors. When antibodies of the appropriate Isotype bind to antigens, they can activate the *classical pathway* of complement, which leads to the elimination of the pathogen by the various mechanisms. Soluble immune complexes of antigen and antibody also fix complement and are cleared from the circulation via complement receptors on red blood cells. Most classes of *antibody* are distributed by diffusion from their site of synthesis, but specialized transport mechanisms are required to deliver antibodies to luminal epithelial surfaces, such as those of the lung and intestine. The distribution of antibodies is determined by their Isotype, which can limit their diffusion or enable them to engage specific transporters that deliver them across epithelia.

3.2.1   IgG

IgG is the major serum Ig making up 85% of the total amount in adults. IgG antibodies are large molecules of about 150 kDa composed of four peptide chains. It is a tetrameric quaternary structure. (Table 3.2).

Table 3.2 Receptors for IgG

Receptor	Present on	Interacts with
Fcr R_1 (CD 64)	Monocytes Neutrophils	IgG_1, IgG_3, IgG_4
Fcr R_2 (CD 32)	Neutrophils Eosinophils	IgG_1, IgG_3
Fcr R_3 (CD 16)	Neutrophils NK cells	IgG_1, IgG_3

As an IgG molecule has got two identical antigen binding sites, it is called divalent.

IgG participates in most of the immunological reactions such as precipitation, complement fixation and neutralization of toxin and viruses.

It is the only immunoglobulin that passes through placenta and provides natural passive immunity to new-born. Ig is not formed in the foetus in any significant amount.

IgG has a longest half-life amongst all the Igs which is about 23 days.

In the human IgG molecule, the heavy chain (gamma chain) exists in four different forms and on this basis IgG has been classified as IgG_1, IgG_2, IgG_3 and IgG_4, which can be identified with specific antisera able to detect differences in the Fc fragment of the heavy chains

In human serum, the four IgG subclasses are distributed as IgG_1 (65%), IgG_2 (23%), IgG_3 (8%) and IgG_4 (4%).

Immunological response to bacterial polysaccharide is predominantly made by the IgG_2 production.

IgG is one of the major activators of classical complement pathway, particularly IgG_1 and IgG_3.

IgG has cellular receptors – Fcr R_1, Fcr R_2, Fcr R_3 which bind, recruit and activate cells such as polymorphous, macrophages and NK cells,

FcR receptor is also responsible for active process of placental transfer from mother to foetus.

3.2.2   Immunoglobulin A

IgA is the principal Ig that appears in the seromucous secretions such as milk, saliva, tears, nasal fluids sweat, colostrum's and in secretions of respiratory, intestinal and genital tracts.

Their content in serum is about 150-250 mg/100 mL and constitutes about 10 to 13% of serum Ig.

The molecular weight of IgA monomer is 1, 50,000 Daltons or 150 kD, sedimentation coefficient is 6.85, and half-life is 6-8 days. Since IgA molecules express morphological diversity in different locations, the secretory IgA is much larger than serum IgA.

IgA is largely synthesized locally by plasma cells and only a little amount may be derived from serum. IgA production requires B cells help and special mucosal stimulation to promote production of secretory IgA.

IgA is dimerised within the epithelial cells of glands. Intestines and the respiratory tract with a cysteine rich polypeptide called J (joining) chaining.

The linkage occurs between J chains and Fc fragment. The dimeric IgA combines with another protein. Secretory component, synthesized by local epithelial cells and then the complex is transported across the cytoplasm and secreted into body fluids.

Although IgA does not fix complement, but it is capable of activating the alternate complement pathway and is also an effective opsonin with F_{cR} on monocytes and neutrophils.

3.2.3   IgM

Antibodies of the IgM class make up 5 to 10% of the Abs in serum.

IgM forms polymers where multiple immunoglobulins are covalently linked together with polypeptide "J" chain and disulfide bonds, mostly as a pentamer but also as a Hexamer. IgM has a molecular mass of approximately 970 kDa (in its pentamer form).

The large size of the molecule prevents IgM from moving about as freely as IgG does so IgM Abs generally remain in blood vessels without entering the surrounding tissue.

IgM is the predominant type of antibody involved in the response to the ABO blood group antigen on the surface of red blood cells.

It is effective in aggregating Ags and in reactions involving complement, and it can enhance the ingestion of target cells by phagocytic cells, as does IgG.

IgM offers protection against *"bacteraemia"*, its deficiency may lead to septicaemia.

IgM is particularly important for immunity against the polysaccharide Ags present on the exterior of pathogenic bacteria.

IgM also promotes phagocytosis and bacteriolysis through its complement activation activity.

3.2.4   Immunoglobulin D

IgD is the least well characterized of the immunoglobulins from functional aspect. IgD was first detected by Rose and Fahey (1965) in myeloma protein. It is a 7s monomer present is a concentration of about 3 mg/100mt serum (less than 1% serum AgIG) and mostly intravascular in distribution.

Nearly all the IgD is present, together with IgM, on the membranes of a proportion of unstimulated B lymphocytes of blood and serve as recognition receptors for Ags. It has a monomeric structure similar to that of IgG. Their function is to signal the B cell to start antibody production upon antigen binding.

3.2.5   Immunoglobulin E

IgE is discovered by Ishizaka (1996) in serum of patients with certain types of allergies. Based upon the observation that allergic responses typically affect the skin, gut, and respiratory tract, the major sites of parasitic invasion, it is thought that IgE evolved as a defence against parasitic infestation. Helminthes stimulate a vigorous IgE production, including parasite-specific IgE antibody.

They play a very key role in early recognition of foreign material ("gate keeper function") or a general potentiating of the immune system response by the improved antigen presentation. Actually, allergy triggered by IgE may be considered a beneficial function of the host; the typical allergic reactions of mucus secretion, sneezing, itching, coughing, bronchoconstriction, tear production, inflammation, vomiting and diarrhoea are all mechanisms that expel allergenic proteins from the body.

IgE is a 8s molecule with a short half-life of 2.3 days. It constitutes less than 1% of the total immunoglobulin.

Although IgE is typically the least abundant isotype-blood serum IgE levels in a normal ("non-atopic") individual are only 0.05% of the Ig concentration.

Clearly bound to Fc receptor on most cells and found in insignificant amount in normal serum.

IgE molecules bind tightly by their Fc regions to receptors on mast cells and basophils, specialized cells that participate in allergic reactions shown in Fig. 3.2.

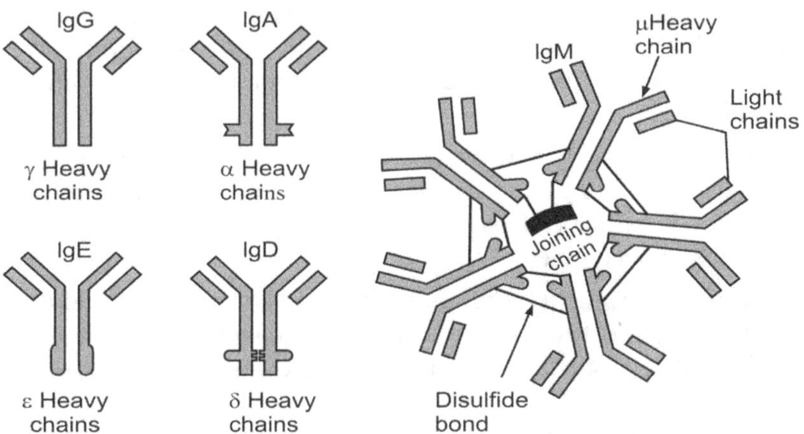

Fig. 3.2 Figures of different immunoglobulins

3.2.6   Antigens-Antibody Reactions

♦ The antigen-antibody reaction depends on non-covalent interactions including hydrogen bonds, ionic bonds, hydrophobic interactions and Vander Waals interactions.

♦ Antigen-antibodies combine with each other specifically and in observable manner.

♦ The reactions between antigens and antibodies serve several purposes.

1. In the body, they form the basis of antibody mediated immunity in infectious diseases, or of tissue injury in some types of hypersensitivity and auto immune diseases.

2. In the laboratory, they help in the diagnosis of infections, and of non-infectious antigens such as enzymes.

3. This reaction can be used for detection and quantification of either antigens or antibodies.

Features of Antigen-Antibody Reaction

1. **Affinity:** Antibody affinity is the strength of the reaction between a single antigenic determinant and a single combining site on the antibody. It is the sum of the attractive and repulsive forces operating between the antigenic determinant and the combining site of the antibody.

2. **Avidity:** Avidity is a measure of the overall strength of binding of an antigen with many antigenic determinates and multivalent antibodies. Avidity is influenced by both the valence of the antibody and the valence of the antigen.

3. **Specificity:** Specificity refers to the ability of an individual antibody combining site to react with only one antigenic determinant or the ability of a population of antibody molecules to react with only one antigen.

4. **Cross reactivity:** Cross reacting refers to the ability of an individual antibody combining site to react with more than one antigenic determinant or the ability of a population of antibody molecules to react with more than one antigen.

♦ There is no denaturation of antigen or antibody during the reaction.

♦ Both antigens and antibodies participate in the formation of agglutinates or precipitates.

Antigen-Antibody reactions conducted in vitro are known as serological reactions.

3.2.7   Precipitation Reactions

The reaction of soluble antigens with IgG or IgM antibodies to form large interlocking aggregates is called precipitation reaction.

- The precipitations formed by antibodies are known as precipitins.
- The precipitation reactions occur in two stages
- Rapid interactions within a second between antigen and antibodies and formation of complex.
- Slow rate of reaction completing even within a few minutes or hours and forming lattices from antigen-antibody complexes.
- When antibodies and antigens are in proper ratio, precipitation reactions normally occur.
- When there is excess amount of either of two, no visible precipitate is formed. One can produce the optimal ratio of these two by putting antigens and antibody adjacent to each other and waiting for their diffusion together.
- In precipitation test, a precipitation ring appears which display the creation of optimal ratio. This zone is known as zone of equivalence precipitation can take place in liquid media or in gel.

Mechanism of Precipitation

According to lattice hypothesis concept, multivalent antigens combine with bivalent antibodies in varying proportion, depending on the antigen-antibody ratio in the reacting mixture.

Precipitation results when a large lattice is formed consisting of alternating antigen and antibody molecules. This is possible only in the zone of equivalence.

In the zones of antigen or antibody excess, the lattice does not enlarge, as the valencies of the antibody and the antigen are fully satisfied.

Application of Precipitation Reaction

The precipitation test may be carried out as either a qualitative or quantitative test.

♦ It is very sensitive in the detection of antigens and as little as 1 mg of protein can be detected by precipitation tests.

♦ It finds forensic application in the identification of blood and seminal stains, and in testing for food adulterants.

The following types of precipitation and flocculation tests are in common use.

1. **Ring test:** This is the simplest type of precipitation test, consists of layering the antigen solution over a column of antiserum in a narrow tube.

    ♦ A precipitate form at the junction of the two liquids.

    e.g., Ascoli's themo precipition test, grouping of streptococci by the Lancefield technique.

2. **Slide test:** When a drop each of the antigen and antiserum are placed on a slide and mixed by shaking, floccules appear.

    E.g.: VDRL test for syphilis

3. **Tube test:** A quantative tube flocculation test is employed for the standardisation of toxins and toxoids.

    ♦ Serial dilutions of the toxin/toxoid are added to the tubes containing a fixed quantity of the antitoxin. The amount of toxin or toxoid that flocculates optimally with one unit of the antitoxin is defined as an LF dose.

    E.g.: Kahn test for syphilis.

4. **Immuno diffusion (precipitation in gel):** Immuno diffusion tests are performed in a gelled agar medium.

    ♦ The reaction is visible as a distinct band of precipitation, which is stable and can be stained for preservation.

    ♦ Immuno diffusion also indicates identity, cross reaction and non-identity between different antigens.

Different modifications of the test are available

1. **Single diffusion in one dimension:** The antibody is incorporated in agar gel in a test tube and the antigen solution is layered over it.

    ♦ The antigen diffuses downward through the agar gel, forming a line of precipitation that appears to move downwards. This is due to the precipitation formed at the advancing front of the antigen, and is dissolved as the concentration of antigen at the site increases due to diffusion.

♦ The number of bands indicates the number of different antigens present.

2. **Double diffusion in one dimension:** The antibody is incorporated in gel, the column of plain agar in placed above it.

♦ The antigen is layered on top of this.

♦ The antigen and antibody move towards each other through the intervening column of plain agar and form a band of precipitate where they meet at optimum proportion.

3. **Single diffusion in two Dimensions:** The antiserum is incorporated in agar gel poured in flat surface.

♦ The antigen is added to the wells cut on the surface of the gel. It diffuses radially from the well and forms ring shaped bands of precipitation concentrically around the well.

♦ The diameter of the halo gives an estimate of the concentration of the antigen.

♦ This method is employed for the estimation of the immunoglobulin classes in sera and for screening sera for antibodies to influenza viruses, among others.

4. **Double diffusion in two dimensions:** In test wells are cut, into which a purified antiserum (a serum containing antibodies) is added, and to each surrounding well, soluble form of test antigens are added.

♦ Thereafter, a line of visible precipitate is formed between the wells where after diffusion optimal ratio of antigen-antibody is formed.

♦ Through this test the presence of antibodies in the serum against more than one antigen at a time can be demonstrated.

♦ We can also find out the identical, partially identical and different types of antigens through this test.

♦ A special variety of double diffusion in two dimensions is the Elek test for toxigenicity in *Diphtheria bacilli*.

♦ When *Diphtheria bacilli* are streaked at right angles to a filter paper strip carrying the antitoxin implanted on a plate of suitable medium, arrowhead shaped lines of precipitation appear on incubation, if the bacillus is toxigenic.

5. **Immuno electrophoretic:** This method involves the electrophoretic separation of a composite antigen in its constituent proteins, followed by immune diffusion against its antiserum, resulting in separate precipitin lines.

   ♦ The technique is performed on agar or agarose gel, on a slide, with an antigen well and antibody trough cut on it.

   ♦ Antigen well filled with human serum.

   ♦ Serum separated by electrophoresis

   ♦ Antiserum trough filled with antiserum to whole human serum.

   ♦ Serum and antiserum allowed to diffuse into agar.

   ♦ Precipitin lines form for individual serum proteins.

   ♦ It is useful for testing the normal and abnormal proteins in serum and urine.

3.3   Electro Immunodiffusion

The development of precipitin lines can be speeded up by electrically driving the antigen and antibody.

Methods Include

1. Counter immune electrophoretic (counter current immune electrophoresis)

2. One dimensional single electro immunodiffusion (rocket electrophoresis)

1. **Counter Current Immuno Electrophoresis:** (counter immune electrophoresis (CIE)) antibody in a gel, but also uses electrophoresis for their rapid movement.

   ♦ The principle of CIE is based on the movement of antigens and antibodies to opposite poles after applying electric current in buffers of correct electric strength and pH, because some of the antigens and antibodies have the opposite charges.

   ♦ If a reaction occurs, a precipitation line appears within an hour.

   ♦ By using this method protein can be separated within an hour.

♦ CIE is useful for the diagnosis of bacterial meningitis and the other diseases.

2. One dimensional single electro immunodiffusion (rocket electrophoresis):

♦ In this method the antiserum to the antigen to be quantitated is incorporated in agarose and gelled on the glass slide.

♦ The antigen, in increasing concentrations, is placed in wells punched in the set gel.

♦ The antigen is then electrophoresed into the antibody containing agarose

♦ The pattern of immunoprecipitation resembles a rocket hence the name rocket electrophoresis.

♦ The main application of this technique is for quantitative estimation of antigens.

3.3.1   Agglutination Reaction

Agglutination is the process of linking together of antigens by antibodies and the formation of visible aggregates given in Fig. 3.3.

♦ Agglutination reaction involve particulate antigens i.e., soluble antigens adhering to particles.

♦ Agglutination reactions are very sensitive, readable and available in several varieties.

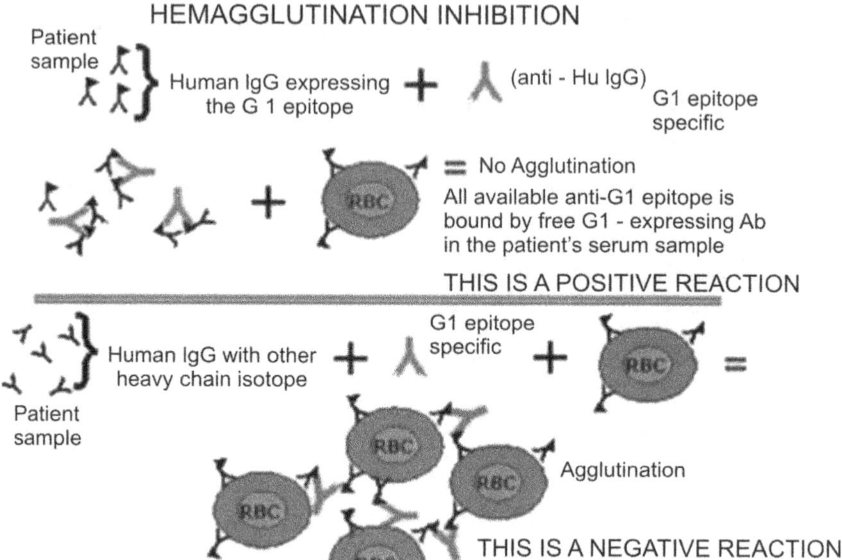

Fig. 3.3 Schematic representation of Hemagglutination reactions

1. *Direct Agglutination Test*

♦ Direct agglutination test diagnoses antibodies against a large number of cellular antigens such as RBC's, bacteria and fungi.

♦ This test is carried out in plastic microtiter plates that have several small shallow wells. Each well acts as small test tube.

♦ Each well contains an equal amount of particulate antigen (e.g., RBC's) but the amount of antibodies in the serum is serially diluted in successive wells so that their concentration may be half of the previous well.

♦ If one starts with more antibodies, more dilutions will be required to lower the amount to a point at which agglutination does not occur. This is the measure of titer or concentration of serum antibody.

♦ In a positive reaction, agglutination occurs, and sufficient antibodies are present in the serum to link the antigen together. This results in the formation of antibody-antigen mat which sinks to bottom of well.

♦ In the negative reaction, agglutination does not occur and insufficient antibodies are present to cause the linking of antigens.

2. ***Indirect (passive) Agglutination Tests***: These types of diagnostic tests are very rapid particularly for the detection of streptococci.

- If the antigen are adsorbed onto particles (e.g., RBC, latex beads), soluble antigens can respond to agglutination test.

- Antibody reacts with the soluble antigen adhering to the particles.

- Therefore, the particles agglutinate with each other as these do in the direct agglutination tests.

- The Weil-Felix reaction for serodiagnosis of typhus fever is a heterophile agglutination test and is based on the sharing of a common antigen between typhus *rickettsiae* and some strains of proteus bacilli.

3.3.2   Complement Fixation Test (CFT)

A group of 20 or more serum proteins are collectively known as complement. The complement system is an enzyme cascade. During reaction, the complement binds to antigen-antibody complex and is used up or fixed.

The phases in the complement cascade are

- Recognition

- Activation amplification

- Membrane attack

Complement Action Steps:

- Lysis of foreign cells

- Increased vascular permeability

- Lysis of bacteria

- Neutrophil activation and chemotaxis

- Mast cell degranulation

- Smooth muscle contraction

- Localization of complexes in germinal centres

- Opsonization and phagocytosis of bacteria.

- This process of complement fixation may be used to measure even very small amount of antibody that does not produce a visible reaction such as precipitation or agglutination. Therefore, it is necessary to use indicator system.

- The test requires patient's serum, test antigen, complement from Guinea pig and antibodies of sheep RBCs to determine whether sheep RBC's may be lysed by Guinea pig complement.

The test is accomplished in two stages:

Stage 1: The patient's serum is heated at 56 °C for 30 minutes so that the complement should be inactivated.

- The heated serum is diluted and then added to known amount of specific antigen and complement.

- The test antigen may correspond to the diseases.

E.g., If a patient is suffering from a disease caused by *streptococci* the test antigen would be streptococcal antigen.

If the patient's serum contains antibodies against *streptococci*, the test antigen will form complement sequence. This mixture is again incubated for about 30 minutes. At this point, no antigen-antibody reaction occurs

Stage 2: The complement fixed by antigen-antibody reaction is detected by an indication system. This system consists of sheep RBC's containing specific antibodies attached to their surfaces.

- When these are added to complement, haemolysis of RBC's occur that impart changes in colour of the mixture. This shows that the complements have not been fixed during the first stage; therefore, these become available to cause haemolysis. This indicates that the patient has no streptococcal pneumonia.

- However, if the Guinea pig complements are destroyed, they would not be able to cause the lysis of RBC's.

- If the complements are fixed (by antigen-antibody reaction) during the first stage, this indicates that the patient has the infection of streptococci.

- The classical example of CFT is the Wassermann reaction, a method for the serodiagnosis of syphilis.

- The test consists of two steps.

- In the **first step**, the inactivated serum of patient is incubated at 37 °C for one hour with the Wassermann antigen and a fixed amount (two units) of Guinea pig complement.

- If the serum contains syphilitic antibody, the complement will be utilized during antigen antibody interaction.

- If the serum does not contain the antibody, no antigen-antibody reaction occurs and the complement will be left intact.

- The **second step** includes the testing for complement in the post incubation mixture this will indicate whether the serum had antibodies or not.

- This is followed by adding sensitized cells (sheep erythrocytes coated with 4MHD hemolysin), and incubating at 37 °C for 30 minutes.

- Lysis of the erythrocytes indicates that complement was not fixed in the first step and therefore, the serum did not have the antibody (–ve CFT).

- Absence of erythrocyte lysis indicates that the complement was used up in the first step and, therefore the serum contained the antibody (+ve CFT)

Indirect complement fixation test: The test is set up in duplicate and after first step, the standard antiserum known to fix complement is added to one set.

- If the test serum contained antibody, the antigen would have been used in the first step and therefore the standard antiserum added subsequently would not be able to fix complement therefore in the indirect test, haemolysis indicates a positive result.

Coagulating complement absorption test: For systems which do not fix guinea pig, an alternating method is the coagulating complement absorption test. (Fig. 3.4 & Table 3.3 (a), (b) & (c)).

- This uses horse complement which is non haemolytic. The indicator system is sensitized sheep erythrocytes mixed with bovine serum.

- Bovine serum contains a β-globulin component called conglutinin, which acts as antibody to complement.

- Therefore, conglutinin causes agglutination of sensitized sheep erythrocytes (conglutination) if they have combined with complement.

♦ If the horse complement had been used up by the antigen-antibody interaction in the first step, agglutination of sensitized cells will not occur.

Table 3.3 (a) Complement Fixation Assay Test Phase

Complement Fixation Assay Test Phase	
Positive serum- Antibodies	**Negative serum- no Antibodies**
Antigen	Antigen
Complement	Complement
AG-AB complex formed	No Ag-Ab complex
Complement used up	Complement NOT used up

Table 3.3 (b) Complement Fixation Assay Indicator phase

Complement Fixation Assay Indicator phase	
Positive Test phase - No complement	Negative test phase- Complement
Indicator system, Sheep RBCs, Anti sheep RBCs	Indicator System- Sheep RBCs, Anti Sheep RBC's
Result-NO LYSIS of RBCs. CLOUDY	Result- LYSIS of RBCs, CLEAR

Table 3.3 (c) Advantages and Disadvantages of CFT

Advantages of CFT	**Disadvantages of CFT**
Reagents easily available	Indirect test
Semi quantitative or quantitative	Need adequate controls
Wide application	Reagents unstable
Extensively sensitive	Quantitation time consuming, cannot be automated

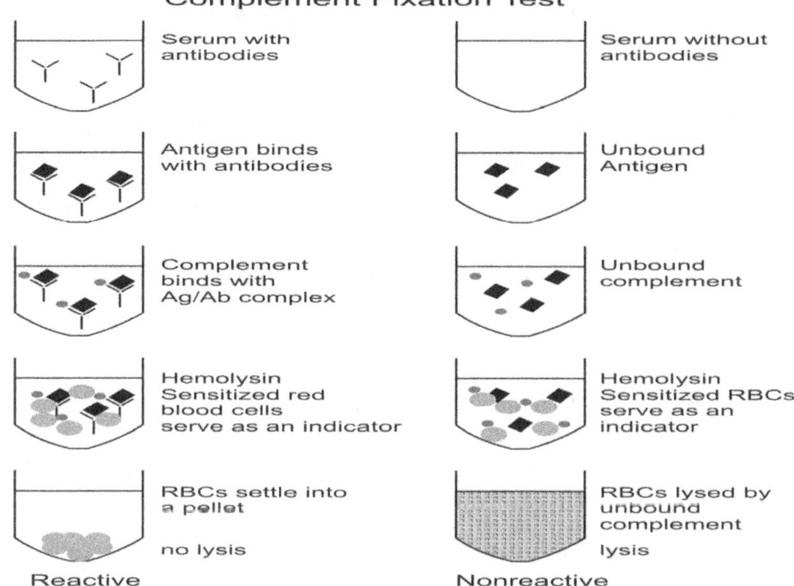

Fig. 3.4 Complement fixation test

3.3.3   Opsonization

The name 'opsonin' was given to a heat liable substance present in fresh normal sera, which facilitated phagocytosis. This factor was subsequently identified as complement.

- Opsonisation is a phenomenon of adsorption of certain antibodies or complement ($c_3 - c_5$ complex) especially c_{3b} onto the surface of foreign material that result in stimulation in phagocytosis.

- Opsonization is also known as immune adherence.

- Opsonization is also one of the main antigen-antibody reactions associated with humoral antibodies.

- The two main opsonin's (complement and certain antibodies) stimulate phagocytosis.

- The complement stimulates T-cells to process for cell mediated immunity and release histamine from leukocytes, which in turn increases the capillary permeability and smooth muscle contraction.

◆ 'Opsonic index' is used to study the progress of resistance during the course of disease.

◆ Opsonic index is defined as the ratio of the phagocytic activity of the patient's blood for a given bacterium, to the phagocytic activity of blood from a normal individual.

◆ It was measured by incubating fresh citrated blood with the bacterial suspension at 37 °C for 15 minutes and estimating the average number of phagocytosed bacteria per polymorphonuclear leukocyte (phagocytic index) from stained blood films.

3.3.4   Radio-immuno Assay (RIA)

◆ A variety of tests have been devised for the measurement of antigen and antibodies using labelled reactants.

◆ The term binder-ligand assay has been used for these reactions.

◆ The substance whose concentration is to be determined is termed as analyte or ligand. The binder protein which binds to the ligand is called the binder.

◆ RIA permits the measurement of analyte up to pictogram (10^{-12} gm) quantities.

◆ RIA has versatile applications in various areas of biology and medicine, including the quantitation.

◆ There are two methods of measuring RIA: the liquid phase and the solid phase RIA's.

1. **Liquid phase RIA:** The liquid phase RIA is based on competitive binding of radiolabelled antigen and unlabelled antigen, to a high affinity antibody.

◆ The antigen labelled with I is mixed with such a concentration of antibody that can just saturate the antibody.

◆ Therefore, the increasing amount of antigen (unlabelled) of unknown concentration is added.

◆ The two types of antigens now compete for available sites of the antibody.

♦ The antibody does not differentiate the labelled antigen from unlabelled one.

♦ Upon gradually increasing concentration of unlabelled antigen, the labelled antigen could be displaced from the binding sites available on antibody.

♦ The labelled antigens are made free in the solution.

♦ The amount of labelled antigen in solution is measured, and the concentration of unlabelled antigen can be determined.

2. **Solid phase RIA:** In solid phase RIA, either antigen or antibody is immobilized on a solid phase matrix. It is simple and easy in handling as compared to liquid phase RIA.

3.3.5   Neutralization Reaction

The neutralization reactions are the reactions of antigen-antibody that involve the elimination of harmful effects of bacterial exotoxins or a virus by specific antibodies.

♦ This neutralizing substance i.e., antibodies are known as antitoxins.

♦ This specific antibody is produced by a host cell in response to a bacterial exotoxin or corresponding toxoid (inactivated toxin).

♦ The antitoxin reacts with exotoxin and neutralizes it.

♦ These antitoxins can be artificially induced in animals such as horses.

♦ Thus, the antitoxin of animal sources in turn can be injected into human who provides a passive immunity against a toxin present in human body produced by the pathogen causing diphtheria, tetanus etc.

♦ Neutralization of animal viruses can be demonstrated in three systems - animals, eggs and tissue culture.

Toxin neutralization: Bacterial toxins are good antigens and induce the formation of neutralising antibodies which are important in protection against and recovery from diseases such as diphtheria and tetanus.

♦ Neutralisation tests in animals consist of injecting toxin-antitoxin mixtures and estimating the least amount of antitoxin that prevents death or disease in the animals.

3.3.6   Enzyme Immuno Assays (EIA)

The term enzyme immunoassay is used for all assays based on the measurement of enzymes labelled antigen, hapten or antibody.

EIAs are of 2 basic types: homogeneous and heterogeneous.

In homogeneous EIA, there is no need to separate the bound and free fractions so that the test can be completed in one step, with all reagents added simultaneously.

The EIA test can be used only for assay of haptens such as not microbial antigens and antibodies.

e.g., Enzyme multiplied immunoassay technique (EMIT), is simple method for small molecule drugs such as opiates, cocaine, and barbiturates amphetamine in serum.

Heterogeneous EIA requires the separation of the free and bound fraction either by centrifugation or by absorption on solid surfaces and washing.

It is therefore a multi-step procedure, with reagents added sequentially.

e.g., ELISA

3.3.7   Enzyme Linked Immunosorbent Assays (ELISA)
ELISA Principle Basis and Extension

Enzyme-linked Immunosorbent Assays (ELISAs) combine the specificity of antibodies with the sensitivity of simple enzyme assays, by using antibodies or antigens coupled to an easily-assayed enzyme.

ELISAs can provide a useful measurement of antigen or antibody concentration. There are two main variations on this method: The ELISA can be used to detect the presence of antigens that are recognized by an antibody or it can be used to test for antibodies that recognize an antigen.

A general ELISA is a five-step procedure:

1. Coat the microtiter plate wells with antigen;

2. Block all unbound sites to prevent false positive results;

3. Add primary antibody (e.g., rabbit monoclonal antibody) to the wells;

4. Add secondary antibody conjugated to an enzyme (e.g., anti-mouse IgG);

5. Reaction of a substrate with the enzyme to produce a colored product, thus indicating a positive reaction.

There are many different **Error! Hyperlink reference not valid.**. One of the most common types of ELISA is "sandwich ELISA".

Buffer Preparation

1. Bicarbonate/carbonate coating buffer (100 mM):

   Antigen or antibody should be diluted in coating buffer to immobilize them to the wells:

   - 3.03 g Na_2CO_3

   - 6.0 g $NaHCO_3$

   - 1000 ml distilled water,

   - pH 9.6

2. PBS:

   - 1.16 g Na_2HPO_4

   - 0.1 g KCl

   - 0.1 g K_3PO_4

   - 4.0 g NaCl (500 ml distilled water)

   - pH 7.4

3. Blocking solution:

   - Commonly used blocking agents are 1% BSA, serum, non-fat dry milk, casein, gelatin in PBS.

4. Wash solution:

   - Usually PBS or Tris -buffered saline (pH 7.4) with detergent such as 0.05% (v/v) Tween20 (TBST).

5. Antibody dilution buffer:

   - Primary and secondary antibody should be diluted in 1x blocking solution to reduce non-specific binding.

Protocol of sandwich ELISA test:

1. Before the assay, both antibody preparations should be purified and one must be labeled.

2. For most applications, a polyvinylchloride (PVC) microtiter plate is best; however, consult manufacturer guidelines to determine the most appropriate type of plate for protein binding.

3. Bind the unlabeled antibody to the bottom of each well by adding approximately 50 μL of antibody solution to each well (20 μg/mL in PBS). PVC will bind approximately 100 ng/well (300 ng/cm^2). The amount of antibody used will depend on the individual assay, but if maximal binding is required, use at least 1 μg/well. This is well above the capacity of the well, but the binding will occur more rapidly, and the binding solution can be saved and used again.

4. Incubate the plate overnight at 4 °C to allow complete binding.

5. Wash the wells twice with PBS. A 500 mL squirt bottle is convenient. The antibody solution washes can be removed by flicking the plate over a suitable container.

6. The remaining sites for protein binding on the microtiter plate must be saturated by incubating with blocking buffer. Fill the wells to the top with 3% BSA/PBS with 0.02% sodium azide. Incubate for 2hr to overnight in a humid atmosphere at room temperature.

7. **Note:** Sodium azide is an inhibitor or horseradish peroxidase. Do not include sodium azide in buffers or wash solutions if an HRP-labeled antibody will be used for det*ection*.

8. Wash wells twice with PBS.

9. Add 50 μL of the antigen solution to the wells (the antigen solution should be titrated). All dilutions should be done in the blocking buffer (3% BSA/PBS). Incubate for at least 2 hr at room temperature in a humid atmosphere.

10. Wash the plate four times with PBS.

11. Add the labeled second antibody. The amount to be added can be determined in preliminary experiments. For accurate quantitation, the second antibody should be used in excess. All dilutions should be done in the blocking buffer.

12. Incubate for 2 hr. or more at room temperature in a humid atmosphere.

13. Wash with several changes of PBS.

14. Add substrate as indicated by manufacturer. After suggested incubation time has elapsed, optical densities at target wavelengths can be measured on an ELISA plate reader.

Note: Some enzyme substrates are considered hazardous, due to potential carcinogenicity. Handle with care and refer to Material Safety Data Sheets for proper handling precautions.

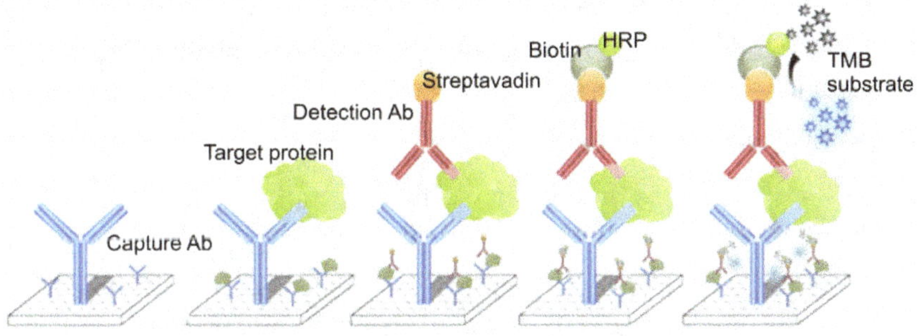

Fig. 3.5 ELISA Test

3.4   Hypersensitivity

The term hypersensitivity refers to the injurious consequences in the sensitized host, following contact with specific antigens.

- Hypersensitivity is concerned with what happens to the host as a result of the immune reaction.

- Hypersensitivity reactions can be divided into four types: type I, type II, type III and type IV, based on the mechanisms involved and time taken for the reaction.

3.4.1   Type I Hypersensitivity

(Anaphylactic, IgE or regain dependent):

♦ Antibodies ('cytotropic' IgE antibodies) are fixed on the surface of tissue cells (most cells and basophiles) in sensitised individuals.

- The antigen combines with the cell fixed antibody, leading to release of pharmacologically active substances (vasoactive amines) which produce the clinical reaction.

- Type I hypersensitivity is also known as immediate anaphylactic hypersensitivity.

- In this type of hypersensitivity, the $1°$ immune response will be normal effect is seen only in $2°$ immune response.

- Instead of IgA or IgD culprit antibody such as IgE is released.

- IgE will also attack phagocytic cell of the host and degranulation occurs.

Mechanism of Anaphylaxis

- IgE molecule are bound to surface receptors on mast cells and basophils.

- These cells carry large number of such receptors called F_c ER receptors, analogous to TCR receptors on T cell surface.

- IgE molecules attach to these receptors by their F_c end.

- The antigen molecules combine with the cell bound IgE, bridging the gap between adjacent antibody molecules.

- This cross-linking increases the permeability of the cells to calcium ions and leads to degranulation, with release of biologically active substances contained in the granules.

- The manifestations of anaphylaxis are due to pharmacological mediators, which are of two kinds.

- Primary mediators which are preformed contents of mast cell and basophil granules (histamine, serotonin, eosinophil chemotactic factor, haparin etc)

Secondary mediators which are newly formed upon stimulation by mast cells, basophils and other leucocytes (slow reacting substance of anaphylaxis,

- prostaglandins, platelet activating factor and cytokines such as IL3, IL4, IL5, IL6, Gm-csF)

Anaphylactoid Reaction: Intravenous injection of peptone, trysin and certain other substances provokes a clinical reaction resembling anaphylactic shock. This is termed 'anaphylactoid' reaction'.

♦ Type I hypersensitivity reaction usually takes 15-30 minutes from the time of exposure to the antigen.

e.g., wheeze (whistling sound during night times)

Asphyxia (breath lessness)

Asthma

Vomiting

Diarrhoea

3.4.2   Type II Hypersensitivity

♦ These reactions involve a combination of IgG (or rarely IgM) antibodies with the antigenic determinants on the surface of cells leading to cytotoxic or cytolytic cffccts.

♦ Examples are lysis of red cells caused by ant erythrocyte antibodies in autoimmune anaemias and haemolytic disease of the new-born.

♦ The reaction time is minutes to hours.

♦ Alternatively, a free antigen or hapten may be absorbed on cell surfaces.

♦ Subsequently reaction of the combined antigen or hapten with its corresponding antibody leads to cell damage.

♦ In some Type II reactions, the antibody combines with cell surface receptors and disrupts normal function, either by uncontrolled activation (eg: Graves diseases) or by blocking (e.g.: *Myasthenia gravis*)

♦ Diagnostic tests include detection of circulating antibody, the tissues involved and the presence of antibody and complement in the lesion (biopsy) by immunofluorescence.

♦ Treatment involves anti-inflammatory and immunosuppressive agents.

3.4.3   Type III Hypersensitivity

♦ Type III hypersensitivity is also known as immune complex hypersensitivity.

♦ The reaction may be general (eg: serum sickness) or may involve individual organs including skin (e.g., systemic lupus erythematosus, Arthus reaction), kidneys (e.g., lupus nephritis), lungs (e.g., Aspergillosis), joints (e.g., rheumatoid arthritis) or other organs.

♦ The reaction may take 3-10 hours after exposure to the antigen (as in Arthus reaction).

♦ **Arthus reaction:** Arthus (1903) observed that when rabbits were repeatedly injected subcutaneously with normal horse serum, the initial injections had no local effect but with later injections, there occurred intense local reaction consisting of oedema, indurations and haemorrhagic necrosis. This is known as the Arthus reaction and it's a local manifestation of generalised hypersensitivity.

♦ The tissue damage is due to formation of antigen-antibody precipitates causing complement of antigen-antibody of inflammatory molecules activation and release of inflammatory molecules.

♦ The Arthus reaction can be passively transferred with sera containing precpitating antibodies (IgG, IgM) in high *titres*.

♦ Serum sickness: This is a systemic form of Type III hypersensitivity

♦ This appeared, 7-12 days following a single injection of a high concentration of foreign serum such as the diphtheria antitoxin.

♦ The pathogenesis is the formation of immune complexes (consisting of the foreign serum and antibody to it that reaches high enough titers by 7-12 days) which get deposited on the endothelial lining of blood vessels in various parts of the body, causing inflammatory infiltration.

Treatment includes anti-inflammatory agents.

3.4.4   Type IV Hypersensitivity

♦ Type IV hypersensitivity is also known as cell mediated or delayed type hypersensitivity.

♦ The classical example of this hypersensitivity is tuberculin (montoux) reaction which peaks 48 hours after the injection of antigen (PPD or old tuberculin).

♦ The lesion is characterized by indurations and erythema.

♦ In delayed hypersensitivity, the interaction between antigens and T-cells occur.

♦ The reaction is not induced by circulating antibodies but by sensitised T cells (Tdth, Th1, Th2, Tc) which, on contact with the specific antigen, release cytokines that cause biological effects on leucocytes, macrophages and tissue cells.

♦ Delayed hypersensitivity cannot be passively transferred by serum but can be transferred by lymphocytes or the transfer factor.

♦ Two types of delayed hypersensitivity are recognized the tuberculin (infection) type and the contact dermatitis type.

Tuberculin (Infection) Type

♦ When a small dose of tuberculin is injected intradermally in an individual sensitised to tuberculoprotein by prior infection or immunisation, an indurated inflammatory reaction develops at the site within 48-72 hr.

♦ In unsensitised individuals, the tuberculin injection provokes no response.

♦ The tuberculin test therefore provides useful indication of the state of delayed hypersensitivity (cell mediated immunity) to the bacilli.

Contact Dermatitis Type

♦ Delayed hypersensitivity sometimes results from skin contact with a variety of chemical – metals such as Nickel and chromium, simple chemicals like dyes, picrylchloride, dinitrochlorobenzene, drugs such as penicillin and toiletries.

♦ Sensitisation is particularly liable when contact is with an inflamed area of skin and when the chemical is applied in an oily base.

♦ Antibiotic ointments applied on patches of dermatitis frequently provoke sensitisation.

♦ The substances involved are in themselves not antigenic but may acquire antigenicity on combination with skin proteins.

♦ Sensitisation requires percutaneous absorption.

♦ Langerhans cells of the skin capture locally applied hapten, along with the modified tissue proteins, and migrate to the draining lymph nodes where they present the processed antigen along with MHC molecules to T cells.

♦ The sensitised T cells travel to the skin site, where on contacting the antigen they release various lymphokines.

♦ Contact with the allergen in a sensitised individual leads to ' contact dermatitis', the lesions varying from macules and papules to vesicles that break down, leaving behind raw weeping area typical of acute eczematous dermatitis.

♦ Hypersensitivity is detected by the 'patch test'

♦ The allergen is applied to the skin under an adherent dressing.

♦ Sensitivity is indicated by itching appearing in 4-5 hours, and local reaction which may vary from erythema to vesicle or blister formation, after 24-28 hours.

3.4.5   Allergenic Extracts

Allergenic extracts comprise a large group of products that are unique compared to other biologics and conventional pharmaceuticals.

♦ A specific license is required for their manufacture, and they are available mainly from specialty companies.

♦ Allergenic extracts are relatively crude drugs by contemporary standards.

♦ Allergenic extracts are concentrated solutions or suspensions of allergens used for the diagnosis and treatment of allergic diseases.

Handling

♦ Allergenic extracts usually are designated as being aqueous or glycerinated products.

♦ Normal saline or similar isotonic electrolyte solution is the diluent.

♦ The preparations are normally buffered to pH 8 and contain phenol (0.4%) as a preservative.

♦ The most common measures of allergenic potency are by weight/volume and the protein nitrogen unit.

♦ Weight/volume is the weight of allergic substance extracted pre volume of extracting fluid.

For example: A 1: 50 extract is prepared by extracting 1 g of substance with 50 mL of solvent and decimal dilutions of this extract provide 1:500, 1:5000 etc concentrations.

♦ One protein nitrogen unit represents 0.01 mcg of total protein nitrogen in the product.

♦ A typical allergenic substance contains multiple allergenic molecules and epitopes of varying potency, and there is significant chemical and biological variation with different lots of the substance.

♦ The potency of these products is expressed in terms of allergy units or bioequivalent allergy units.

3.4.6   Examples of Allergenic Extracts

1. ***Pollen extract:*** Pollen is a fine yellowish powder that is transported from plant to plant by the wind, by birds, by insects or by other animals. The spread of pollen helps to fertilize plants and can mean misery for seasonal allergy with symptoms like sneezing, nasal congestion, runny nose, watery eyes, itchy throat and eyes wheezing etc., Some of the plants producing such allergic pollens from which allergenic extracts are prepared are Alfalfa, barley, canary grass, dandelion, eucalyptus, hazelnut, juniper, mustard, palm, ryegrass, etc.

2. ***Fungal extract:*** Airborne fungal spores occur in greater concentrations than pollen grains. Immunoglobulin E-specific antigens (allergens) on airborne fungal spores induce type I hypersensitivity (allergic) respiratory reactions in sensitized atopic subjects, causing rhinitis and/or asthma. Some of the fungal and mould extracts used are *Alternaria, candida, epidermaphyton, fusarium, mucor, penicillium species, rhizopus, sacchromyces* etc.

3. ***Dust extracts:*** Dust allergies may trigger asthma symptoms, such as wheezing, coughing, tightness in the chest and shortness of breath. Dust Allergy symptoms are sneezing, runny or stuffy nose, and red, itchy or teary eyes wheezing, coughing, tightness in the chest and shortness of breath Itching. Some of the dust allergy triggers are dust mites, Cockroaches, Mold, Pollen, Pet hair, feathers etc.

4. ***Insect allergen extracts:*** The insect allergy occurs due to bite, sting, and inhalation of insect parts mainly of the order *–Hymenoptera*. For biting insects, the optimal allergens source may be the salivary

glands. Some examples of allergic insect extracts are Fire ant, black ant, housefly, wasps, yellow jacket bee, hornet, fire ant, honeybee, moth, mites, mosquitoes, fruit fly, cockroach, caddis fly, etc.

5. *Food allergy*: Food allergy is an immune-based disease. A group of the eight major allergenic foods is often referred to as the Big-8 and comprises milk, eggs, fish, crustacean shellfish, tree nuts, peanuts, wheat and soybean. The symptoms of food allergy are asthma, rhinitis, headache, urticaria etc.

6. *Seasonal Allergies*: **Spring Allergies:** As the trees start to bloom and the pollen gets airborne, allergy sufferers begin their annual ritual of sniffling and sneezing in spring.
Summer Allergies: Many of the allergic triggers that can make us miserable in the spring persist into summer.
Fall Allergies: The allergy triggers might be slightly different, but they can be just as misery-inducing as the flower pollen that fills the air in the spring and summer.
Winter Allergies: Allergic reactions, mainly due to cold weather, mainly affecting skin and lips.

7. *Pet Allergies*: Allergy to proteins and glycoproteins from animal sources is an important public health problem affecting both children and adults. Some of the pets causing allergic reactions are dogs, cats, etc

8. *Latex Allergy*: Type IV hypersensitivity are due to latex additives. Allergic reactions to latex may be serious and can very rarely be fatal. People who are at higher risk for developing latex allergy include Health care workers and others who frequently wear latex gloves, people who have had multiple surgeries such as children with spina bifida, People who are often exposed to natural rubber latex, including rubber industry workers etc.,

9. *Drug Allergy*: In Drug allergy, the reaction is triggered by certain medicaments like penicillin, Aspirin and other NSAIDs such as Ibuprofen, Anticonvulsants, and drugs related to Monoclonal antibody therapy, Chemotherapy etc. Patch tests help to confirm the etiology of the cutaneous adverse drug reactions involving delayed hypersensitivity mechanisms.

10. *Miscellaneous inhalant extracts*: Besides above sources, there are number of other miscellaneous substances causing allergies like Hairs

from various sources such as human, camel, cat, rabbit fur, wool, Bird feathers such as from chicken, pigeon, duck etc. and Algae, gum acacia, jute, silk, tobacco etc.

3.4.7   Classification of Vaccines

Vaccines are preparations of antigenic substances that are administered for the purpose of inducing in the recipient a specific and active immunity against the infective agent or toxin produced by it.

Bacterial Vaccines: Bacterial vaccines are either sterile suspensions of live or killed bacteria or sterile extracts of derivatives of bacteria. Most vaccines against bacterial infections are effective at preventing disease Reactions can occur after vaccinations Vaccines are available against tuberculosis, diphtheria, tetanus, pertussis, *Haemophilus influenzae* type B, cholera, typhoid, and *Streptococcus pneumoniae.*

Bacterial toxoids: Bacterial toxoids are toxins or material derived therefrom, the toxicity of which has been reduced to a very low level or completely eliminated by chemical or physical means without destroying their immunizing potency. Examples are Tetanus toxoid, Botulism toxoid.

Viral and rickettsial vaccines: Viral and rickettsial vaccines are suspensions of viruses or rickettsiae and are prepared from infected tissues or blood obtained from artificially infected animals, from cultures in fertile eggs, or from cell or tissue cultures. Examples of viral vaccines are Hepatitis A & B vaccines, Influenza vaccine, MMR vaccine, Poliomyelitis vaccine, rabies vaccine, rotavirus vaccine, yellow fever vaccine etc. and *Rickettsia rickettsii* vaccine is an example of rickettsial vaccine.

Antisera (Immunosera): Antisera are native (unconcentrated) sera or preparations from native sera containing specific immunoglobulins that have prophylactic or therapeutic action when injected into persons exposed to or suffering from a disease caused by a specific micro-organism. Examples are snake venom antiserum, scorpion venom antiserum, tetanus immune-human globulin etc.

There are several different types of vaccine available and with new technology, there will be further additions. The body response to a vaccine depends on the type of vaccine being administered. The more similar a vaccine is to the natural disease, the better the immune response to the vaccine.

3.4.8 The following is the fate of most Vaccines Injected directly into Muscle Tissue

1. Vaccine antigen disassociates from adjuvant (i.e., Aluminium hydroxide).

2. Cells of the non-specific immune system (i.e., Macrophages and dendritic cells) recognize the antigen as foreign and engulf it. These cells then chop the antigen into smaller fragments and display these on their cell surfaces.

3. The dendritic cells move through the lymphatic system to a local lymph node where specific T cells and B cells, which recognize the fragments of antigen generates a specific immune response.

4. Other components in the vaccine such as the adjuvant and preservative, if present, are absorbed into the blood where they circulate and are excreted in the stools and urine.

3.4.9 There are Two Basic Types of Vaccines based on the Properties of Antigens

(i) Live attenuated Vaccines

(ii) Inactivated Vaccines.

The characteristics of live and inactivated vaccines are different, and these characteristics determine how the vaccine is used.

Live Attenuated Vaccines: are produced by modifying a disease-producing ("wild") virus or bacteria in a laboratory. The resulting vaccine organism retains the ability to replicate (grow) and produce immunity, but usually does not cause illness. Live attenuated vaccines include live viruses and live bacteria. Reduction of virulence is known as attenuation and can be achieved by passage through unfavourable hosts, repeated cultures in artificial media, growth under high temperature or in the presence of weak antiseptics, desiccation, or prolonged storage in culture.

Properties of Live Attenuated Vaccines

Live vaccines are derived from "wild," or disease-causing, virus or bacteria.

These wild viruses or bacteria are attenuated, or weakened, in a laboratory, usually by repeated culturing.

Unlike live antigens, inactivated antigens are usually not affected by circulating antibody.

Inactivated vaccines may be given when antibody is present in the blood (*e.g.*, In infancy, or following receipt of antibody-containing blood products).

Inactivated vaccines always require multiple doses. In general, the first dose does not produce protective immunity, but only "primes" the immune system. A protective immune response develops after the second or third dose.

The immune response to an inactivated vaccine is mostly humoral, little or no cellular immunity results.

Antibody titers against inactivated antigens diminish with time. As a result, some inactivated vaccines may require periodic supplemental doses to increase, or "boost," antibody titers.

Examples of currently available inactivated vaccines are limited to inactivated whole viral vaccines (influenza, polio, rabies and hepatitis A). Whole inactivated bacterial vaccines include Pertussis, Typhoid, Cholera, and Plague. "Fractional" vaccines include subunits (Hepatitis B, Influenza, Acellular Pertussis), and Toxoids (Diphtheria, Tetanus).

- The measles vaccine used today was isolated from a child with measles disease in 1954.

- Almost 10 years of serial passage on tissue culture media were required to transform the wild virus into vaccine virus.

- Live attenuated vaccines must replicate (grow) in the vaccinated person.

- A relatively small dose of virus or bacteria is given to stimulate an immune response.

- Anything that either damages the live organism in the vial (e.g., Heat, light), or interferes with replication of the organism in the body (circulating antibody) can cause the vaccine to be ineffective.

- They are generally effective with one dose, except those administered orally.

Disadvantages: Live attenuated vaccine virus could theoretically revert back to its original pathogenic (disease-causing) form. This is known to happen only with live (oral) polio vaccine.

◆ Due to interference from circulating antibody to the vaccine virus, active immunity may not develop from a live attenuated vaccine.

◆ Antibody from any source (e.g., transplacental, transfusion) can interfere with the growth of the vaccine organism and lead to a poor response or no response to the vaccine (also known as vaccine failure).

◆ May cause severe or fatal reactions as a result of uncontrolled replication (growth) of the vaccine virus, with immunodeficient persons (e.g., From leukaemia, treatment with certain drugs, or HIV infection).

◆ The measles vaccine virus seems to be more sensitive to circulating antibody. Polio and rotavirus vaccine viruses are least affected.

◆ They are labile, and can be damaged or destroyed by heat and light.

◆ They must be handled and stored carefully.

Examples of currently available live attenuated viral vaccines include Measles, Mumps, Rubella, Varicella, Yellow fever, Influenza (intranasal) and Oral polio vaccine. Bacterial vaccines include BCG and Oral Typhoid vaccine.

3.5   Inactivated Vaccines

These vaccines can be composed of either whole viruses or bacteria, or fractions of either: Fractional vaccines are either protein-based or polysaccharide-based. Protein-based vaccines include toxoids (inactivated bacterial toxin), and subunit or subvirion products. Most polysaccharide-based vaccines are composed of pure cell-wall polysaccharide from bacteria. Conjugate polysaccharide vaccines are those in which the polysaccharide is chemically linked to a protein. This linkage makes the polysaccharide a more potent vaccine.

These vaccines are produced by growing the bacteria or virus in culture media, then inactivating it with heat and/or chemicals (usually formalin). In the case of fractional vaccines, the organism is further treated to purify only those components to be included in the vaccine (e.g., The polysaccharide capsule of *pneumococcus*). Inactivated vaccines are not alive and cannot replicate. The entire dose of antigen is administered in the injection. These vaccines cannot cause disease from infection, even in an immune deficient person.

3.5.1 Polysaccharide Vaccines

Polysaccharide vaccines are a unique type of **inactivated subunit vaccine** composed of long chains of sugar molecules that make up the surface capsule of certain bacteria. Pure polysaccharide vaccines available include: pneumococcal, meningococcal, and *Salmonella typhi*. The immune response to a pure polysaccharide vaccine is typically T-cell independent, which means that these vaccines are able to stimulate B-cells without the assistance of T-helper cells.

Properties of polysaccharide vaccines

T-cell independent antigens, including polysaccharide vaccines, are not consistently immunogenic in children < 2 years of age.

Young children do not respond consistently to polysaccharide antigens, probably because of immaturity of the immune system. Repeated doses of most inactivated protein vaccines cause the antibody titer to go progressively higher, or "boost."

Repeat doses of polysaccharide vaccines do not cause a booster response.

Antibody induced with polysaccharide vaccines has less functional activity than that induced by protein antigens, because the predominant antibody produced in response to most polysaccharide vaccines is IgM and little IgG is produced.

3.5.2 Conjugate Vaccines

In the late 1980s, it was discovered that the problems with polysaccharide vaccines could be overcome through a process called conjugation. Conjugation changes the immune response from T-cell independent to T-cell dependent, leading to increased immunogenicity in infants and antibody booster response to multiple doses of vaccine.

Examples of conjugated polysaccharide vaccine were for *Haemophilus influenza type b (Hib)*.Also now available are conjugate vaccines for pneumococcal disease and meningococcal disease.

3.5.3   Recombinant Vaccines

Vaccine antigens may also be produced by genetic engineering technology. These products are sometimes referred to as recombinant vaccines. There are four genetically-engineered vaccines that are currently available:

♦ Hepatitis B vaccines are produced by insertion of a segment of the hepatitis B virus gene into the gene of a yeast cell. The modified yeast cell produces pure hepatitis B surface antigen when it grows.

♦ Human papillomavirus vaccines are produced by inserting genes for a viral coat protein into either yeast (as the hepatitis B vaccines) or into insect cell lines. Viral-like particles are produced and these induce a protective immune response.

♦ Live typhoid vaccine (Ty21a) is *Salmonella typhi* bacteria that have been genetically modified to not to cause illness.

♦ Live attenuated influenza vaccine (LAIV) has been engineered to replicate effectively in the mucosa of the nasopharynx but not in the lungs.

3.6   Vaccine Preparations

3.6.1   Polio Vaccine

Vaccine: Vaccines are preparations of live or killed micro-organisms or their products used for immunization.

♦ Sabin polio vaccine is an example of live attenuated vaccine preparation.

♦ Salk polio vaccine is an example of killed vaccine preparation.

♦ Salk's killed polio vaccine is a formalin inactivated preparation of the three types of polioviruses grown in monkey kidney tissue culture. Standard virulent strains are used.

- The three types of polioviruses are grown separately in monkey kidney cells.

- Viral pools of adequate titer are filtered to remove cell debris and clumps, and inactivated with formalin (1:4000) at 37 °C for 12-15 days.

- Stringent tests are carried out to ensure complete inactivation and freedom from extraneous agents.

- The three types are then pooled and after further tests for safety and potency, issued for use.

- Killed vaccine is given by injection. It is therefore called inactivated or injectable polio vaccine.

- Three doses given 4-6 weeks apart constitute the primary vaccination, to be followed by a booster six months later.

- The first dose should be given to babies after the age of six months to ensure that immune response is not impaired by residual maternal antibodies.

- Immunity can be sustained by booster doses every 3-5 years thereafter.

- An enhanced potency IPU produced in human diploid cells induces better seroconversion following two subcutaneous doses, 4-8 weeks apart.

- A third dose may be given 6-12 months later

3.6.2   Live Polio Vaccine (Sabin's Polio Vaccine)

- Sabin's vaccine strains were developed by plaque selection in monkey kidney tissue culture.

- Attenuated strains for live vaccine should possess the following criteria

1. Should not be neurovirulent as tested by intraspinal inoculation in monkeys.

2. Should be able to set up intestinal infection following feeding and should induce an immune response.

3. Should be stable and should not acquire neurovirulence after serial enteric passage.

4. Should possess stable genetic characteristics (markers) by which they can be differentiated from the wild virulent strains.

Live polio vaccine is administered orally and is therefore known as oral polio vaccine (OPV)

♦ It is prepared by growing the attenuated strains in monkey kidney cells.

♦ Very stringent precautions are taken to ensure freedom from extraneous agents like SV40 and B virus.

♦ After tests for neurovirulence, genetic stability and potency, the vaccine is issued either in the monovalent or trivalent form, in pleasantly flavored syrup.

♦ The use of molar $MgCl_2$ or sucrose stabilizes the vaccine against heat inactivation, particularly under tropical conditions.

♦ The vaccine is usually given in the trivalent form, it can be given to young infants, as the maternal antibody has little effect on intestinal infection.

♦ Theoretically, a single dose is sufficient to establish infection and immunity but in practice three doses are given at 4-8 week intervals, to ensure that all three types of the vaccine virus multiply in the intestine.

♦ The shelf life of the vaccine at 4-8 °C is four months and a + – 20 °C is two years.

3.6.3   BCG Vaccine

BCG, the tuberculosis vaccine, is an attenuated strain of *M. bovis.*

♦ Immunoprophylaxis is by intradermal injection of the live attenuated vaccine developed by Chalmette and Guerin (1921), the Bacillus Chalmette Guerin or BCG.

♦ Injection of BCG in animals induces self-limit infection, with multiplication and dissemination of the bacillus in different organs and production of small tubercles.

♦ Within a few weeks the bacilli stop multiplying although they survive in the tissues for long periods. This gives rise to delayed hypersensitivity and immunity.

♦ BCG vaccine be administered to babies by intradermal injection on the deltoid immediately after birth, or as early as possible thereafter, before the age of 12 months.

♦ The vaccine need not be administered after the age of two years.

♦ BCG induces a nonspecific stimulation of the immune system providing some protection against leprosy and leukaemia.

♦ BCG grows under high bile salts and the gene responsible for causing infection is inactivated.

3.6.4   Bacterial Toxins

There are two kinds of Bacterial toxins.

1. **Exotoxins**: So-called because they diffuse freely through the bacterial cell wall into the medium in which the organisms are growing.

2. **Endotoxins**: So-called because they are retained within the bacteria and are freed only when the cells die and start to disintegrate.

3.6.5   Exotoxins

They have the following characteristics:

(i) They are the products of the metabolism of actively growing bacteria.

(ii) They are produced mainly by Gram +ve bacteria.

(iii) They are water soluble and can pass into the surrounding medium. This provides a means of separating toxin from the cells, since the latter can be removed on a bacteria – proof filter through which the toxin containing medium will pass.

(iv) Chemically, they are high molecular weight proteins and some are enzymes, they are relatively thermostable and lose activity at about 60 °C

(v) They are extremely toxic to the body. *Botulinus toxin*, produced by clostridium botulinum, an organism responsible for a food poisoning, is the most toxic substance known.

When exotoxin producing bacteria grow in the body the toxins are carried in the blood stream to all parts, the most serious consequences of infection are due to the effects of the toxins rather than the damage to the tissues invaded by the bacteria. *e.g.,* In diphtheria, the causative organism grows in the throat producing a membrane that may cause asphyxiation.

The general effects of exotoxins are often caused on the nervous system and the heart.

e.g., Tetanus exotoxin is neurotoxin and causes severe muscular spasms.

Other toxins cause death of tissues (neuro toxins) intestinal damage (enterotoxins), haemolysis, haemolysins, destruction of WBC (leucocidins).

Exotoxin producing bacteria include clostridium botulinum, clostridium tetani (tetanus) clostridium perfringens, septicum, welchii (gas gangrene) and coryne bacterium diphtheriae (diphtheria).

Exotoxins are soluble, heat-labile proteins that are usually released into the surroundings as the bacterial pathogen grows given in Table 3.4.

♦ In general, exotoxins are produced by gram-positive bacteria, although some gram-negative bacteria also make exotoxins.

♦ Exotoxins are usually synthesized by specific bacteria that often have plasmids or prophages bearing the toxin genes.

♦ They are associated with specific diseases and often are named for the disease they produce (e.g., the diphtheria toxin)

♦ Exotoxins are among the most lethal substances known; they are toxic in microgram-per-kilogram concentrations (e.g., *batulinum toxin*), but are typically heat labile, inactivated at 60-80 °C.

♦ Exotoxins are proteins that exert their biological activity by specific mechanisms.

♦ As proteins, the toxins are highly immunogenic and can stimulate the production of neutralizing antibodies called antitoxins.

♦ The toxin proteins can also be inactivated by formaldehyde, iodine and other chemicals to form immunogenic toxoids (for e.g., tetanus toxoid)

♦ The tetanus vaccine is a solution of tetanus toxoid.

♦ Exotoxins can be grouped into four types based on their structure and physiological activities.

1. One type is the AB toxin, which gets its name from the fact that the portion of the toxin (B) that binds to a host the enzyme activity that causes the toxicity.

2. A second type, which also may be an AB toxin, consists of those toxins that affect a specific host site (nervous tissue neurotoxins), the intestine (enterotoxins), general tissues (cytotoxins) by acting extracellular or intracellular on the host cells.

3. A third type does not have separable A and B portions and acts by disorganizing host cell membranes. Examples include the leukocidins, hemolysins and phospholipases

4. A fourth type is the superantigen that acts by stimulating T cells directly to release cytokines.

3.6.6   Endotoxins

They have the following characteristics

(i)   They are structural elements of bacteria.

(ii) They are contained in most bacterial cells but greatest amounts are found in Gram –ve bacteria.

(iii) They are not excreted into the surrounding medium and are liberated only when the cells die or disintegrate.

(iv) They are complexes of phospholipid, polysaccharide, protein, most of them are thermostable.

(v)   They are much less toxic.

(vi) Endotoxin producing bacteria include *Vibrio chlolerae* (cholera), *Pasteurella pestis* (plague), *Salmonella typhi* (typhoid), *Salmonella paratyphi* (p-typhoid), *Bordetella pertussis* (whooping cough).

♦ Gram-negative bacteria have *Lipopolysaccharide* (LPS) in the outer membrane of their cell wall that, under certain circumstances, is toxic to specific hosts. This LPS is called an endotoxin because it is bound to the bacterium and is released when the microorganism lyses given in Table 3.4.

♦ Bacterial endotoxins are

(a)   Heat stable

(b) Toxic (nanogram amounts)

(c) Weakly immunogenic

(d) Generally similar, despite source

(e) Usually capable of producing general systematic effects: fever (pyrogenic), shock, blood coagulation, weakness, diarrhoea, inflammation, intestinal haemorrhage with endotoxins resulted in complications-even death-to patients.

♦ Endotoxins can be problematic for individuals and firms working with cell cultures and genetic engineering. The result has been the development of sensitive tests and method to identify and remove these endotoxins.

♦ Most firms have set a limit of 0.25 endotoxin units, 0.025 ng/mL, or less as a release standard for their drugs, media or products.

♦ Endotoxins can initially activate Hageman factor (blood clotting factor XII), which in turn activates up to four humoral systems: coagulation, complement, fibrinolytic, and kininogen systems.

♦ Removal of endotoxins presents more of a problem than their detection.

♦ Those present on glassware or medical devices can be inactivated if the equipment is heated at 250 °C for 30 minutes.

Table 3.4 Differences between Exotoxin and Endotoxin

Exotoxin	Endotoxin
Excreted by organisms	Integral part of cell wall
Excreted by both Gram positive and Gram-negative bacteria	Found mostly in Gram-negative bacteria
Chemically polypeptide	Lipopolysaccharide complex
Relatively unstable, heat labile (60 °C)	Relatively stable, heat tolerant
Highly antigenic, neutralized by antitoxin	Weakly immunogenic, antibodies are antitoxic
Can be toxoid	Cannot be toxoid
Highly toxic, fatal in μg quantities	Moderately toxic
Usually binds to specific receptors	Specific receptors not found
Not pyrogenic usually	Fever by induction of interleukin1 (IL-1) production.
Located on extra chromosomal genes (e.g. plasmids)	Located on chromosomal genes

3.7   Toxoids

The toxoids, used as vaccines are toxins that have been incubated with formalin. This treatment completely destroys their toxic properties without causing significant loss of antigenic qualities.

Toxoids are of three types:

(i) Diphtheria vaccine

(ii) Tetanus vaccine

(iii) Staphylococcus toxoid

(iv) Diphtheria Vaccine

Preparation of Toxin

A suitable strain of *Corynebacterium diphtheria* is grown on a liquid medium and must not be made with broth prepared from horse muscle.

Horse muscle must not be used because the presence of horse protein in the toxin and toxoid preparation made from it, might sensitize the recipient to horse serum and make dangerous the subsequent injection of sera, which are made in horses.

After incubation under optimal conditions until toxin production has reached a satisfactory level, the bulk of organisms are removed on paper pulp and the filtrate is sterilized using fibrous pads or ceramic candles.

Conversion of Toxin to Toxoid

Formaldehyde solution (formalin) is added and the mixture incubated at 37°C until the toxicity has been removed which takes 2-3 weeks. The resulting material is known as Formal toxoid (FT).

It was an excellent antigen but it often causes severe reactions in adults.

3.7.1   Preparation of other forms of Toxoid

(i) **Toxoid – antitoxin floccules (TAF):** If suitable amounts of toxoid and antitoxin are mixed, floccules are obtained that contain almost all the antigenic activity and when separated, washed are free from contamination with broth and metabolites. This product is known as toxoid anti toxin floccules and causes fewer reactions.

Neutralized product has no significant activity because neither toxoid nor antitoxin is damaged when they combine. Therefore, the combination can dissociate under suitable conditions.

e.g., after the floccules have been injected into the body, leaving the toxoid free to stimulate antibody production.

Therefore, the following method of preparation is used:

80 units of antitoxin are added to 100 units of toxoid i.e., the toxoid is slightly neutralized.

After leaving for about three weeks to allow the floccules to form and settle, the supernatant liquid is decanted.

The floccules are then washed with saline, by decantation, until the washings are colourless and resuspended in saline containing a bactericide.

Advantages

1. It is especially valuable for adults, who are much more sensitive than young children to the reaction causing constituents of immunological preparation.

2. It is a weaker antigen; therefore, two doses must be given because it contains diphtheria antitoxin, which is made from horse serum.

Disadvantages

Slight risk of sensitization.

(ii) **Alum Precipitated Toxoid (APT):** This preparation from slow absorption of precipitated toxoids from the site of injection and slow excretion from the body led to increased antigenic activity. Its development was made to make purer toxoids.

High quality of formal toxoid is treated with charcoal to remove

(a) Colouring matter

(b) Non-specific impurities that might cause reactions.

After filtration, to remove charcoal, a suitable concentration of alum is added. This reacts with bicarbonate phosphate and protein impurities in the toxoid to produce a precipitate containing $Al\ (OH)_2$ phosphate. The toxoid is adsorbed onto this mineral carrier.

The precipitate is washed and suspended in saline containing a bactericide provides a depot in tissues from which the antigen is slowly released to give a prolonged stimulus.

Advantages

1. APT produces much higher antibody levels than FT and TAF and therefore two doses are sufficient.

2. It is free from sensitizing horse protein and contains toxoid of improved purity.

Disadvantages

1. Adults and older children may show local reactions to the carrier.

2. There is a slight risk of provoking paralytic poliomyelitis in the limb in which the injection is given.

3. Inspite of its high efficiency it has been largely replaced by combined prophylactics because they are more convenient.

(iii) **Purified Toxoid Aluminium Phosphate (PTAP):** The main difference between PTAP and APT is that it contains a much purer form of toxoid. This is obtained:

   (a) By using a semi-synthetic medium in the preparation of the toxin, to exclude as much non-specific material as possible.

   (b) By a complicated purification of the toxoid involving the use of Mg $(OH)_2$ to precipitate colour, phosphate and some protein, ammonium sulphate and cadmium chloride as protein precipitants.

The separation of much of the unwanted protein reduces the reactions, but also removes the impurities that give a precipitate with alum.

Therefore, it is necessary to use a preformed carrier i.e., pure hydrated aluminium phosphate.

Advantages

1. PTAP is an excellent antigen due to its depot effect.

2. Toxoid is very pure and can be freeze dried.

3. It is very stable.

4. The production of batches of uniform potency is greatly facilitated.

Disadvantages

1. It carries the small risk of provocative poliomyelitis.

(iv) Purified Diphtheria Formal Toxoid in combined Prophylactics:
The Ministry of Health recommends that children should be immunized against four infectious diseases (diphtheria, tetanus, pertussis and poliomyelitis) during the first year of life.

It is customary to use a combined vaccine containing either diphtheria, tetanus and pertussis antigens or these 3+ poliomyelitis antigens.

Purified diphtheria formal toxoid (FT) can be used successfully in these preparations because it is less active alone than any of the three adsorbed forms its effect is potentiated by the presence of dead pertussis bacteria which appear to act like alum salts, as an adjuvant.

3.7.2   Tetanus Toxoid

♦ A sterile preparation of the formaldehyde-treated products containing growth of *Clostridium tetani*.

♦ It contains a non-phenolic preservative. It should be stored 2 $^\circ$ to 8 $^\circ$C and not be allowed to freeze.

♦ A sterile preparation of plain tetanus toxoid precipitated or adsorbed by alum, aluminium hydroxide or aluminium phosphate adjuvant.

Tetanus is caused by *Clostridium tetani*, an anaerobic gram-positive, endospore forming rod.

♦ Prevention of tetanus involves the use of the tetanus toxoid.

♦ The toxoid, which incorporates an adjuvant (aluminium salts) to increase its immunizing potency, is given routinely with diphtheria toxoid and pertussis vaccine.

♦ An initial dose is normally administered a few months after birth, a second dose 4 to 6 months later, and finally a reinforcing dose 6 to 12 months after the second injection.

♦ Another booster is given between the ages of 4 to 6 years.

♦ For many years, booster doses of tetanus toxoid were administered every 3 to 5 years.

◆ However, that practice has been discontinued since it has been shown that a single booster dose can provide protection for 10 to 20 years.

◆ Serious hypersensitivity reactions have occurred when too many doses of toxoid were administered over a period of years.

◆ Booster doses are generally given when an individual has sustained a wound infection and only if it has been 10 or more years since the previous dose.

◆ Control measures for tetanus are not possible because of the wide dissemination of the bacterium in the soil and long survival of its spores.

◆ Prevention depends on active immunization with toxoid, proper care of wounds contaminated with soil, prophylactic use of antitoxin

3.8   Official Vaccine Storage Conditions and Stability

The correct storage and handling of vaccinations has helped to reduce the prevalence of vaccine-preventable diseases. Vaccines that are exposed to temperatures outside of the authorised ranges can lose their efficacy, effectiveness, and protection. Good immunisation practises are founded on the foundation of vaccine management, which includes correct storage and handling methods. Vaccines must be carefully preserved from the time they are made until they are given out. Manufacturers, distributors, public health personnel, and health-care providers all have responsibility for ensuring vaccination quality and maintaining the cold chain.

3.8.1   Chain of Custody

A suitable cold chain is a temperature-controlled supply chain that encompasses all equipment and processes used in the transportation, storage, and handling of vaccines from the moment they are manufactured until they are administered.

The cold chain's components:

Each of the three primary components of the cold chain must work together to ensure safe vaccination shipment and storage:

- Transportation and storage equipment
- Well-trained people
- Well-organized management procedures

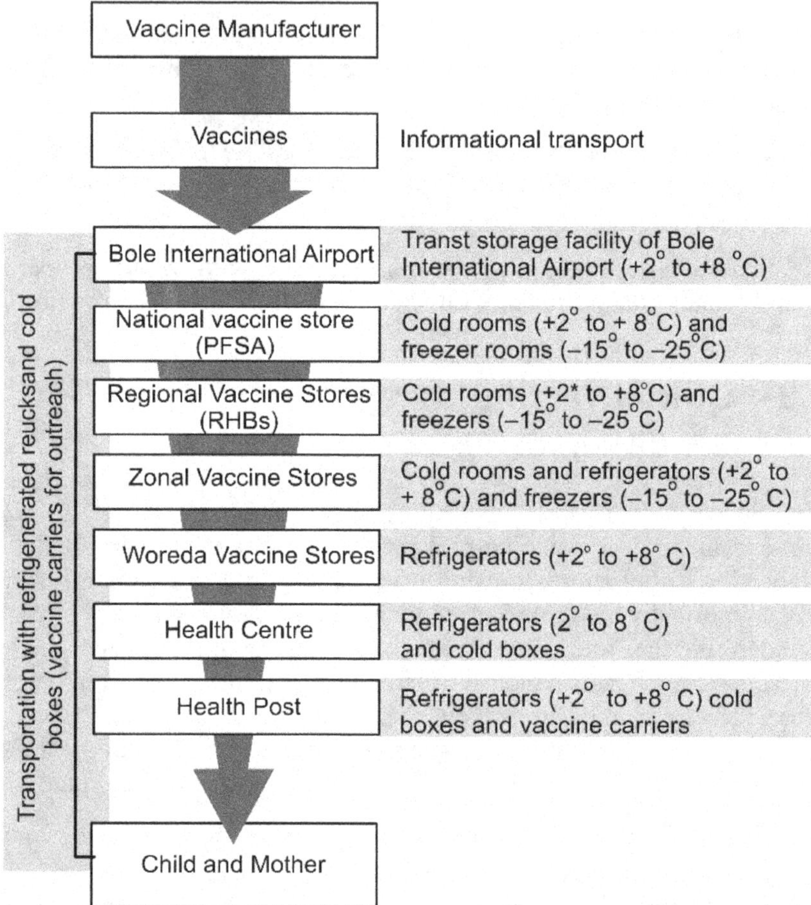

Fig. 3.6 Schematic representation of Components of Cold Chain

Every institution should have clear written policies for routine and emergency vaccine storage and handling that are updated at least once a year. These policies and procedures should be in written and easily accessible to all employees as a reference.

Cold chain equipment

Refrigerators, cold boxes, vaccine carriers, ice packs, and foam pads are examples of popular cold chain equipment used in Health Posts.

3.8.2   Refrigerators

A refrigerator is a device that cools things down. Refrigerators at health care facilities can run on electricity, kerosene, paraffin, bottled gas, or solar energy. Electric refrigerators are typically the least expensive to operate and repair. For keeping vaccinations and freezing and storing ice packs, different refrigerators have varying capacity.

n the refrigerated compartment of a Health Post, one month's supply of vaccinations and diluents should be able to be stored.

♦ A minimum supply of vaccinations and diluents of one to two weeks (i.e. an additional 25 percent of the standard stock).

♦ Fully frozen ice-packs (strong, specifically constructed plastic bottles carrying frozen water) that have been in the freezer compartment for at least 24 hours.

Frozen ice packs should not be placed in the main refrigerator section They may cause the temperature to drop too low, causing the freeze-sensitive vaccines to be destroyed.

3.8.3   Vaccine Carriers and Cold Boxes

A cold box is an insulated container that can be coated with 'conditioned' ice packs to keep vaccinations and diluents cool but not frozen while being transported from the health centre or to outreach sites. When the refrigerator is out of commission or being defrosted, or if vaccines are being transported in a vehicle for a few days by mobile vaccination teams, cold boxes can be utilised for brief durations of vaccine storage (from two to seven days, depending on the manufacturer).

The size of the cold boxes is pretty enormous. Instead, a smaller insulated container known as a vaccination carrier can be used at the Health Post level. Vaccine carriers are additionally lined with conditioned ice packs to keep vaccines and diluents cold during transportation from the health centre's collection store or on trips to outreach sites, as well as for temporary storage during Health Post immunisation sessions. They're smaller than cold boxes and easier to carry when walking, but they only keep cold for 36–48 hours with the top closed as shown in Fig 3.7.

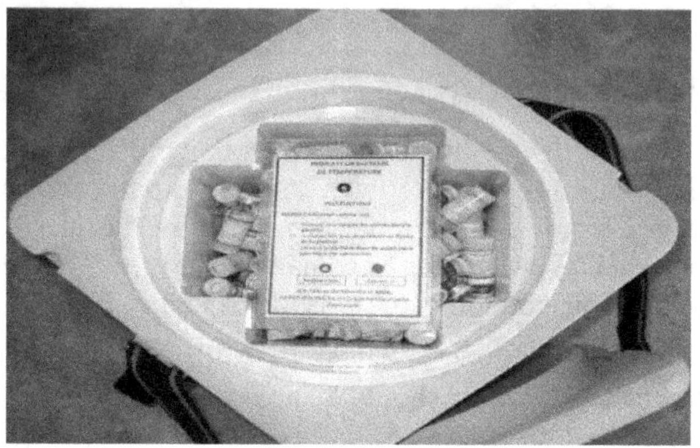

Fig. 3.7 Vaccine Carriers and Cold Boxes

3.8.4   Ice-packs

Ice-packs are flat, rectangular plastic bottles filled with water and kept refrigerated or frozen before being used in vaccination carriers and cold boxes. For a cold box or vaccine carrier, the amount of ice packs required varies.

Every Health Post should carry at least two sets of ice packs, one frozen or refrigerated and the other conditioned for use in a cold box or vaccine carrier, for each of their cold boxes and vaccine carriers.

Putting ice packs in the freezer:

Maintaining the efficacy of vaccinations requires adequate freezing and conditioning of ice packs. Follow these instructions to freeze ice packs.

♦ Fill the ice packs halfway with water, leaving about 20% air space at the top, and tighten the cap.

♦ Squeeze each ice pack upside down to ensure that it does not leak.

♦ Place the ice packs vertically in the freezer section of the refrigerator, touching the evaporator plate with the surface of each ice pack, and close the door.

♦ Freeze ice packs for at least 24 hours to ensure they are completely solid. They should be ready to use after 24 hours.

♦ Return the melted ice packs to the freezer as soon as possible after each immunisation session.

♦ Store any additional unfrozen ice packs that don't fit in the freezer in the main refrigerator compartment's bottom section. This allows the water in the chilled ice packs to freeze fast when placed in the freezer, as well as keeping this portion of the refrigerator cool in the event of a power outage.

Ice packs that have been pre-chilled and chilled water packs that have been pre-chilled

Conditioned ice packs have been thoroughly frozen before being taken out of the freezer and placed at room temperature for a brief period of time (it may take over 30 minutes if the room is cold). Allow the frozen ice packs to lie out at room temperature until the ice melts and water forms. Shake each ice pack and listen for the sound of water moving within to see if it has been thoroughly conditioned. This keeps the ice packs from freezing the vaccines within a cold box or vaccine carrier, causing freeze-sensitive vaccines to be damaged.

Several vaccinations are harmed more severely by freezing than by heat, according to studies conducted in many countries on cold chain temperatures. When shipping freeze-sensitive vaccinations like pentavalent, PCV10, and TT, it's critical to utilise appropriately conditioned ice packs or cold-water packs.

Chilled water packs can be manufactured by nearly filling ice-pack containers or standard plastic water bottles with water and storing them in the refrigerator's main compartment for around 24 hours. Chilled water packs may be more efficient than conditioned ice packs because freezing and conditioning ice packs takes more electricity, gas, or kerosene, as well as more time. Furthermore, if frozen ice-packs are not properly conditioned, they may expose freeze-sensitive vaccines to damage during transport in vaccine carriers or cold boxes.

3.8.5   Pads made of Foam

A foam pad is a soft foam layer that sits on top of conditioned ice packs in a cold box or vaccination carrier. To allow vaccination vials to be put into the pad, several cuts in the foam have been made. The foam pad can be used as a temporary lid to keep unopened vaccines within the carrier cool during immunisation sessions, as well as a surface to grip and protect opened vaccine vials and keep them cool. When vaccines are inserted in the foam pad above the ice packs in the vaccine carrier, they are protected from heat damage during an immunisation session as shown in Fig 3.7 and 3.8

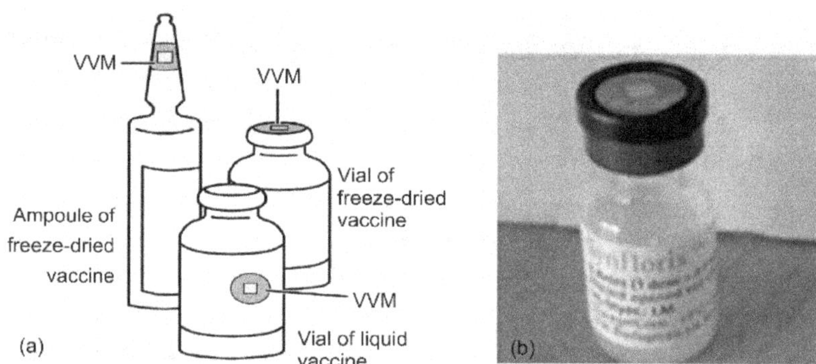

Fig. 3.8 Storage of vaccines

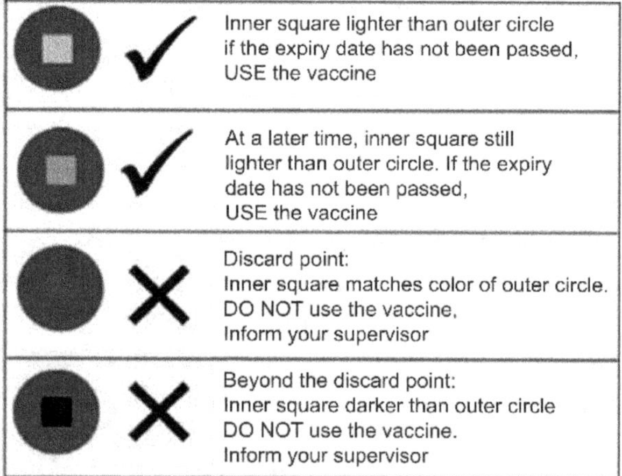

Fig. 3.9 Precaution indications of vaccines

(a) Vaccine Vial Monitors (VVMs) on the neck of an ampoule, or on the label or cap of a vaccine vial

(b) A vial of liquid PCV10 vaccine (Synflorix) with the VVM on the cap

Do not use vaccines that have reached the discard point, even if they have not passed their expiry date.

3.8.6   Heat activates VVMs, but Cold does not!

VVMs respond to heat and do not detect exposure to cold temperatures. The VVM cannot tell you if a vaccination has been frozen and has lost its efficacy. So, even though the VVM says the vaccination hasn't been exposed to heat, the vaccine could still be frozen. As a result, it's critical to ensure that freeze-sensitive vaccines haven't been frozen before utilising them. As mentioned below, inspect the freeze indicator.

3.8.7   Indicators of Freeze

Freeze indicators are devices that track how long vaccinations have been exposed to freezing temperatures. Freeze indicators arc included in batches of freeze-sensitive EPI vaccinations (pentavalent, PCV10, and TT), as well as other freeze-sensitive vaccines like HepB that could be used to protect healthcare personnel. The freeze-tag is the most frequent sort of freeze indicator. This is an irreversible temperature indication that tells if a product has been frozen, such as a vaccine. It's made up of an electrical temperature sensor and a liquid crystal display (LCD). The freeze-tag is working properly when a small blinking dot of light appears in the corner of the display as shown in Fig 3.10

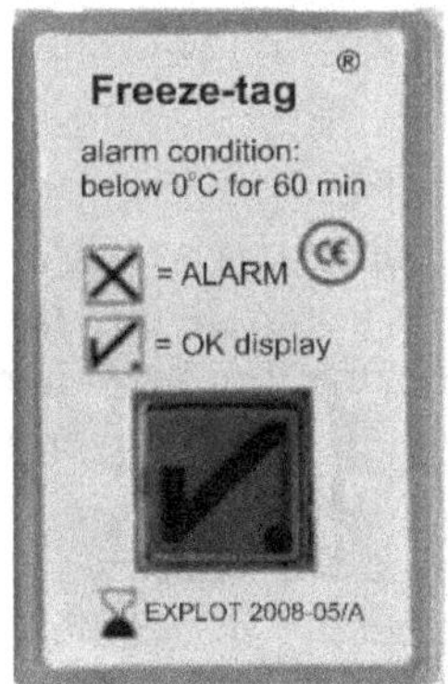

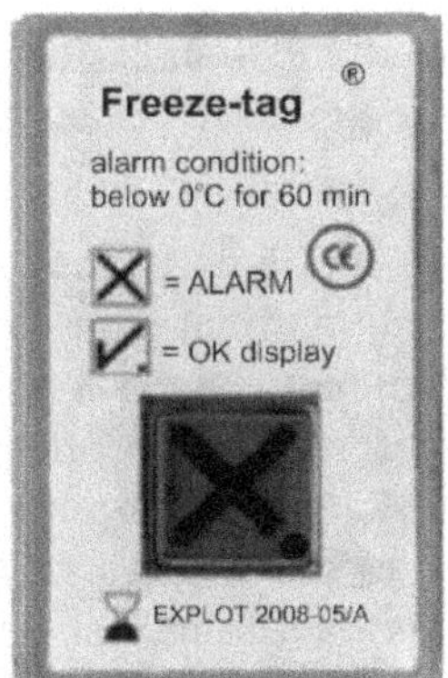

Fig. 3.10 Indicators of Freeze tag

Freeze-tags showing:

(a) 'good status' display;

(b) 'alarm status' display

The display will change from 'good status' to 'alert status' if the freeze-tag is exposed to a temperature below 0°C (with a range of + 0.3 ° C and –0.3 ° C) for more than 60 minutes (with a range of 57 to 63 minutes).

Vaccines that have been frozen may have been destroyed and should be tested using the shake test, as detailed below.

3.8.8   The Shake Tests

The shaking test is used to determine whether freeze-sensitive vaccinations (pentavalent, PCV10, TT, or HepB) have been destroyed by exposure to freezing temperatures. Follow the instructions below to perform the shake test:

Step 1: Make a frozen control vial as follows: Take a vial of vaccine from the same manufacturer, with the same type and batch number as the vaccination you want to test. Allow the vial to defrost after freezing until the contents are solid (at least 10 hours at –10°C). The frozen control vial is this. Make a distinct mark on the vial so that it can be easily identified and is not accidentally used.

Step 2: Select a test vial Take a vial (or several vials) of vaccination from the batch you think was frozen. This appears to be a frozen test vial.

Step 3: Shake the test and control vials: Shake the suspicious frozen test vial and the frozen control vial together vigorously for 10–15 seconds in one hand.

Step 4: Allow the vials to rest: Place both vials side by side on a table and do not move them any farther. Without being frozen, a freeze-sensitive vaccine appears as a uniformly hazy liquid. When you leave the vaccine to rest after vigorous shaking, it tends to create flakes that quickly settle at the bottom of the vial to form sediment. The sedimentation rate is the rate at which the flakes settle. It's worth noting that some vials have huge labels that obscure the contents. It's tough to see the sedimentation process because of this. In such circumstances, observe sedimentation by turning the control and test vials upside down and look for sedimentation in the bottle necks.

Step 5: Compare the vials: For a maximum of 30 minutes, observe the difference in sedimentation rates in the frozen control and suspected frozen test vials. Compare the sedimentation rates of both vials by holding them up to the light. If the vaccine in the suspected test vial has a far slower sedimentation rate than the vaccine in the frozen control vial, the test vaccine was most likely not frozen and can be utilised. If the sedimentation rate in the suspicious test vial and the frozen control vial is similar, the vaccine should not be used since the test vial has most likely been damaged by freezing.

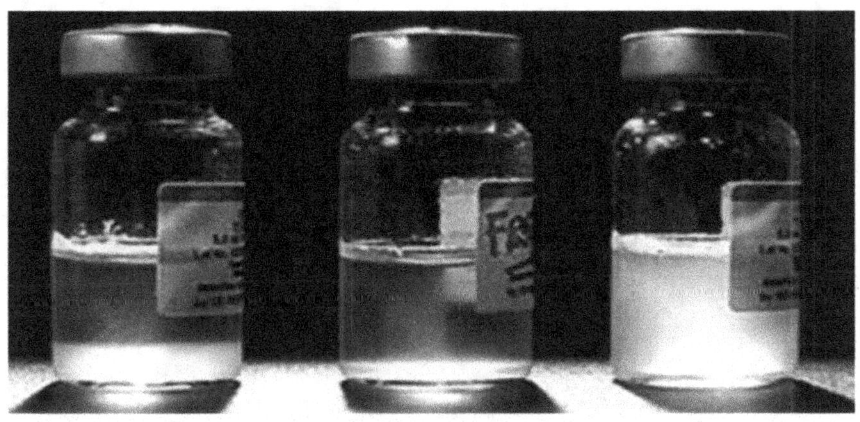

Frozen test vial   Frozen control vial   Non-frozen test vial

Fig. 3.11 Frozen test

With the light behind them, three vials of liquid freeze-sensitive vaccine: (left) A sediment has settled to the bottom of a frozen test vial after vigorous shaking; (centre) a frozen control vial whose sedimentation rate can be compared to that of a suspected frozen test vial; (right) a non-frozen test vial with a uniformly cloudy appearance, indicating that the vaccine has not been damaged by freezing as shown Fig 3.11

All vaccines with the following features should be shaken before use:

- Vaccines packed in boxes with a freeze indicator that is found to be activated.

- Refrigerator temperature records that show the temperature has dropped below +2°C.

- If you suspect the vaccines were frozen by accident, such as by placing them too close to the freezer plate in the refrigerator or by touching frozen ice-packs.

The vaccination must be discarded if it fails the 'shake test' If a liquid vaccine vial is already frozen solid, there is no need to do a shake test; simply discard it. Also, any vials with white lumps of sediment stuck to the glass that won't dissolve after vigorous shaking should be discarded. If a pentavalent vaccine is subjected to freezing below 0°C, this can happen.

3.8.9   Thermometers

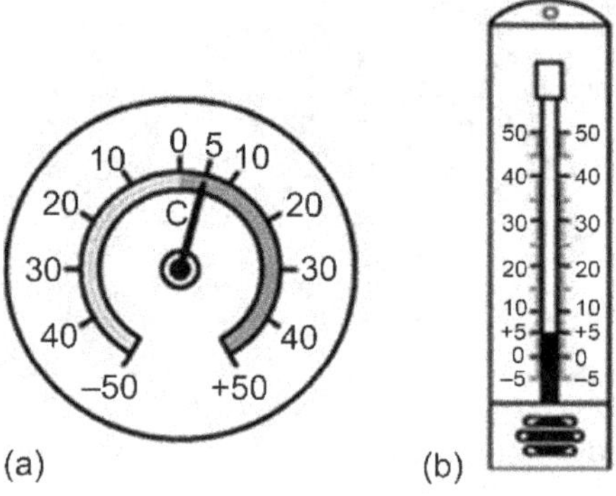

Fig. 3.12 Schematic representation of Thermometers

(a) Dial thermometer, and (b) stem thermometer.

A thermometer is a device that measures the temperature of your cold chain equipment, such as a refrigerator, a cold box, or a vaccine carrier. It allows you to set the temperature to the proper range for vaccination storage and transportation.

A dial or a stem (bulb) thermometer can be used to monitor the temperature of the equipment at a Health Post. On a dial thermometer, the needle moves around the scale, pointing to plus (+) numbers when it's warmer and minus (−) numbers when it's colder; on a stem (or bulb) thermometer, coloured fluid in the bulb moves up the scale as it gets warmer and down the scale as it gets colder; on a digital thermometer, the needle moves around the scale, pointing to plus (+) numbers when it's warmer and minus (−) numbers when it's cold.

Cold chain equipment loading:

To keep the temperature of the vaccines and diluents within the refrigerators, cold boxes, and vaccine carriers within the appropriate range, they must be properly filled. All health professionals in a Health Post should be able to monitor the cold chain equipment and know what to do if the temperature rises or falls too quickly.

Refrigerators for vaccines are designed in a variety of ways.

A thermostat is standard on all electric refrigerators. The thermostat is a device that detects temperature changes and activates switches that control the cooling equipment to keep the refrigerator compartments at the proper temperature. If the temperature of the refrigerator is discovered to be too high or too low when you check the thermometer, you can adjust the thermostat setting. The size of the flame in a gas or kerosene refrigerator can be changed.

There are a few tips that should be followed to guarantee that your immunizations are stored properly in the refrigerator.

Recommendations for storing vaccinations in the fridge

- Avoid repeatedly opening and closing the refrigerator door, as this raises the temperature inside.

- Vaccines should not be stored on the door shelves. The temperature in this section of the refrigerator is too warm for vaccine storage, and when the door is opened, the door shelves are exposed to room temperature immediately.

- Discard any vaccinations that are expired (beyond their expiration date), have VVMs that have reached or exceeded their discard point, or have been reconstituted for more than six hours.

- Do not refrigerate reconstituted vaccines (BCG, measles) or PCV10 vials that have been opened. They should be thrown away at the end of the immunisation session or six hours later, whichever comes first.

- Make sure the refrigerator isn't overly crowded. To allow air to circulate around the vaccines and diluents and keep them cool, about half of the total area inside should be kept empty.

- Vaccines, diluents, and ice packs should be maintained in a refrigerator that is separate from other materials. If your Health Post only has one refrigerator and you need to store other heat-sensitive goods in it, such as medications, ointments, serum, and blood samples, make sure you clearly identify them and place them on a different shelf from the vaccines and diluents.

- Refrigerators come in a variety of shapes and sizes. Some front-loading freezers have only one door and a second freezing compartment on the inside. Others have two distinct chambers, each with its own set of doors as shown in Fig 3.13.

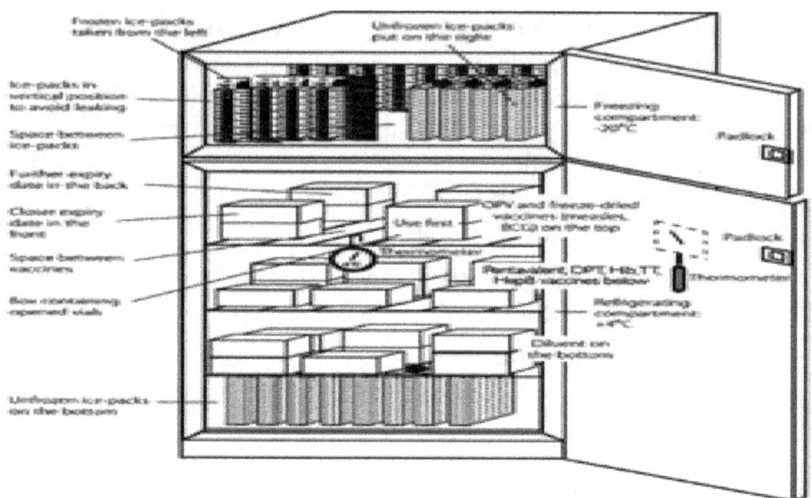

Fig. 3.13 Front-loading refrigerator with separate freezing compartment on top

The following is how the two compartments should be used:

- Vaccines and diluents are stored in the main compartment (the refrigerator), where the temperature should be kept between +2°C and +8°C.

- Ice packs are frozen in the top compartment (the freezer). This compartment will be between –15°C and –20°C if the refrigerator is working properly.

- For multi-dose vaccines that have been opened or unopened vials that have been taken out for an immunisation session but not used, look for the 'use first' box. These vials should be used first, followed by others.

- PCV10 vaccine should not be refrigerated once opened; it is a liquid vaccine with no preservative, and any remaining vaccine in the two-dose vial should be discarded after six hours or at the completion of the immunisation session, whichever comes first.

- Vials with longer expiry dates are kept in the back, while those with shorter expiry dates are kept in the front. Vaccines being loaded into a refrigerator

❖ The following guidelines should be followed when loading a vaccination refrigerator.

- Freeze ice packs and keep them in the freezer compartment.

- Store all vaccines and diluents in the refrigerator compartment; diluents can be stored at room temperature if space is limited.

- Chilling diluents in the refrigerator for several hours before using them to reconstitute BCG or measles vaccines is critical.

- Arrange the vaccination boxes so that air can circulate between them.

- Keep boxes of freeze-sensitive vaccinations (pentavalent, PCV10, TT, and HepB) away from the freezer, refrigeration plates, and the refrigerator's side or bottom linings, where they could accidentally freeze.

- On the bottom shelf of a front-loading refrigerator, keep melted ice packs or plain plastic water bottles filled with cooled water. These keep the temperature cool in the event of a power outage.

- Keep vaccines in places that are acceptable for the type of refrigerator you're using. Vaccines should be stored as follows in a front-loading refrigerator with the freezing compartment on the top:

- On the top shelf, OPV and freeze-dried vaccines (BCG and measles).

- All other vaccinations are located on the intermediate shelves; diluents are located on the bottom shelf.

- The freezing section of certain refrigerators is lined with ice packs. An ice-lined refrigerator is one of these. In this case, all vaccines should be put in the refrigerator's basket in the following order:

- Only the measles vaccination, BCG, and OPV are kept at the bottom.

- Top-only freeze-sensitive vaccinations (pentavalent, PCV10, TT, and HepB).

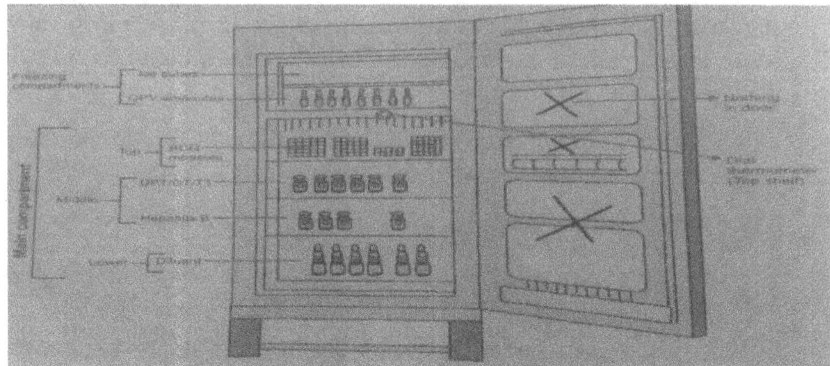

Fig. 3.14 Schematic representation of storage of vaccines in Refrigerator

- Loading vaccine carriers and cold boxes before an immunisation session, it's critical to follow the processes for loading vaccines into cold boxes and vaccine carriers.

- Take all of the frozen ice-packs needed from the freezer compartment of the refrigerator and close the door at the start of the immunisation session day.

- Leave the frozen ice packs at room temperature until the ice melts and water forms. This is crucial because freeze-sensitive vaccinations can be destroyed by freezing if the ice packs are too cold.

- Shake each ice pack and listen for the sound of water moving around the ice within to verify if it has been correctly prepared. Ice packs that have started to melt are referred to as conditioned ice packs.

- Place conditioned ice packs on all four sides of the cold box or vaccine carrier, as well as on the cold box's bottom. Chilled water in ordinary plastic bottles can also be utilised. Place the vaccinations and diluents in the cold box or carrier's centre.

- Place a foam cushion on top of the conditioned ice packs in vaccination carriers. Place conditioned ice packs on top of vaccines in cold boxes.

- Tightly close the cold box or vaccine carrier's lid. It's then ready to go to the immunisation appointment. Keeping cold chain equipment at the proper temperature.

- It's critical to keep your cold chain equipment at the right temperature, and to modify the temperature of your vaccine refrigerator if it's too hot or too cold. Heat and freeze sensitivity are present in all vaccinations. As a result, it's critical to keep an eye on the refrigerator's temperature to ensure that the immunizations don't get too hot or too cold.

- For vaccine storage, a temperature range of +2°C to +8°C is suitable.

You'll need a thermometer and a temperature chart to keep track of the temperature in your refrigerator, which should be taped to the outside of the door.

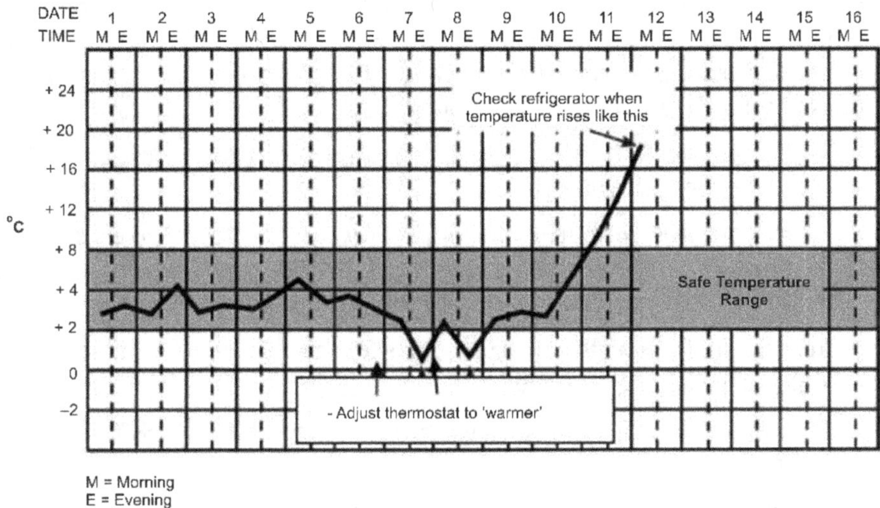

Fig. 3.15 Temperature Chart

- Temperature chart depicting the safe temperature range and dangerous ranges that necessitate thermostat adjustments or checking that the refrigerator is in good operating order.

- The temperature of the refrigerator was around +2°C in the morning of the 7th day of the month, which is within the permitted temperature range, according to the temperature chart. There was no need for any adjustments.

- The temperature had dropped to below +1°C in the evening, which is outside the permitted range. The thermostat should have been set to a "warmer" setting as shown in Fig 3.15.

3.8.10   Refrigerators that run on Kerosene or Gas

Increase or decrease the amount of the flame in a kerosene or gas refrigerator to alter the temperature. Reduce the size of the flame to raise the temperature within the main refrigerator compartment if it is too low. Because a smaller flame provides less cooling, the temperature in the fridge will rise. Increase the size of the flame to lower the refrigerator temperature if it is too high. A larger flame produces greater cooling, lowering the temperature in the refrigerator. After regulating the flame, monitor the temperature change often – around every 15 minutes – until the temperature remains stable between +2°C and +8°C, ensuring that it does not climb too high or fall too low.

If the temperature in your electric refrigerator drops too low (below +2°C), take the following steps:

- Adjust the thermostat so that the arrow points to a lower number, such as 4, if the thermostat dial previously set to 5. The refrigerator will become warmer as a result of this.

- Inspect freeze-sensitive vaccines to see if they've been harmed by the cold. The shake test is used to do this.

❖ If the temperature in the refrigerator rises above +8°C, do the following steps:

- Check to see if the refrigerator is operational. If not, make sure the power supply is turned on. After a power outage or after putting a new batch of vaccine into the refrigerator, do not immediately adjust the thermostat to a colder setting. The immunizations may freeze if the refrigerator becomes too cold.

- Change the thermostat's dial to a higher number, for example, if the dial was set to 3, change it to 4. The refrigerator will become cooler as a result of this.

- Check to see whether ice is stopping cold air from accessing the refrigerator compartment from the freezing chamber. It may be required to defrost the refrigerator if it has been clogged with too much ice (remove the ice).

- If the temperature in the refrigerator cannot be maintained between +2°C and +8°C, keep vaccines in another location, such as a vaccine carrier, and have the refrigerator fixed as soon as feasible.

- Keeping cold boxes and vaccination carriers at the proper temperature Maintaining the proper temperature in cold boxes and vaccine carriers is just as critical as maintaining the proper temperature in your refrigerator.

❖ Follow the steps below to accomplish this:

- Fill the cold box or vaccination carrier with enough conditioned (melting) ice packs or chilled water bottles.

- Keep the refrigerated box or vaccination carrier in the shade – never in direct sunlight.

- Only open the lid of your cold box or vaccine carrier when withdrawing a vaccination, and then close it immediately afterward.

- During immunisation sessions, place the foam pad atop the conditioned ice packs to contain vials.

❖   If the ice packs have entirely melted, proceed as follows:

- Discard all reconstituted vaccine vials (BCG and measles).

- Check the vaccinations' VVM status and place those that can still be used in a refrigerator at the proper temperature as soon as possible.

- Put them in the 'use first' box and utilise them first at your next immunisation appointment.

3.9   Live Vaccines

Heat is a problem for live vaccines. MMRV, varicella, and zoster vaccines must be kept frozen in a freezer at 5°F (-15°C) or below until used. Heat affects the MMRV, varicella, and live vaccinations. When zoster vaccinations are withdrawn from the freezer, they quickly degrade. MMR vaccination (measles, mumps, and rubella) is usually kept in the refrigerator, although it can also be kept in the freezer. If you have enough freezer space, the National Centre for Immunization and Respiratory Diseases recommends keeping MMR and MMRV together in the freezer. This may lower the chance of MMRV being stored inadvertently in the refrigerator. Although LAIV and rotavirus vaccines are live viral vaccines, they must be kept in the refrigerator. These vaccines should not be kept in the fridge.

3.10 Inactivated Vaccines

Vaccines that have been inactivated are vulnerable to both extreme heat and ice. Excessive heat and freezing are equally harmful to inactivated vaccinations. They should be kept in the refrigerator between 35- and 46-degrees Fahrenheit (2 and 8 degrees Celsius), with an average temperature of 40 degrees Fahrenheit (5 degrees Celsius). When temperatures outside of this range are reached, vaccine potency is reduced and the risk of vaccine-preventable diseases rises. Inactivated vaccines can withstand a limited amount of heat, but they are cold sensitive and are quickly degraded by freezing temperatures.

3.11 Vaccine Light Sensitivity

Vaccines such as HPV, MMR, MMRV, rotavirus, varicella, and zoster are light sensitive, resulting in potency loss. Light must be kept away from these immunizations at all times. As a result, keep these vaccinations in their original packaging, with the lids on, until they're needed. Light sensitivity causes HPV, MMR, MMRV, rotavirus, varicella, and zoster vaccines to lose their efficacy.

3.12 Lyophilized (Freeze-Dried) Vaccines and Diluents

The diluent for MMR, MMRV, varicella, and zoster vaccines is packaged separately from the lyophilized (freeze-dried) vaccine and can be kept at room temperature or in the refrigerator. Diluents supplied separately from their vaccinations can be stored in the refrigerator door to save space. Diluents can be kept at room temperature or in the refrigerator if they are packaged separately from the vaccinations. Diluents that come packaged with vaccines should be kept in the refrigerator with the vaccines. Diluents (such as ActHIB® and Menomune®) that come packed with vaccines should be kept in the refrigerator with the vaccines.

3.13 Hybridoma Technology

The word hybridoma refers to cells that have fused together due to the fusion of two types of cells: (i) An antibody-producing lymphocyte cell (e.g., a mouse spleen cell vaccinated with sheep red blood cells) and (ii) A single myeloma cell (bone marrow tumour cell) that can reproduce indefinitely. These fused hybrid cells, also known as hybridoma, have the ability to produce antibodies acquired from lymphocytes and can develop indefinitely (immortal) like malignant cancer cells.

When cells of interest fuse with cancer cells using fusogens such as sendaivirus or polyethylene glycol (PEG), the two cells' cytoplasmic membranes fuse to generate heterokaryon, or cells with two distinct nucleuses. The two nucleuses then fused together to generate cybrid or hybrid cells. Hybrid cells combine the nuclear components of both cells while retaining the species' normal chromosomal number due to the loss of an additional chromosome. In cybrid cells, the genetic material of one cell is totally preserved while the genetic material of the other is completely lost, implying that cybrid cells are hybrids in terms of the cytoplasmic component.

A hybrid cell is used to produce vast quantities of antibodies for diagnostic or therapeutic purposes. Injecting a specific antigen into a mouse, extracting an antibody-producing cell from the mouse's spleen, and fusing it with a tumour cell termed a myeloma cell results in hybridoma's. In the laboratory, hybridoma cells can proliferate indefinitely and can be utilised to manufacture a specific antibody indefinitely.

Antibodies, also known as immunoglobulins, are protein molecules produced by an unique type of cell in mammals called B-lymphocytes (plasma cells). Antibodies are part of the body's defence system that protects it from invading foreign substances known as antigens.

Antigen determinants (epitopes) are specific antigen determinants found on each antigen. Complementary determining regions (CDRs) of antibodies are primarily responsible for antibody specificity. B-lymphocytes create a variety of antibodies in response to an antigen (which may have several distinct epitopes). Polyclonal antibodies are antibodies that can respond with the same antigen several times.

The generation of polyclonal antibodies varies and is influenced by factors such as epitopes, immune response, and so on. Polyclonal antibodies have various limitations in terms of therapeutic and diagnostic applications due to their lack of specificity and heterogenic nature.

Monoclonal antibodies (MAb) are antibodies that are directed towards a single antigenic determinant (epitope). Animals were immunised against a specific antigen in the early years, and B-lymphocytes were extracted and cultivated in vitro to produce MAbs. Because culturing normal B-lymphocytes is challenging, and MAb synthesis is short-lived and limited, this strategy was not successful.

The existence of immortal monoclonal antibody-producing cells in nature is intriguing. They're present in people who have multiple myeloma, a type of malignancy (a cancer of B- lymphocytes). It happened in 1975. MAbs were mass produced on a massive scale by George Kohler and Cesar Milstein (Nobel Prize, 1984). In vitro, they were able to successfully hybridise antibody-producing B-lymphocytes with myeloma cells, resulting in a hybridoma.

As a result, B-lymphocytes that have been artificially immortalised can grow endlessly in vitro and create MAbs. Hybridoma cells have myeloma-like growth and multiplication abilities, yet release B-lymphocyte-like antibodies. Hybridoma technology refers to the manufacture of monoclonal antibodies via hybrid cells as shown in Fig. 3.16.

3.13.1 Principle for Creation of Hybridoma Cells

Hat medium selection

Myeloma cells utilised in hybridoma technology can't mnake their own antibodies, thus they can't synthesise them. The fact that mammalian cells may manufacture nucleotides via two separate mechanisms (de novo and salvage) influences HAT selection. Aminopterin, a folic acid analogue, blocks the de novo route in which a methyl or formyl group is transferred from an active form of tetrahydrofolate. When the de novo process is stopped, cells turn to the salvage pathway, which avoids the aminopterin block by directly converting purines and pyrimidines to DNA. Hypoxanthine-guanine phosphoribosyl transferase (HGPRT) and thymidine kinase are enzymes that catalyse the salvage route (TK). A mutation in one of these two enzymes prevents the salvage mechanism from working.

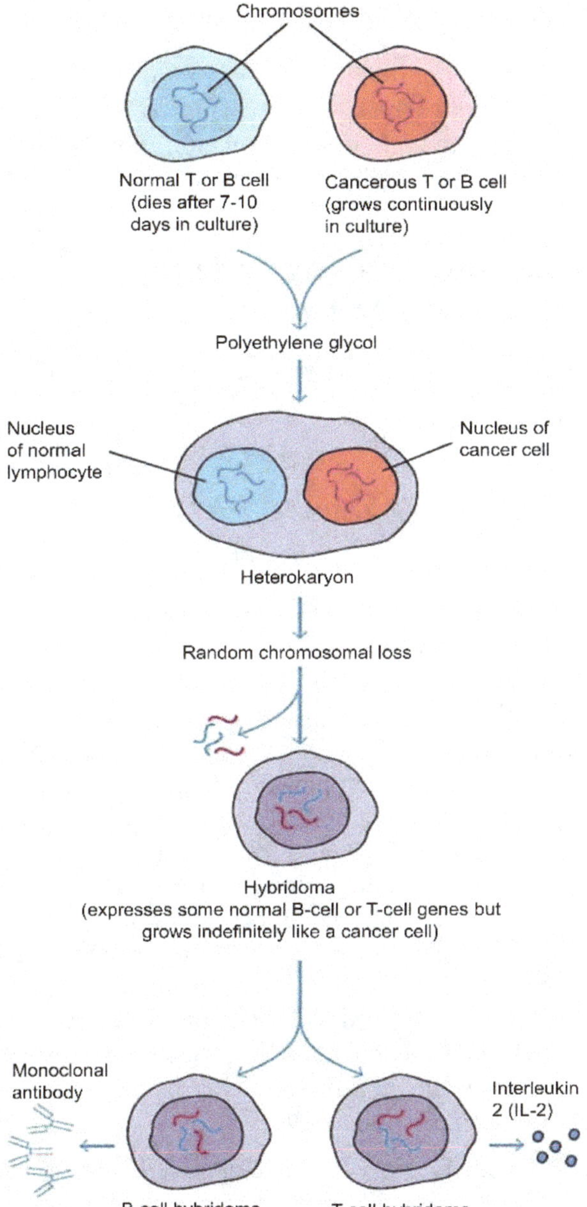

Fig. 3.16 Schematic representation of production of monoclonal antibodies via hybridoma cells

Aminopterin blocks the de novo pathway, while hypoxanthine and thymidine allow growth via the salvage process in HAT media. Only the hybrid cells carry the entire complement of enzymes required for growth on HAT media via the salvage route when two types of cells, one with a mutation in TK and the other with a mutation in HGPRT, are joined. In HAT media, only hybrid cells will develop.

3.13.2 Monoclonal Antibody Production by Hybridoma Technology

Monoclonal antibodies produced in the following steps:

1. Preparation of Cells

2. Fusion of cells

3. Selection of Hybridoma cells

4. Culturing of selected hybridoma cells

5. Screening of culture for antibody production

6. Propagation of screened colony

7. Isolation of antibodies

1. **Preparation of Cells:** Cells must be appropriately prepared in order to produce monoclonal antibodies. Monoclonal antibodies are made from B cell and myeloma cells. B cells' genetic machinery should be changed to Ig+, HGPRT-, and TK+. This is accomplished using a procedure known as site guided mutagenesis. These B cells are obtained from mice that have been injected with the antigen of interest, and they also have the ability to produce antibodies against that antigen. Myeloma cells' genetic machinery has been altered to become Ig-, HGPRT+, and TK-. The purpose of genetic alteration is to provide B cells the potential to produce antibodies and to select hybrid cells from the culture following hybridization. Immortality is achieved by using myeloma cells.

2. **Fusion of Cells:** B cells and myeloma cells are prepared separately and then merged using sendaivirus or polyethylene glycol (PEG). Fusogens fuse cells, resulting in fused B cells, myeloma cells, cybrids, and hybrids. There may be some unfused cells in the media.

3. **Selection of Hybrid cells:** After utilising fusogens to fuse the cells, they are placed in a culture medium containing HAT selection media.

Aminopterin prevents the synthesis of new nucleotides. HGPRT and TK are required when de novo synthesis is inhibited so that cells can employ the salvage pathway to generate nucleotides. B cells, myeloma cells, and cybrids cannot survive in the selection medium because one of these enzymes is missing. Hybrid cells with functional HGPRT and TK have been discovered to be capable of growing in selection media. They can also be referred to as being selected in selection.

4. **Culturing of selected hybridoma cells:** After hybridoma cells have been chosen, they are grown in microtiter wells with single hybridoma cells in each well. As a result, a mono clone is formed, which is a collection of cells developed from a single hybridoma cell.

5. **Screening cells for antibody production:** Despite the fact that hybridoma cells survived in the selection medium and formed clones, their potential to produce antibodies has yet to be confirmed. ELISA or RIA assays are used to assess this characteristic. Those clones that are capable of producing the antibody of our choice are allowed to proceed to the next stage of monoclonal antibody manufacture.

6. **Propagation of screened clones:** It's just growing or permitting selected clone cells to develop in vitro or in vivo, as the case may be. Clone cells are cultivated in tissue culture flasks with appropriate medium in the invitro procedure. The rate of production is found to be between 10 and 100 micrograms per millilitre. Select clones are injected into the peritoneal cavity of histocompatibility mice and allowed to proliferate and manufacture antibodies in the Invivo approach. Antibody production is measured in milligrammes per millilitre.

7. **Isolation of antibodies:** Before being employed for a number of reasons, monoclonal antibodies may need to be separated and purified. The cultures may be treated to cell fractionation for antibody protein enrichment prior to final purification. Antibodies may be secreted in the periplasm of E. coli, which can be exploited for antibody enrichment, simplifying further purification. Alternatively, antibodies can be isolated from medium-derived cell homogenate or cell detritus. Antibodies can be purified using one of two methods: I ion exchange chromatography, or (ii) antigen-affinity chromatography as shown in Fig 3.17.

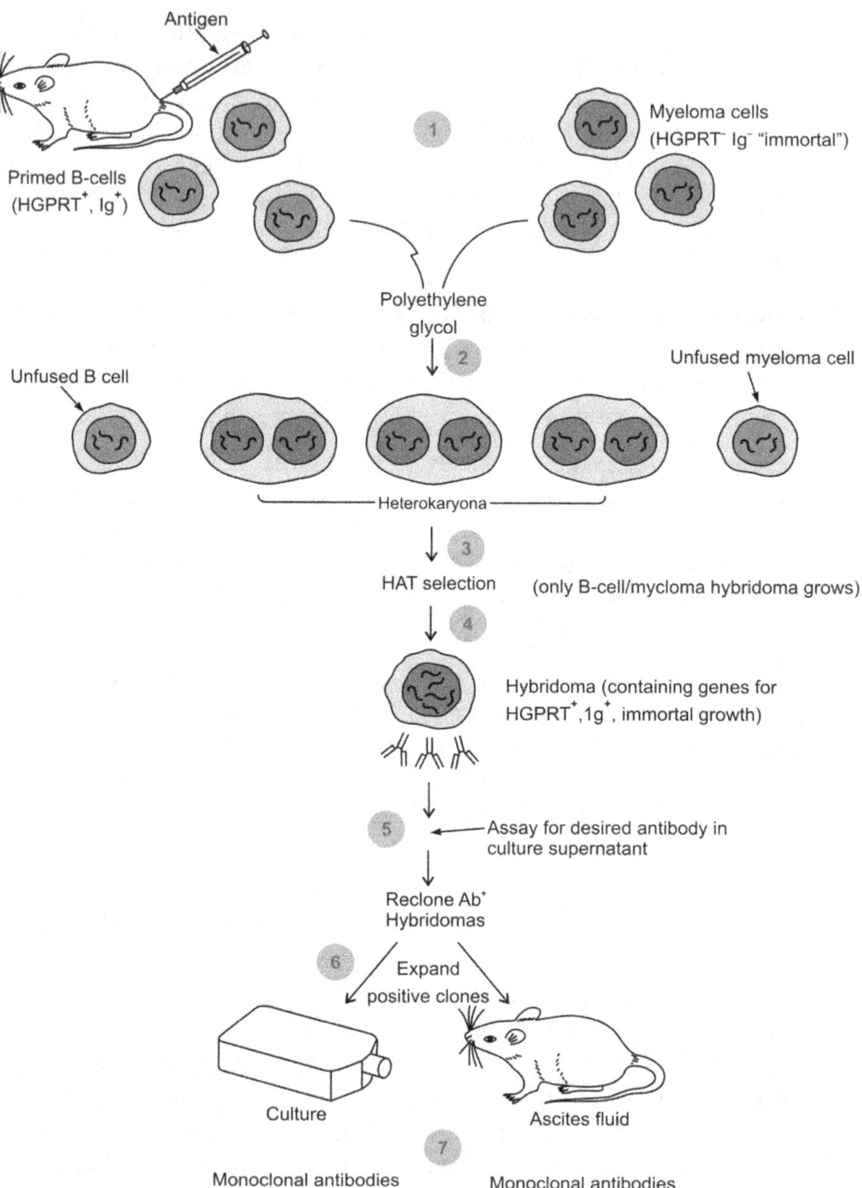

Fig. 3.17 Schematic representation of production of Monoclonal antibodies

3.13.3   Types of Monoclonal Antibodies

Following are the different types of monoclonal antibodies:

A. Immunotoxins

B. Chimeric Immunotoxins

C. Humanized antibodies

D. CDR grafted antibodies

E. Heterconjugate antibodies

A. **Immunotoxins:** It is a compound of antibodies and toxins such as ricin, diphtheria toxin, and others, which are poisons connected to immunoglobins at their Fc region. Tumours are the primary target of immunotoxins. When immunotoxins for a specific tumour cell were delivered, antibodies helped them reach the target cell. It is taken up by tumour cells via endocytosis after their adhesion to tumour cells. Toxins interfered with cellular metabolism, and cells died as a result. Toxins are targeted to specific tumour cells thanks to the use of monoclonal antibodies as shown in Fig 3.18

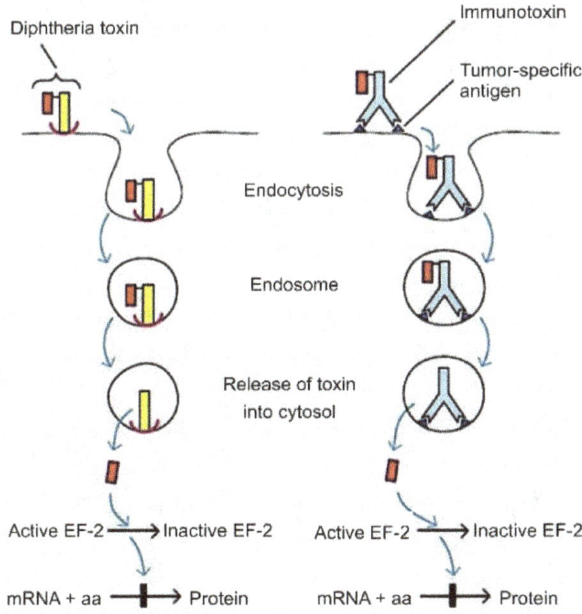

Fig. 3.18 Schematic representation of Immunotoxins

B. Chimeric Immunotoxins: Because, unlike Immunotoxins, toxin replaces one of the constant area domains of Ig, particularly the carboxy terminal domain of the H chain, the word chimaera is employed. Cancers can also be treated with it. It has a benefit over Immunotoxins in that it does not activate complements, resulting in an inflammatory response, after binding to antigens. Because chimeric Immunotoxins lack the Fc region, this is the case.

C. Humanized antibodies: Antibodies from mice can activate immunogenic reactions against tumours when injected as anti-tumour medicines in humans. Humanized antibodies can help to mitigate this to some extent. Humanized antibodies have a consistent L and H chain region derived from humans and variable L and H chain regions derived from mice. It gets its name from the fact that it contains human gene coding areas. It can also serve as a diagnostic tool as shown in Fig 3.19.

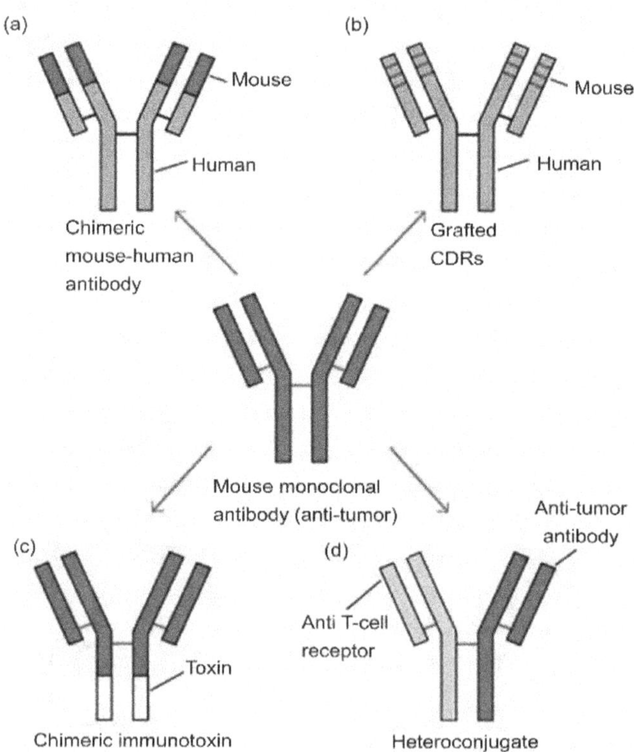

Fig. 3.19 Schematic representation of Humanized antibodies

D. CDR grafted Antibodies: It is a humanised antibody with a hypervariable area of both the light and heavy chains variable region gene that is exclusively derived from mice. The rest of the genes were derived from humans. It is used to treat cancer and acts as an immunosuppressant. Antibodies are usually directed against CD3 or CD4 components in such circumstances. Because the activation of cell-mediated immunity was harmed when these components were prevented.

E. Heterconjugate antibodies: Antibodies with different specificities, i.e., different paratopes with different specificities in a single antibody, are referred to as hetero. Antibodies of this sort are used to treat cancer. One antibody paratope is directed against tumour cells in this situation, while the other is directed against cytotoxic cells, mainly Tc cells. These antibodies bring effective cytotoxic cells close to tumour cells, allowing cytotoxic processes to easily lyse them.

3.13.4   Applications of Monoclonal Antibodies

In clinical medicine, monoclonal antibodies are proving to be very valuable as diagnostic, imaging, and therapeutic reagents. Monoclonal antibodies were originally developed as in vitro diagnostic tools. Products for detecting pregnancy, diagnosing a variety of harmful microbes, measuring medication levels in the blood, matching histocompatibility antigens, and detecting antigens secreted by certain cancers are among the many monoclonal antibody diagnostic assays presently available. In vivo, radiolabelled monoclonal antibodies can detect or locate tumour antigens, allowing enabling an earlier detection of some primary and metastatic malignancies in patients. Monoclonal antibodies against breast cancer cells, for example, are tagged with iodine-131 and injected into the bloodstream to detect tumour spread to regional lymph nodes. Other, less sensitive scanning techniques would miss breast cancer metastases shown by this monoclonal imaging technology.

Mainly monoclonal antibodies applied in two fields namely,

I.   Diagnostic Field

II.   Therapeutic Field

I. Diagnostic Field:

For the following purposes, monoclonal antibodies used:

a. Leucocyte Identification

b. Lymphocyte subset determination

c. HLA typing

d. Viral detection and sub typing

e. Parasitic determination

f. Polypeptide hormone detection

g. Detection of cancer with tumour marker determination

h. Detection of cardiac myosin in cardiac injury

i. Pregnancy detection

In the above-mentioned conditions, the basic principle is production of antibodies against antigen and identification or quantification of antigen and antibody complex.

I. *Therapeutic Field*: There are four different headings available in this field namely,

a. Anti-tumour therapy

b. Immunosuppression

c. Fertility control

d. Drug toxicity reversal

a. **Anti-tumour therapy:** Antibodies against tumour antigen are created in anti-tumour therapy and transformed into Immunotoxins, chimeric Immunotoxins, or Heterconjugate antibodies. When these antibodies are used, they harm tumour cells and slow tumour growth. Anti-tumour antibodies are sometimes referred to as "magic bullets."

b. **Immunosuppression:** Host vs graft rejections are controlled with monoclonal antibodies against TCR, BCR, Co-receptor complex, and cytokines, among other things, after transplantation between partially incompatible individuals. Hypersensitivity reactions are also treated with blocking monoclonal antibodies.

c. **Fertility control:** By producing antibodies against HCG or trophoblast, fertility controlled.

d. Drug toxicity reversal: Toxicity produced by drugs is treated using monoclonal antibodies against drugs, so that the functions of drugs are blocked and effect reversed.

3.13.5   Improvements in Hybridoma Technology

Efforts have been made to enhance the yield of monoclonal antibodies employing hybridoma technology over the last 10-15 years (1980s and 1990s). Among the things that were done as part of this initiative were the following: I As previously stated, polyethylene glycol was used to enhance cell fusions (PEG). (ii) As a fusion partner for the antibody-producing B cells, a continuous cell line (SP2/0) was employed. (iii) Feeder layers containing extra cells to feed newly formed hybridomas were used for optimal growth and hybridoma production; the most common feeder layers included I murine peritoncal cells, (ii) macrophages derived from mouse, rat, or guinea pigs, (iii) extra non-immunized spleen cells, (iv) human fibroblasts, human peripheral blood monocytes, or thymus Other sources of hybridoma growth factors (HGF), such as interleukin-6 (IL-6) generated from human cells, were employed because these feeder cells had some disadvantages, such as depletion of nutrients destined for hybridoma and contamination.

Blood is a constantly circulating fluid that provides nutrition, oxygen, and waste elimination to the body. Blood travels through blood vessels (arteries and veins). Blood products are described as blood components (red cells, platelets, fresh frozen plasma, and cryoprecipitate) created in a blood transfusion centre or plasma derivatives produced in plasma fractionation centres from pooled plasma donations (such as albumin, coagulation factors and immunoglobulins). Plasma derivatives are governed by the Medicines Act, and must be prescribed by a licenced practitioner, just like any other drug.

Transfusions of whole blood are currently uncommon. Because most patients require a single constituent of blood, such as red cells or platelets, blood component therapy makes clinical sense, and the dose may then be tailored. Each component is preserved under optimal conditions (red cells must be refrigerated, platelets do not), allowing for more efficient use of scarce blood donations.

3.14 Collection, Processing and Storage

Objectives

1. To maintain viability and function

2. To prevent physical changes.

3. To minimize bacterial contamination

The required volume of collected blood samples varies depending on a number of parameters, including the length of the study and the intended uses for the samples, but can range from 1 mL to 450 mL in repeated collections. If the goal is to harvest plasma and blood cells, samples must be treated with an anticoagulant to prevent clotting. Stabilizers can be incorporated in the collection device or added to the sample after it has been collected to prevent analytes from breaking down. Blood is generally obtained without anticoagulants when serum is sought.

A mixture of cellular components, colloids, and crystalloids make up whole blood. When centrifugal force is applied, distinct blood components with varied relative density, sediment rate, and size can be separated. Plasma, platelets, leucocytes (Buffy Coat [BC]), and packed red blood cells are the blood components with the highest specific gravity (PRBCs). Each component's functional efficiency is determined by how it is processed and stored. Component therapy must be generally tailored in order to use one blood unit effectively and sensibly.

3.15 Blood Components Concept

Blood is usually transfused to keep tissues oxygenated or to treat bleeding and coagulation problems.

When blood is transfused, what role does each component play?

1. When a patient's red cells are lost due to haemorrhage or anaemia, red cells (erythrocytes) maintain oxygen flow to the tissues.

2. Platelets (thrombocytes) treat thrombocytopenia-related bleeding problems.

3. After a haemorrhage caused by trauma or surgery, plasma is occasionally administered to maintain blood volume.

4. Fresh plasma can be utilised to replace clotting factors and help with abnormal bleeding correction.

5. Plasma can be separated to make derivatives to treat clotting factor abnormalities, immunoglobulins to give short-term immunity, and albumin to cure burns.

6. White blood cells (leucocytes, including granulocytes) are not transfused on a regular basis. They may contain TTIs such as CMV and, on the other hand, cause immunological modulation, both of which are harmful to the patient. Although granulocyte transfusions may have some indications, component therapy tries to limit the number of white cells transfused in general.

The following are some of the benefits of separating whole blood into its constituents:

Blood serves a variety of purposes, as is obvious. There are evident benefits for both the patient and the blood transfusion service when a whole blood unit is processed into particular red cell, plasma, and platelet components:

- A single blood donation can help a number of different patients. This is how you make the best use of a limited resource.

- Patients only get the component(s) required to treat their ailment; components not required by the patient are not transfused (such as white cells or plasma proteins when the patient requires only red cells). Transfusion responses are less likely as a result of this.

- The storage conditions of the items can be optimised by selecting the right additive, temperature, bag type, and other factors to guarantee that each component remains functional for as long as feasible.

3.15.1 Processing Whole Blood into Components

To process whole blood into components a basic understanding of the following is required:

1. Selection of blood donors
2. Sterile systems
3. Blood bag systems
4. Principles of centrifugation
5. Preparation of specific blood components

1. **Selection of blood donors:** A suitable volunteer for whole blood or apheresis collection is chosen based on criteria established by drug control authorities and the National AIDS Control Organization.

2. **Sterile systems:** All blood bags, anticoagulants, and additive solutions must be sterile (free of bacteria or viruses) and pyrogen-free, according to blood bag manufacturers (do not contain endotoxins or micro-organism debris).

The venepuncture site on the donor's arm is properly cleaned before the sterile needle on the end of the blood bag tubing is put into the vein for blood donation. This creates a direct connection between the donor's bloodstream and the sterile blood bag. The tube is shut at the end of the donation, and the contents of the blood bag should be clear of bacterial contamination. When the blood bag is sealed, it is considered a 'closed system,' which is ideal because the product's integrity is preserved.

It is called an 'open system' if the bag is opened at any point after it has been sealed, whether intentionally or accidently (i.e. environmental air, which contains microbial aerosols, could have entered the bag). If a blood bag is accidentally opened, it must be thrown because sterility can no longer be ensured. This is due to the fact that microorganisms can get into any product that has been exposed to the environment. To make a specific blood product, a blood bag is sometimes purposely opened under controlled conditions (e.g., in a laminar flow cabinet). In some situations, the product is given a shorter expiry term, usually up to 24 hours from the time of opening.

Closed blood bag systems are required for the normal processing of blood into components. Individual bags in multiple bag systems are connected by tubing to form a closed system. Because the primary bag is never opened and the entire process occurs in a closed system, the components can be pushed into the associated bags (after centrifugation) without impacting sterility.

3. **Bag systems for blood collection:** Many suppliers offer a wide range of polyvinyl chloride (PVC) plastic blood bag systems. The type of bag to use is determined by the needs of the specific blood service:

- Cost-effectiveness

- Whether units will be handled manually or mechanically

- The level of product storage that will be reached (additive solutions, special plastic bags for platelets)

- Whether filtration (leucodepletion) is necessary

a) **Systems with a single bag:** This is the most basic of the bags. The donation is placed in the bag, which is then sealed with the pilot tubing. The unit is not further processed into components and is transfused as whole blood. An anticoagulant solution is contained in the bag (CPDA). Sodium citrate prevents clotting, whereas citric acid (C), monobasic sodium phosphate (P), dextrose (D), and adenine (A) offer buffers and nutrition for improved red cell survival.

b) **Double bag (two bag system):** The primary bag in a multiple bag system is the bag with anticoagulant into which the donation is taken. This is the same sort of primary bag as the single unit, but a second empty bag is attached in the double bag system (called a transfer or satellite bag). After centrifuging the whole blood, the plasma can be transferred to the associated transfer bag through tubing, resulting in two components: a red cell concentrate suspended in plasma (in the primary bag) and plasma (in the transfer bag).

c) **Triple bag (three bag system):** Only the addition of a transfer bag distinguishes a triple bag from a double bag. There is still another empty transfer bag attached to the first transfer bag once plasma has been divided into it. This arrangement is used to extract Cryoprecipitate from fresh frozen plasma or to make platelet concentrates from platelet rich plasma.

d) **Quadruple (quad) bag (four bag system):** A quad bag system is similar to a triple bag system, but it includes an additional bag carrying red cell additive solution. It's commonly used in automated systems to make: • Red cell concentrates (RCC), which have had the white cells removed and to which additive solution has been added.

e) **Top and bottom bag:** This is a three-bag system built specifically for automated systems. An empty transfer bag is connected to the top of the primary collection bag, and another transfer bag holding additive solution is connected to the bottom. Following centrifugation, the bag is placed in a blood processing machine, which separates the plasma from the top and the red cells from the bottom, leaving the BC in the primary collection bag. The same three products are made as in the quad bag system:

- ABC layer of white cells and platelets that stays in the primary bag.

- Red cell concentrates (with buffy coat removed and suspended in additive solution) in the bottom transfer bag. This BC can either be discarded or used to make platelet concentrate.

- The transfusion service's management team should decide whether or not to remove BCs from RCCs.

There are certain benefits to removing the BC:

- All of the plasma is removed and stored as fresh frozen plasma, which can be used as is or as a starting material for fractionated products.

- The red cells can be resuspended in a solution designed to provide optimal conditions for red cell storage, such as saline adenine-glucose-mannitol (SAGM).

- The BCs can be utilised to create platelet concentrates.

A quad or top and bottom blood bag system, as well as automated processing equipment, are frequently required to create these advanced products. Where collection and demand are not high enough to justify the system, the cost of bags and machinery may make it unfeasible to execute these operations. In these cases, simpler double or triple bag systems may be more viable as shown in Fig 3.20.

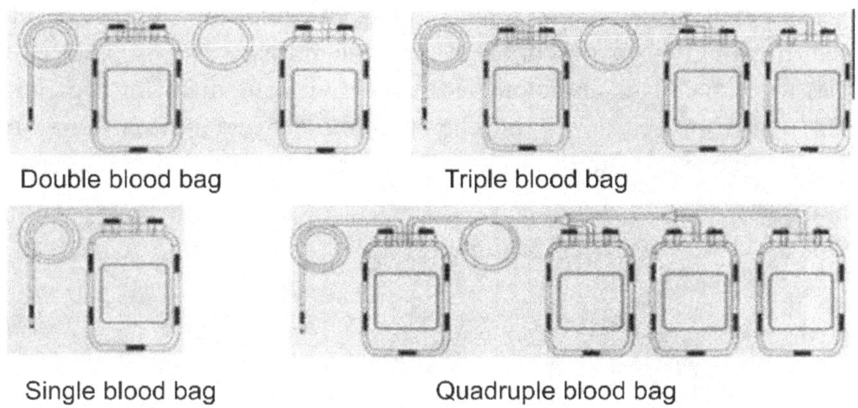

Fig. 3.20 Types of Bag systems for blood collection

4. **Principles of centrifugation:** Blood constituents can be separated because their sizes and densities differ, and when centrifugal force is applied, they sediment at different rates.

The red cells settle at the bottom of the blood bag when whole blood, which is a mixture of cellular components suspended in plasma and anticoagulant, is centrifuged, since they have the highest density (have a bigger mass/weigh more than the other components).

Because white cells and platelets are less thick, they do not settle as quickly and stay in suspension longer. The white cells settle above the red cells as centrifugation continues, and the platelets form a layer above the white cells, leaving the initial suspending fluid (now clear plasma plus anticoagulant) at the top. The separation of components as a result of moderate or hard centrifugation of a unit of whole blood. The speed and duration of centrifugation to be utilised to separate the required component must be chosen. Centrifugation should be halted before platelet sedimentation begins, for example, if platelet rich plasma is required. It would be easier to choose the time to quit if the centrifugation speed was lower for a longer length of time. If cell-free plasma is required, a faster centrifuge speed for an extended period of time will result in clear plasma and densely packed red cells. To acquire the desired components, it is critical to thoroughly assess the best parameters for a good separation for each centrifuge.

The bag system is carefully removed from the centrifuge after centrifugation (to avoid mixing), and the primary bag is placed in a plasma extractor or an automated processing equipment for separation. The bag is pressed down, and the component layers are transferred one by one into one of the transfer bags in the closed system as shown in Fig. 3.21.

Whole blood Unit

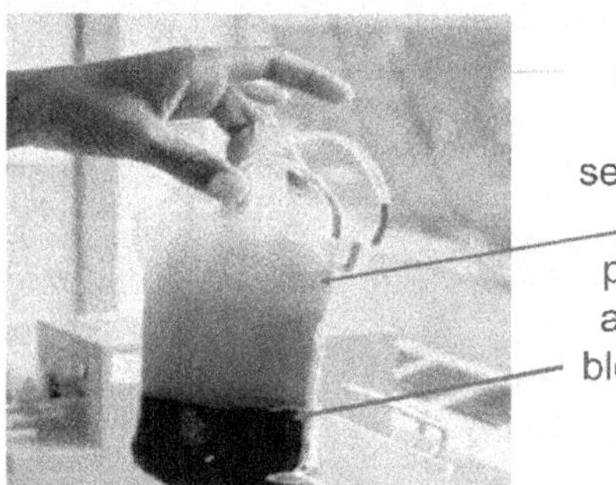

Fig. 3.21 Whole blood Unit

5. **Preparation of specific blood components:** Blood components can be manufactured in a variety of methods, depending on the needs of the transfusion service and the resources available (donors, personnel, disposables, funding and space).

3.15.2 Substitutes for Plasma

Any liquid that is used to replace blood plasma, usually a saline solution with serum albumins; plasma substitutes are dextran's or other preparations. These compounds do not increase the capacity of blood to carry oxygen; rather, they simply replace the volume. Dehydration is also treated using them.

Due to limited sources of plasma, the high expense of creating the dried form, and the risk of transmitting serum hepatitis, researchers looked for nonhuman origin alternatives that may temporarily restore blood volume while the receiver restored the lost protein. (Refer Chapter 5)

Characteristics of a Perfect Plasma Substitute

- A viscosity similar to plasma, with the same colloidal osmotic pressure as whole blood.

- A molecular weight that prevents molecules from diffusing freely through capillary walls.

- Complete and final elimination from the body.

- Toxicity-free, e.g., no impairment of renal function.

- Antigenicity, pyrogenicity, and perplexing effects on essential assays like blood grouping and erythrocyte morphology are all eliminated. Rate of sedimentation

- In solution, isotonicity equivalent to that of blood plasma.

- Ease of preparation, immediate availability, and low cost in liquid form at normal and sterilising temperatures, as well as during shipping and storage.

Questions

1. Discuss about the structure of immunoglobulins in detail.
2. Describe the Major Histocompatibilty Complex's structure and function.
3. Compile a list of hypersensitivity reactions.
4. Describe immunological stimulations and immune suppressions in detail.
5. Describe the general procedure for making bacterial vaccines.
6. Describe the general procedure for making viral vaccines.
7. Describe the general procedure for preparing taxoids.
8. Describe the general procedure for making antitoxins.
9. Describe the general procedure for making serum immune blood derivatives.

10. Summarize the storage conditions for official vaccines and their stability.

11. Describe Hybridoma technology, production, purification, and uses in detail.

4.1   Blotting Techniques

Blotting is the process of immobilizing nucleic acids or proteins on a solid support, such as nylon or nitrocellulose membranes. The central technique for hybridization research is nucleic acid blotting. Nucleic acid labeling and hybridization on membranes have been used to develop a variety of experimental approaches for studying gene expression, organization, and other topics. Identifying and detecting individual proteins in complicated biological mixes like blood has long been a priority in scientific and medical practice. Identification of defective genes in genomic DNA has become more relevant in clinical research and genetic counseling in recent years.

Unique proteins and nucleic acid sequences are identified using blotting techniques. They've been fine-tuned to be exceedingly specific and sensitive, and they've become valuable instruments in molecular biology and clinical research.

The following are the major steps in blotting:

1. Gel electrophoresis for sample separation

2. Immobilization on a firm surface

3. The probe's attachment to the target

4. Visualization of the target and detection of the target

Southern, northern, and western blotting are the three main blotting techniques that have been developed.

Southern blotting (a technique for detecting DNA) entails immobilizing DNA on a solid substrate and identifying target DNA with a probe DNA.

Northern blotting (for detecting RNA) entails immobilizing mRNA on a solid substrate and identifying the target with DNA probes.

Immobilization of proteins on a solid support is followed by target identification using specific antibodies as probes in Western blotting (which is used to detect proteins).

4.1.1 Southern Blotting

Principle: E.M. Southern invented the approach in 1975. It is used to determine the existence of a specific DNA fragment in a sample. A single gene or a portion of a bigger chunk of DNA, such as a viral genome, can be detected. Hybridization is the key to this strategy.

Hybridization: Creating a double-stranded DNA molecule from a single-stranded DNA probe and single-stranded target patient DNA.

Hybridization has two key characteristics

❖ The reactions are particular; probes will only bind to targets that have the same sequence as them. In a combination of millions of related but non-complementary molecules, the probe can discover one target molecule.

❖ The DNA that will be studied, such as an organism's entire DNA, is extracted.

❖ High-molecular-weight DNA strands are cut into smaller fragments by restriction endonucleases, which are then electrophoresed on an agarose gel to sort them by size. If the DNA fragments are greater than 15 kb, the gel should be depurinated with an acid, such as weak HCl, before blotting. This breaks the DNA into smaller pieces, allowing for more efficient transfer from the gel to the membrane. The DNA gel is placed in an alkaline solution (including NaOH) to denature the double-stranded DNA if alkaline transfer methods are utilized. Denaturation in an alkaline environment may increase the negatively charged DNA's adherence to a positively charged membrane, splitting it into single DNA strands for later hybridization to the probe, and destroying any leftover RNA in the DNA.

❖ A nitrocellulose (or nylon) membrane is placed on top of (or below) the gel, depending on the transfer direction. The gel is given an even amount of pressure (either using suction, or by placing a stack of paper towels and a weight on top of the membrane and gel),

❖ To ensure that the gel and membrane make good and even contact. The DNA is moved from the gel to the membrane via buffer transfer by capillary action from a region of high-water potential to a region of low water potential (usually filter paper and paper tissues); ion exchange interactions bind the DNA to the membrane due to the negative charge of the DNA and the positive charge of the membrane.

❖ To permanently attach the transferred DNA to the membrane, the membrane is baked in a vacuum or conventional oven at 80 °C for 2 hours, or subjected to ultraviolet radiation (nylon membrane).

The membrane is then subjected to a hybridization probe, which is a single DNA fragment with a specified sequence that is used to determine the presence of the target DNA. The probe DNA is labeled to make it detectable, which is commonly done by adding radioactivity or tagging it with a fluorescent or chromogenic dye. Excess probe is rinsed from the membrane after hybridization, and the pattern of hybridization is observed on X-ray film by autoradiography in the case of a radioactive or fluorescent probe, or by developing color on the membrane in the case of a chromogenic detection method.

Note that the probe's hybridization to a specific DNA fragment on the filter membrane indicates that this fragment contains complementary DNA sequence to the probe. By transferring DNA from an electrophoresis gel to a membrane, the labelled hybridization probe can easily bind to the size-fractionated DNA. The number of sequences (e.g., gene copies) in a genome can be determined using Southern blots using restriction enzyme-digested genomic DNA. On a Southern blot, a probe that hybridizes only to a single DNA segment that hasn't been cut by the restriction enzyme will yield a single band, however when the probe hybridizes to several highly similar sequences, multiple bands are likely to appear (e.g., those that may be the result of sequence duplication Increased specificity and decreased hybridization of the probe to sequences that are less than 100 percent identical can be achieved by changing the hybridization conditions (e.g., raising the hybridization temperature or decreasing the salt concentration).

Southern Blotting Applications

❖ Southern blots are utilized in a variety of applications, such as gene discovery and mapping, evolution and development studies, diagnostics, and forensics.

❖ Southern blots allow researchers to identify a restriction fragment's molecular weight and compare relative quantities in different samples.

❖ Southern blots are used in DNA fingerprinting, genetic engineering, and forensic science to detect the presence of a specific bit of DNA in a sample and to analyze the genetic patterns that emerge in a person's DNA for tests such as: –Paternity testing –Personal identity

❖ Determination of sex Southern blotting is a definitive test for genetically modified organisms to guarantee that a specific piece of DNA with a known genetic sequence has been successfully incorporated into the host organism's genome.

❖ Congenital hereditary illnesses, such as congenital adrenal hyperplasia, are diagnosed (CAH).

Determine whether there are any mutations, deletions, or gene rearrangements.

- Leukemias

- HIV-1 and infectious illness diagnostics

- Used in the prognosis of cancer and the prenatal detection of hereditary problems

4.1.2   Blotting in the Western Hemisphere

Western blotting is a common method for detecting and analyzing proteins based on their propensity to bind to certain antibodies. Towbin, et al. created this technique in 1979, and it has since become one of the most widely employed in life science research.

Principle: A protein sample is electrophoresed on an SDS-PAGE and electro transferred to a PVDF or nitrocellulose membrane in this analytical procedure. Specific primary and secondary enzyme labelled antibodies are used to detect the transferred protein. Antibodies bind to epitopes, which are specific amino acid sequences Antibodies can detect specific proteins among a group of many because amino acid sequences differ from one protein to the next. As a result, in a cell lysate containing thousands of distinct proteins, a single protein can be identified and its abundance evaluated using western blot analysis. Proteins are first differentiated from one another by their size. Antibodies are employed to detect the protein of interest in the second step. Finally, the antibody/protein combination is seen using a substrate that reacts with an enzyme as shown in Fig 4.1.

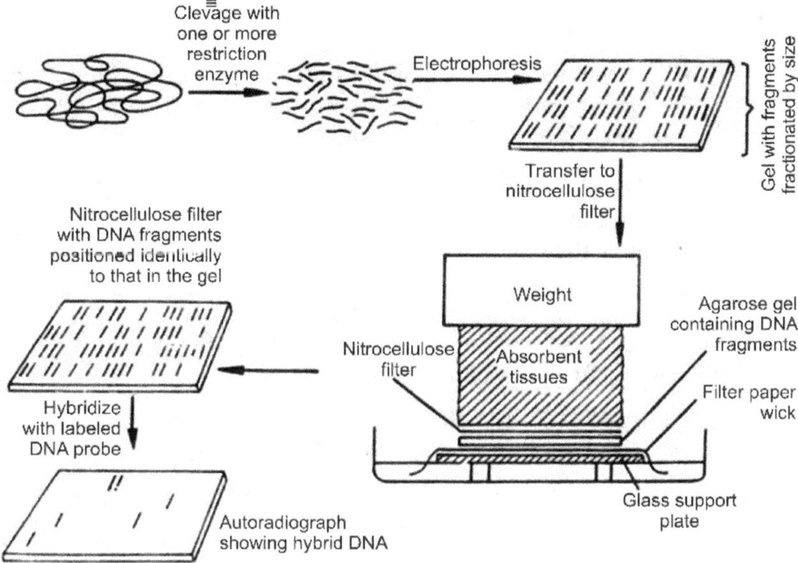

Fig. 4.1 Schematic representation of western blot analysis

Procedure

o   Samples can be collected from entire tissue or from cell culture. Solid tissues are often mechanically broken down using a blender (for larger sample volumes), homogenizer (for lower amounts), or sonication.

o   To stimulate cell lysis and solubilize proteins, a variety of detergents, salts, and buffers can be used. Protease and phosphatase inhibitors are frequently used to keep the sample from being digested by its own enzymes.

o   To minimize protein denaturation, tissue preparation is frequently done at low temperatures. To separate different cell compartments and organelles, a mix of biochemical and mechanical procedures, such as various forms of filtration and centrifugation, can be used.

1. **Gel electrophoresis:** Gel electrophoresis is used to separate the proteins in a sample. Isoelectric point (pI), molecular weight, electric charge, or a combination of these parameters can be used to separate proteins.

- The proteins may then be separated electrophoretically on a polyacrylamide gel.

- Typically utilizing the SDS-page approach, which entails lowering proteins first to eliminate disulphide interactions (i.e., converting S-S bridges to -SH SH- sulphydryl groups).

- Proteins migrate to the positively charged end of the gel in different ways depending on their molecular weight (KDa). Smaller proteins travel quicker through this mesh, separating the proteins according to their size.

- Increasing the concentration of acrylamide in the gel improves the resolution of lower molecular weight proteins.

- Samples are loaded into the gel's wells. A marker or ladder, which is a commercially available combination of proteins with predetermined molecular weights dyed to generate visible, colored bands, is normally designated for one lane.

- Proteins migrate into the gel at varying speeds when voltage is supplied throughout the length of it.

- Within each lane, these varied rates of progress (different electrophoretic mobilities) split into bands.

Apply a nylon membrane to a polyacrylamide gel:

- To make the proteins accessible to antibody detection, they are transferred from the gel to a nitrocellulose or polyvinylidene difluoride membrane (PVDF).

- The membrane is placed on top of the gel, followed by a stack of filter papers. The entire stack is submerged in a buffer solution that, through capillary action, travels up the paper, carrying the proteins with it.

- Electro blotting is a method of transferring proteins that uses an electric current to draw proteins from a gel into a PVDF or nitrocellulose membrane.

- The proteins travel from the gel to the membrane while retaining their structure. The proteins are exposed on a thin surface layer for detection as a result of this "blotting" process.

- Both membrane types were chosen for their ability to bind non-specific proteins (i.e. binds all proteins equally well). Protein binding relies on both hydrophobic and charged interactions between the membrane and the protein.

- Nitrocellulose membranes are less expensive than PVDF membranes, however they are significantly more fragile and do not withstand repeated probing.

Antibodies that attach to the membrane are blocked:

- Because the membrane was chosen for its propensity to bind protein, and because both antibodies and the target are proteins, precautions must be made to avoid membrane interactions with the antibody employed to detect the target protein.

- Non-specific binding is blocked by immersing the membrane in a dilute solution of protein - commonly Bovine serum albumin (BSA) or non-fat dry milk (both of which are affordable) - with a small amount of detergent such as Tween 20.

- The protein in the dilute solution binds to the membrane in all of the areas where the target proteins haven't. As a result, when the antibody is introduced, there is no place on the membrane for it to adhere to anything other than the precise target protein's binding sites. This decreases "noise" in the Western blot's final product, resulting in clearer results and fewer false positives.

- Complementary antibody binding (and reporter enzyme binding) to validate the presence of a certain protein:

- Antibodies specific to proteins adhering to the membrane are retrieved and used to bind to them.

- These are 'primary antibodies,' which are adhered to the membrane for a few hours before being rinsed away. Secondary antibodies,' which have reporter enzymes attached, can bind to species-specific locations on primary antibodies (i.e. detection is a two-step process).

- The reporter enzyme confirms antibody-protein binding by driving a colorimetric reaction and producing a colour when exposed to an appropriate substrate as shown in Fig 4.2

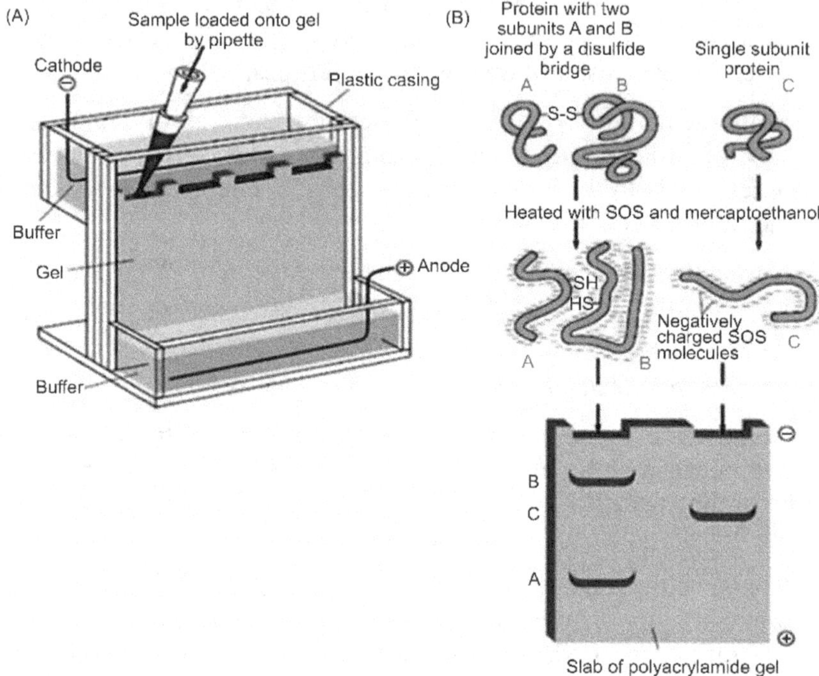

Fig. 4.2 Antibodies that attach to the membrane are blocked

4.1.3   Western Blotting Applications

➢ A Western blot is used in the confirmatory HIV test to detect anti-HIV antibodies in a human serum sample. Proteins from known HIV-infected cells are isolated and blotted on a membrane, after which the serum to be tested is incubated with the primary antibody; free antibody is washed away, and a secondary anti-human antibody linked to an enzyme signal is added. The proteins to which the patient's serum carries antibody are subsequently indicated by the stained bands.

➢ A Western blot can also be used to diagnose Bovine spongiform encephalopathy (BSE, popularly known as "mad cow disease").

Western blotting is used in several Lyme disease tests

Table 4.1 Comparison of blotting techniques

	Southern blotting	**Northern blotting**	**Western blotting**
Molecule detected	DNA (ds)	mRNA (ss)	Protein
Gel electropho resis	Agarose gel	Formaldehyde agarose gel	Polyacrylamide gel
Blotting method	Capillary transfer	Capillary transfer	Electric transfer
Probes	DNA Radioactive or nonradioactive	cDNA, cRNA Radioactive or nonradioactive	primary antibody
Detection system	Autoradiography Chemiluminescent Colorimetric	Autoradiography Chemiluminescent Colorimetric	Chem iluminescent Colorimetric

4.2   Eukaryote Genetic Organization

The genome contains all of an organism's genetic information. It is either encoded in DNA or, in the case of many viruses, in RNA. The genome is made up of both genes and non-coding DNA sequences. The total collection of genes, as well as all other functional and nonfunctional DNA sequences in an organism with a haploid set of chromosomes, is referred to as the genome. Structural genes, regulatory genes, and non-functional nucleotide sequences are all included. All living creatures' genomes are made up of DNA and represent their hereditary material.

Prokaryotic cells are prokaryotic cells. In the nucleoid area of the cell cytoplasm, genomic DNA forms a single circular chromosome devoid of basic proteins. DNA is connected with basic proteins (histones) in Eukaryotic cells, forming lengthy chromatin fibers. During cell division, chromatin fibers form a network that is encased in a double-layered nuclear envelop and condenses into chromosomes.

The size of a genome

Despite the fact that the basic physical architecture of all eukaryotic nuclear genomes are similar, one key trait differs significantly between organisms. The smallest eukaryotic genomes are less than 10 megabytes in length, while the largest are over 100,000 megabytes. The entire amount of DNA contained within one copy of a genome is referred to as genome size. The formula 1 pg. = 978 Mb = 978000000 can be used to relate genome size to molecular mass.

The C-value conundrum

The smallest eukaryotes, like fungi, have the smallest genomes, while larger eukaryotes, like vertebrates and flowering plants, have the biggest. This may appear to make sense because one would anticipate an organism's complexity to be proportional to the number of genes in its genome - higher eukaryotes require larger genomes to accommodate the additional genesis

Table 4.2 Comparative genome sizes of organisms

Organism	Size (bp)	Gene number	Average gene density	Chromosome number
Homo sapiens (human)	3.2 billion	−25.000	1 gene /100.000 bases	46
Mus musculure (mouse)	2.6 billion	−25,000	1 gene /100.000 bases	40
Drosophia malanogaster (fruit fly)	1.37 million	13.000	1 gene / 9,000 bases	8
Arabidopsis thaliana (Plane)	100 million	25.000	1 gene / 4000 bases	10
Caenorhabditis elegance (roundworm)	97 million	19.000	1 gene / 5000 bases	12
Saccharomyces cerevisiae (yeast)	12.1 million	9000	1 gene / 2000 bases	32
Escherichia coli (bacteria)	4.6 million	3200	1 gene / 1400 bases	1
H. influenza (bacteria)	1.8 million	1700	1 gene / 1000 bases	1

However, the correlation is far from exact: if it were, the yeast S. cerevisiae's nuclear genome, which is 0.004 times the size of the human nuclear genome at 12 Mb, would be anticipated to contain just 0.004 35 000 genes, or just 140. The total number of DNA bases in the genome is the C-value (per haploid set of chromosomes). The amount of DNA necessary to generate all of the proteins produced by the organism, or their position in the food chain, is not proportionate.

The nuclear genome is divided into chromosomes, each of which contains a set of linear DNA molecules. There are at least two chromosomes in every eukaryote investigated, and the DNA molecules are always linear. At this level of eukaryotic genome organization, the only variable is chromosome number, which appears to be unrelated to the organism's basic characteristics as shown in Fig 4.3.

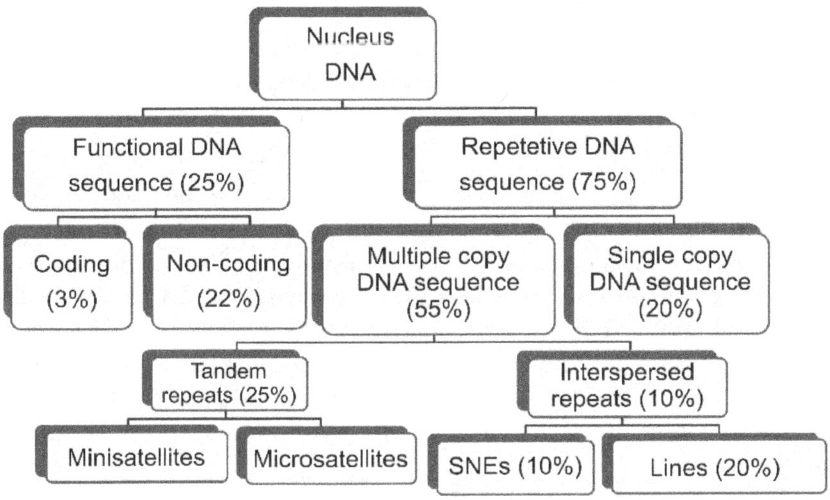

Fig. 4.3 Classification of nuclear genome into various categories

DNA chromosomal packaging: Chromosomes are substantially shorter than the DNA molecules they contain. To fit a DNA molecule into its chromosome, a highly ordered packaging machinery is required. Several groups tested nuclease protection on chromatin (DNA-histone complexes) that had been carefully removed from nuclei using procedures that preserved as much of the chromatin structure as feasible in 1973-74.

In a nuclease protection experiment, the complex is exposed to an enzyme that breaks the DNA at locations where it is not 'protected' by protein attachment. The positions of the protein complexes on the original DNA molecule are indicated by the sizes of the resultant DNA pieces. Purified chromatin was subjected to a restricted nuclease treatment. In the nucleus, DNA is generally found in conjunction with histone proteins; the DNA–histone complex is referred to as "chromatin." Chromatin's structure can vary in response to diverse cellular metabolic needs. Chromatin can be thought of as a series of structural components known as "nucleosomes." The nucleosome core particle is made up of an octamer of histones and the DNA that surrounds it. Each of the histones H2A, H2B, H3, and H4 has two molecules in the histone octamer. In around 1.75 turns, DNA wraps around the octamer in a left-handed supercoil, enclosing about 150 bp.

Histone H1 is a linker histone that physically binds adjacent nucleosome core particles with linker DNA (the DNA between two nucleosome core particles).

The length of linker DNA differs depending on the species and cell type. The nucleosome core particle and linker DNA on both sides of the core usually contain between 180 and 200 base pairs of DNA.

There are numerous layers of organization and compaction of chromatin between the nucleosome unit structure and the metaphase chromosomal structure with two chromatids. The nucleosomes are compacted into a 30 nm solenoid fibre structure called a 30 nm fibre; the 30-nm solenoid fibres are compacted into a 300-nm filament; and ultimately, the 300-nm filaments are compacted into a 700-nm chromosome. When the chromosomes duplicate during cell division, a 1,400-nm metaphase chromosome with two chromatids of 700 nm each is formed.

During interphase, the time between nuclear divisions, the 30 nm fibre is most likely the most common kind of chromatin in the nucleus. When the nucleus divides, the DNA takes on a more compact form of packaging, resulting in the highly condensed metaphase chromosomes that can be seen under a light microscope and have the look of a chromosome. Metaphase chromosomes are formed after DNA replication has occurred in the cell cycle, and each one includes two copies of its chromosomal DNA molecule. The centromere, which is located in a precise location on each chromosome, holds the two copies together. Individual chromosomes can thus be distinguished by their size and the position of the centromere in relation to the telomere

- When chromosomes are dyed, they reveal even more distinct characteristics. There are a variety of staining procedures available, each of which produces a unique banding pattern for each chromosome. This means that an organism's chromosomes can be represented as a karyogram, with each one portrayed as a banded appearance. The terminal region, often known as the telomere, is an important portion of the chromosome. Telomeres are crucial because they mark the ends of chromosomes, allowing the cell to distinguish between a natural end and an artificial end caused by chromosome breakage - a vital necessity because the latter must be repaired while the former cannot. Hundreds of copies of a repeating motif make up telomeric DNA., 5 -TTAGGG-3 in humans, with a small expansion of the double-stranded DNA molecule's 3 terminus as shown in Fig 4.4.

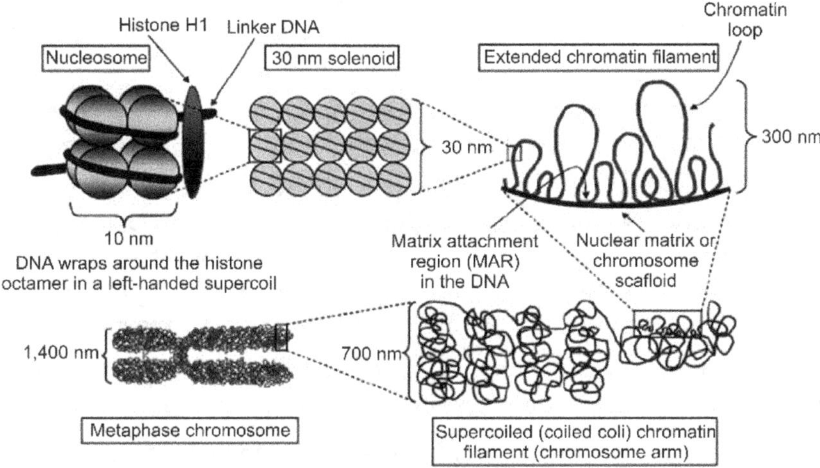

Fig. 4.4 Nucleosome to Chromosome

4.2.1   Analysis of Chromatin from Human Nuclei for Nuclease Protection

A nuclease enzyme is used to delicately purify chromatin from nuclei. The nuclease treatment is done under restrictive circumstances, so the DNA is only cut once in each of the linker sections between the bound proteins on average. The DNA fragments are tested by agarose gel electrophoresis after the protein has been removed, and they are found to be 200 bp in length, or multiples thereof. The nuclease treatment is then completed, digesting all of the DNA in the linker regions. All of the remaining DNA pieces are 146 bp long.

Functional DNA content of the genome accounts for 25% of the nuclear genome and contains both coding and non-coding genes. When chromosomes are dyed, the banding patterns that result determine their uneven distribution. The dyes utilized in these processes bind to DNA molecules, but with a preference for specific base pairs in most cases. Giemsa, for example, prefers DNA sections with a high concentration of A and T nucleotides. The AT-rich sections of the genome are assumed to be the dark G-bands in the human karyogram. Because the genome's base composition is 59.7% A + T, the dark G-bands must have AT concentrations that are significantly higher than 60%. Because genes usually have an AT content of 45-50 percent, cytogeneticists hypothesized that there would be fewer genes in dark G-bands. When the draught genome sequence and the human karyogram were compared, this prediction was validated.

The isochore model of genome structure provides the second line of evidence pointing to unequal gene distribution.

According to this hypothesis, vertebrates and plants (and probably other eukaryotes) have genomes that are mosaics of DNA segments, each of which is at least 300kb long and has a uniform base composition that differs from the surrounding segments. Experiments using genomic DNA segments of about 100 kb support the isochore concept.

dyes that bind selectively to AT- or GC-rich areas, and density gradient centrifugation to separate the pieces

When this experiment is performed on human DNA, five fractions are seen, each indicating a separate isochore type with a distinct base composition: two AT-rich isochores, designated L1 and L2, and three GC-rich classes, designated H1, H2, and H3. H3, the last of them, is the least common in the human genome, accounting for about 3% of the total while containing almost 25% of the genes. This shows that genes are not uniformly distributed throughout the human genome. The genes in an organism can be categorized in two ways: one based on their function, and the other based on the specific domain of the protein for which the gene codes. The second technique is more instructive and superior since it demonstrates that a specific genome specifies a number of protein domains that are not found in other animals' genomes, including numerous domains involved in cell adhesion, electric couplings, and nerve cell proliferation.

Multigene families - clusters of genes with the same or similar sequence - have been recognized as frequent aspects of many genomes since the beginning of DNA sequencing.

The rRNA genes are instances of 'simple' or 'classical' multigene families, which have identical or almost identical sequences in all members. These families are thought to have formed as a result of gene duplication, with the individual members' sequences being kept similar through an evolutionary process. Other multigene families, which are more common in higher eukaryotes than lower eukaryotes, are referred to as 'complex' because the individual members, while similar in sequence, differ enough for the gene products to have diverse features.

4.2.2   The DNA Content of Genomes with Repetitive Sequences

Repetitive DNA is found in all organisms and makes up a significant portion of the genome in some, including humans. There are many different forms of repetitive DNA, and multiple categorization schemes have been developed to classify them. They are as follows:

Tandemly repeated DNA is a typical component of eukaryotic genomes, although it is found far less commonly in prokaryotic genomes. Because DNA fragments containing tandemly repeated sequences form 'satellite' bands when genomic DNA is fractionated by density gradient centrifugation, this type of repetition is also known as satellite DNA. Because the satellite bands contain repeating DNA segments, they have GC contents and buoyant densities that differ from the genome as a whole. Satellite bands in eukaryotic DNA density gradients are segments made up of extended series of tandem repeats, perhaps hundreds of kb in length.

A single genome can have numerous different forms of satellite DNA, each with its own repeat unit, which can range from 5 to 200 bp. In human DNA, there are at least four distinct repeat types in the three satellite bands. The alphoid DNA repeats found in the centromere regions of chromosomes are one kind of human satellite DNA. Although satellite DNA is found throughout the genome, the majority of it is found at centromeres, where it may perform a structural purpose, such as serving as binding sites for one or more of the particular centromeric proteins. Alternatively, the centromere's repetitive DNA content could reflect the fact that it is the final section of the chromosome to be replicated.

4.2.3   DNA from Satellites

Two more forms of tandemly repeated DNA are classified as 'satellite' DNA, although not appearing in satellite bands on density gradients. Minisatellites and microsatellites are the two types of satellites.

Microsatellites form clusters of up to 150 bp in length, with repeat units of up to 25 bp; minisatellites form clusters of up to 20 kb in length, with repeat units of up to 25 bp; and minisatellites form clusters of up to 20 kb in length, with repeat units of up to 25 bp. Telomeric DNA is one form of minisatellite DNA. In addition to telomeric minisatellites, several eukaryotic genomes contain a variety of additional minisatellite DNA clusters, many of which are towards the ends of chromosomes, but not all of which are. The roles of the remaining minisatellite sequences are unknown. Microsatellites have an equally enigmatic function. Many microsatellites are variable, which means that the amount of repeat units in the array varies between species members. This is because when a microsatellite is duplicated during DNA replication, 'slippage' can occur, resulting in the insertion or, less frequently, deletion of one or more of the repeat units. No two people have the exact same combination of microsatellite length variants; if enough microsatellites are studied, each person's genetic profile can be determined. Genetically identical twins are the lone exception. Although genetic profiling is well-known as a forensic tool, identifying criminals is a relatively simple use of microsatellite variability. The fact that a person's genetic profile is inherited in part from the mother and in part from the father is used in more advanced technique. This indicates that microsatellites can be used to determine familial links and population affinities in animals and plants other than humans.

Tandemly repeated DNA sequences are assumed to have formed either through replication slippage, as explained for microsatellites, or through DNA recombination mechanisms. Rather than isolated repeat units distributed throughout the genome, each of these events are likely to result in a network of linked repeats. Interspersed repeats must have developed through a separate method., One that can cause a duplicate of a repeat unit to emerge in the genome at a different site than the original sequence. Transposition is the most common mechanism for this to happen, and most interspersed repetitions have inherent transpositional activity.

There are two types of transposition: one that uses an RNA intermediary and the other that does not. Retro transposition is the version that involves an RNA intermediate. Three phases make up the basic mechanism:

1. **The usual transcription process produces an RNA copy of the transposition.**

- The RNA transcript is transcribed into DNA in the second step. The reversal of the regular transcription process, converting RNA to DNA, necessitates the use of a particular enzyme known as reverse transcriptase.

- Often, a gene within the transposon codes for reverse transcriptase, which is translated from the RNA copy generated in step 1.

- The transposon's DNA copy integrates into the genome, perhaps back into the same chromosome as the originating unit or into a different chromosome entirely. As a result, there are now two copies of the transposon in the genome, each at a distinct location.

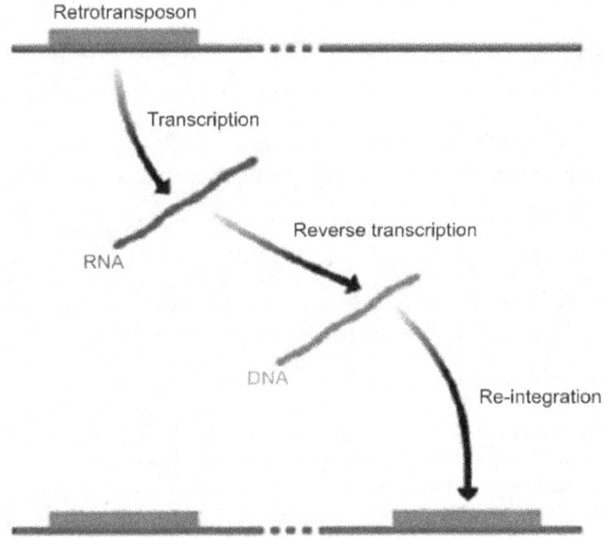

Fig. 4.5 RNA copy of the transposition

- RNA transposons, also known as retroelements, are found in the genomes of eukaryotes but have yet to be detected in prokaryotes.

- Retroviruses that are produced in the body (ERVs)

- Endogenous retroviruses (ERVs) are retroviral genomes that have been integrated into the chromosomes of vertebrates. Some are still active and may direct the creation of foreign viruses at some point throughout a cell's existence.

- However, the majority of them are long-dead relics that can no longer create viruses. These inactive sequences are genome-wide repeats that are incapable of proliferating further.

2. **Retro transpositions:**

- Retrotransposons, like ERVs, are found in nonvertebrate eukaryotic genomes (e.g., plants, fungi, invertebrates, and microbial eukaryotes), not vertebrate genomes.

- In some genomes, the number of copies of retrotransposons is very high, and there are many different forms of retrotransposons. The Ty3 / gypsy family (Ty3 and gypsy are instances of this class in yeast and fruit fly, respectively), whose members have the same set of genes as an ERV, and the Ty1/copia family, which lacks the env gene.

- Both types can transpose, but the Ty1/copia group is unable to produce infectious viral particles due to the lack of the env gene.

- Despite the existence of env in the Ty3/ gypsy genome, it was only recently discovered that some of these components may form viruses, indicating that they should be considered non-vertebrate retroviruses.

- Retrotransposons are sometimes discovered in clusters in a genome sequence due to the availability of preferential integration sites for transposing elements, despite the fact that they are technically interspersed elements.

- LTR elements are the three types of retroelements described thus far, as they have long terminal repetitions at either end that aid in the transposition process. LTRs are not present in other retroelements.

- Retropositions are a type of DNA that can be found in animals.

4.2.4   Structures (Long Interspersed Nuclear Elements)

They have a reverse-transcriptase-like gene that is likely involved in retrotransposition. The human element LINE-1, for example, is 6.1 kb in size and has 516,000 copies in the human genome. A LINE has a pol II promoter as well as two open reading frames (ORFs), one for endonuclease and the other for reverse transcriptase. The following is how the LINE action goes: RNA pol II converts LINE DNA to LINE RNA, which is then translated into proteins, which then bind together and rejoin the nucleus.

The reverse transcriptase copies the LINE RNA into LINE DNA, which is inserted into the target DNA, forming a new LINE element there; the endonuclease cuts a strand of the target genomic DNA, often in the intron of a gene; the endonuclease cuts a strand of the target genomic DNA, often in the intron of a gene; the endonuclease cuts a strand of the target genomic DNA, ssthe human genome has three distantly related LINE families: LINE1, LINE2, and LINE3. Only LINE1 (L1) remains operational.

4.2.5   SINEs (Synthetic Intelligence Networks) (Short Interspersed Nuclear Elements)

- They lack a reverse transcriptase gene, yet they can still transpose, most likely by 'borrowing' reverse transcriptase enzymes from other retroelements. SINEs are short (100–400 bp) sequences that include an internal pol III promoter but do not encode any proteins.

- The tRNA and 7SL RNA genes are the source of all currently known SINEs. The 3′end of most nonautonomous SINEs is shared with a resident LINE.

- The Alu element is the only active SINE in the human genome, accounting for approximately 11% of the genome (1 million Alu elements). An RNA intermediary isn't required for all transposons.

- Many are able to transfer DNA to DNA in a more direct method. DNA transposons are less prevalent in eukaryotes than retrotransposons, but they hold a distinct place in genetics because a family of plant DNA transposons has been discovered.

- DNA transposons are far more important than RNA transposons in bacterial genome architecture.

- DNA transposons include the insertion sequences IS1 and IS186, and a single E. coli genome can have up to 20 of them of various forms. Other DNA transposons found in E. coli, as well as those found in prokaryotes in general, include: Tn3-type transposons and composite transposons

4.3   Prokaryote Genetic Organization

The genomes of prokaryotes and eukaryotes are substantially different. The largest prokaryotic and smallest eukaryotic genomes have considerable overlap in size, but bacterial genomes are substantially smaller overall. The E. coli K12 genome, for example, is just 4639 kb in size, two-fifths the size of the yeast genome, and contains only 4405 genes.

4.3.1   Prokaryotic Genome Features

- In eukaryotes and prokaryotes, the physical organization of the genome differs.

- An entire bacterial genome is thought to be contained in a single circular DNA molecule, according to conventional wisdom. Prokaryotes may have additional genes on smaller, circular or linear DNA molecules called plasmids in addition to this one 'chromosome.'

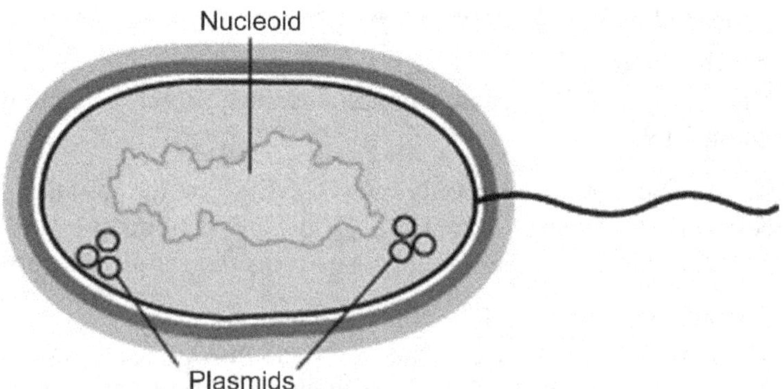

Fig. 4.6 Structure of Prokaryotic Genome

- Plasmids carry genes that code for traits like antibiotic resistance or the capacity to utilize complicated molecules like toluene as a carbon source, but they appear to be unnecessary; a prokaryote can survive fairly well without them. Prokaryotes have a wide range of genome organization, with some having a single-partite genome, such as E. coli, and others being more sophisticated as shown in Fig 4.6.

- Borrelia burgdorferi B31, for example, has a 911-kilobyte linear chromosome. 853 genes are carried, along with 17 or 18 linear and circular polymers that provide another 533 kb and at least 430 genes. Many additional bacteria and archaea now have multipartite genomes.

- The genomes of prokaryotes are even smaller than those of yeast and other lower eukaryotes. For example, thrA and thrB are separated by a single nucleotide, and thrC starts at the nucleotide immediately following the last nucleotide of thrB.

- These three genes make up an operon, which is a collection of genes that work together to carry out a particular metabolic pathway (in this case, the synthesis of the amino acid threonine).

- Operons have been used as model organisms to study how gene expression is controlled. Prokaryotic genes are often shorter than eukaryotic genes, with the average length of a bacterial gene being roughly two-thirds that of a eukaryotic gene, even after the latter's introns have been deleted. Genes from bacteria appear to be slightly longer than those from archaea.

- In the genes found in this section of the E. coli genome, there are no introns. In fact, E. coli has no discontinuous genes at all, and it is widely assumed that this form of gene organization is rare in prokaryotes, with the archaea being the only exception.

- The infrequency of repeating sequences is another trait. The high-copy-number genome-wide repeat families seen in eukaryotic genomes are not found in most bacterial genomes.

4.3.2   The Bacterial Genome's Physical Structure

The majority of prokaryotic genomes are under 5 megabytes, although a few are much larger: B. megaterium, for example, has a massive genome of 30 megabytes. The traditional view has been that the genome of a typical prokaryote is contained in a single circular DNA molecule, which is located within the nucleoid, a featureless area of the prokaryotic cell. This is unquestionably true of E. coli and many other commonly studied bacteria.

4.3.3   'Chromosome' of Bacteria

A prokaryotic genome, like eukaryotic chromosomes, must fit into a small space (the circular E. coli chromosome has a circumference of 1.6 mm, while an E. coli cell is only 1.0 2.0 m) and, like eukaryotes, this is accomplished with the help of DNA-binding proteins that package the genome in an organized manner.

4.3.4   DNA Supercoiling

E. coli DNA supercoils when more turns are added to the double helix (positive supercoiling) or when turns are deleted (negative supercoiling) (negative supercoiling). The torsional tension created by over- or under-winding in a linear molecule is quickly relieved by rotation of the DNA molecule's ends, but a circular molecule with no ends cannot reduce the strain in this way. Instead, the circular molecule replies by looping itself around to create a more compact structure. As a result, supercoiling is an excellent approach to compact a circular molecule into a small space. Supercoiling is important in packaging the circular E. coli genome, according to evidence gained from isolated nucleoids in the 1970s and verified as a characteristic of DNA in living cells in 1981.

Two enzymes, DNA gyrase and DNA topoisomerase I, are assumed to be responsible for supercoiling in E. coli. The two enzymes that are principally responsible for maintaining the supercoiled form, DNA gyrase and DNA topoisomerase I, are found in the protein component of the nucleoid.as well as a group of at least four proteins thought to play a more specialized role in bacterial DNA packaging. The most abundant of these packing proteins is HU, which looks nothing like eukaryotic histones but functions similarly, producing a tetramer around which around 60 bp of DNA is wound. There are roughly 60 000 HU proteins per E. coli cell, enough to cover about one-fifth of the DNA molecule, but it's unclear whether the tetramers are evenly spaced along the DNA or only in the nucleoid's core area as shown in Fig 4.7.

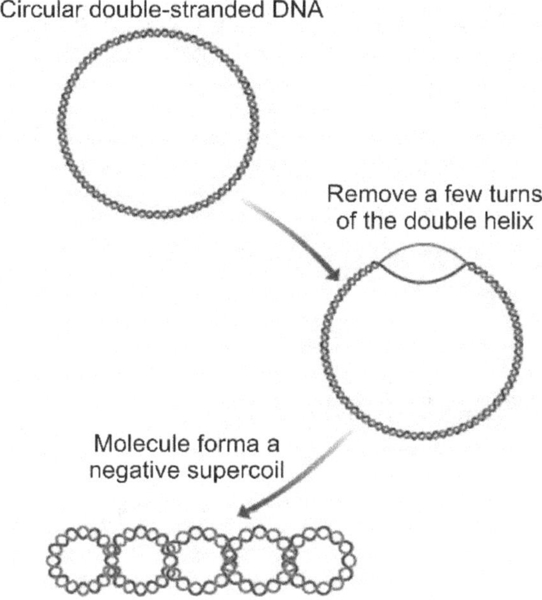

Fig. 4.7 DNA Supercoiling

4.3.5 Negative Supercoiling is caused by Underwinding a Circular Double-Stranded DNA Molecule, as deen in the Diagram

Operon

- An operon is a set of genes in the genome that are close together, with only one or two nucleotides separating the end of one gene from the start of the next. An operon's genes are all expressed as a single unit. In bacterial genomes, this form of organization is widespread.

- The lactose operon, which comprises three genes involved in the conversion of the disaccharide sugar lactose into its monosaccharide parts - glucose and galactose - is a typical E. coli example.

- It was the first operon to be found (Jacob and Monod, 1961). (Figure 2.20A) Because monosaccharides are substrates for the energy-generating glycolytic pathway, the lactose operon's genes transform lactose into a form that may be used as an energy source by E. coli.

- Because lactose is not a common component of E. coli's natural environment, the operon is rarely expressed, and the bacterium does not produce lactose-utilizing enzymes.

- When lactose is present, the operon is activated; all three genes are expressed simultaneously, resulting in coordinated production of lactose-utilizing enzymes.

- This is a classic example of bacterial gene regulation.

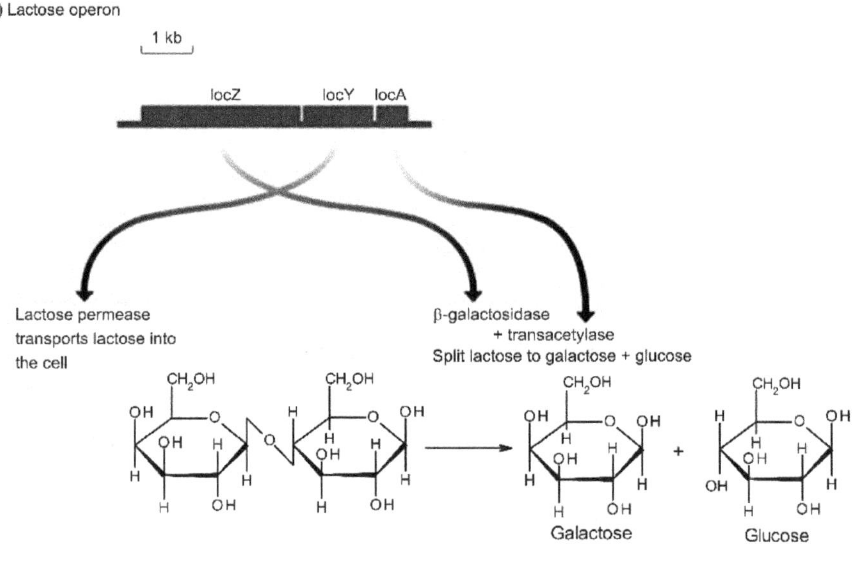

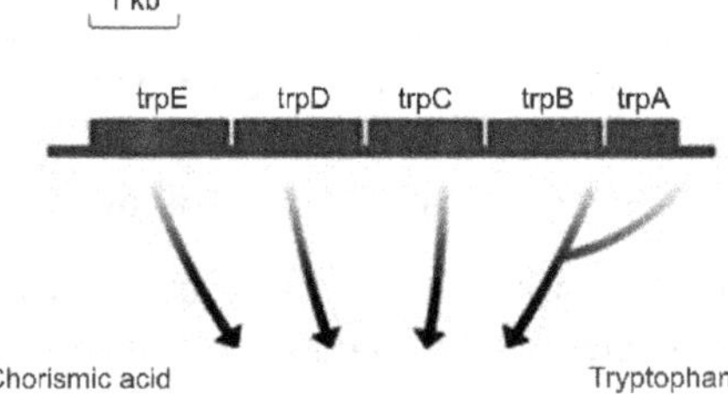

Fig. 4.8 Escherichia coli has two operons

4.3.6   Genomes of Prokaryotes and the Concept of Species

- The problems in applying the species concept to prokaryotes have been highlighted by genome sequencing.

- It's become evident that different strains of the same species can have vastly diverse genome sequences, as well as distinct sets of strain-specific genes.

- A comparison of two strains of Helicobacter pylori, which causes stomach ulcers and other disorders of the human digestive tract, was the first to demonstrate this.

- The genomes of the two strains, which were isolated in the United Kingdom and the United States, are 1.67 Mb and 1.64 Mb, respectively.

- The bigger genome has 1552 genes, whereas the smaller genome has 1495 genes, with 1406 of these genes shared by both strains. In other words, about 6–7% of each strain's gene composition is unique to that strain.

- When other bacterial and archaeal genomes are investigated, the challenges become even more significant.

- It was expected that the same genes would occasionally be found in different prokaryotic species due to the ease with which genes can flow between them, but the magnitude of lateral gene transfer shown by sequencing has surprised everyone.

- The majority of genomes contain a few hundred kb of DNA received directly from another species, and in some cases, the figure is even higher: 12.8 percent of the E. coli K12 genome, or 0.59 Mb, was gained this way.

- The fact that transfer has occurred between quite diverse species, including bacteria and archaea, is a second surprise.

- The thermophilic bacteria Thermatoga maritima, for example, possesses 1877 genes, 451 of which are thought to have come from archaeons.

The transfer of bacteria to archaea in the opposite direction is also common.

- Prokaryotes residing in comparable ecological niches exchange genes with one another to improve their individual fitness for survival in their specific environment, according to the developing picture.

- Many of the Thermatoga genes found in archaeons are thought to have helped this bacterium develop its capacity to survive high temperatures.

- Lateral gene transfer has undoubtedly played a significant role in prokaryote evolution. Bacteria and archaea's evolutionary histories, unlike those of higher creatures, cannot be characterized as a simple branching pattern, but must instead account for horizontal gene flow across species.

- Comparing the sequences of comparable genes in various species in higher creatures can be used to build evolutionary links between those species.

(A) No lateral gene transfer between species

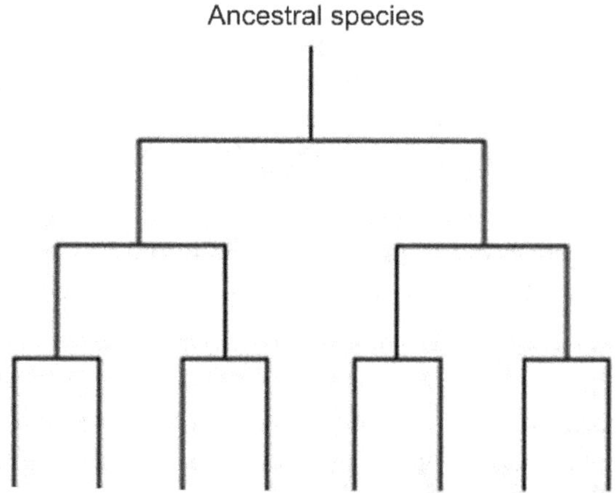

Evolutionary histories of modern species are distinct

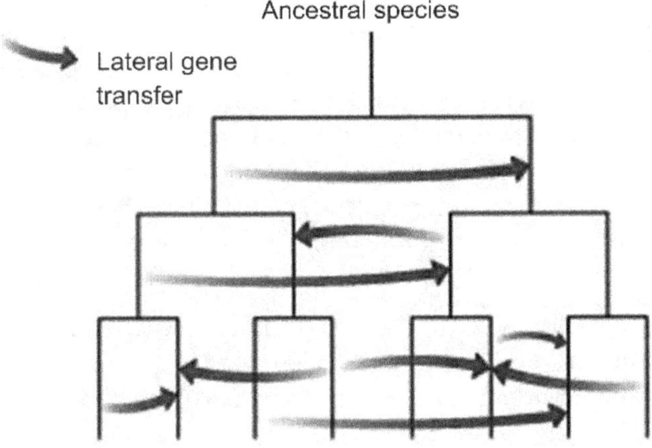

Fig. 4.9 Lateral gene transfer obscures the evolutionary relationships between species

Table 4.3 Genetic arrangement in prokaryotes vs. eukaryotes

Prokaryotic	Eukaryotic
No-nonsense genomes – nearly all coding	Lots of noncoding regions (introns, intergenic regions)
Frequent horizontal gene transfer (HGT)	Less frequent HGT
Circular genome plus plasmids	Distinct linear chromosomes
Streamlined genomes, few repetitive elements	More dispersed regulations
Very rapidly evolving in both sequence and structure	More conservative mode of evolution
Very large population sizes (10^9-10^{10})	Smaller population sizes ($\sim 10^3 - 10^4$)

4.4   Microbial Genetics

Genetic recombination can be referred as the exchange of genetical material between two double strand molecules with identical (a) very similar sequences. In bacteria the genetic information is preserved in a single chromosome and in minichromosome called episomes and plasmids. The chromosome of *Escherichia coli* is a double stranded DNA circle of about 5 million base pairs encoding approximately 5,000 genes. Because there is only one chromosome, each gene (with occasional exceptions) is present in only one copy. Bacteria reproduced by simple fission results in distribution of their genetic material to the two progeny cells equally. They are haploid; a multinucleate do not go through mitotic and meiotic cycle like in eukaryotes. One important consequence of having a haploid genome is that genetic changes have an immediate effect on the phenotype or properties of the bacterial cell.

Bacterial variation can also occur by **horizontal transfer** of genetic material from one cell to another. Consider two cells from different populations: bacterium B has features distinct from those of bacterium A. There are three possible mechanisms for transferring a trait from B to A:

1. **Transformation**, release and uptake of naked DNA from one bacterium (the donor cell) to another bacterium (the recipient cell);

2. **Transduction**, packaging and transfer of bacterial DNA from a donor cell, to recipient cell by bacteriophage, and

3. **Conjugation**, bacterial mating in which cells must be in contact, through a specialized sex pilus.

For all three processes, the transferred DNA must be stably incorporated into the genetic material of the recipient bacterium.

This can occur in two ways:

(i) **Recombination (Table 4.4)**, or integration of the transferred DNA into the bacterial chromosome; or

(ii) **Establishment of a plasmid**, i.e., the transferred material essentially forms a minichromosome capable of autonomous replication.

Mutation and gene transfer work together to accelerate the rate of bacterial evolution. The spontaneous changes required to produce a new function (*e.g.*, antibiotic resistance) may occur at a low frequency. However, once the function has developed it can readily spread to other bacterial populations. The limitation is the probability and efficiency of gene exchange between different bacteria. Under certain conditions, gene exchange is very efficient.

Table 4.4 Recombination Process

Recombination Process	Cell Contact Required	Sensitive to DNase
Transformation	No	Yes
Transduction	No	No
Conjugation	Yes	No

4.4.1   Criteria for Determining the Mode of Recombination in Bacteria

4.4.1.1   Transformation (Gene Exchange between Bacteria)

In 1928 Griffith, an English health officer discovered transformation process initially in pathogenic strains of *Streptococcus pneumonia*. He injected a mouse with a mixture consisting of a few rough (non capsulated and non-pathogenic) pneumococci and large number of heats killed smooth (capsulated pathogenic) cells.

He showed that injecting into mice a mixture of heat killed virulent (smooth) *S. pneumoniae* with a live attenuated (rough) strain led to the development of a live virulent strain, which ultimately killed the mouse. Avery, MacCleod and McCarty purified the transforming substance and identified it as DNA. This experiment was the first to demonstrate that DNA was the genetic material. It was also the first discovery of gene transfer between bacteria. Since then, other bacteria, including certain species of *Haemophilus*, *Bacillus*, *Actinobacillus*, and *Neisseria*, have been found to be naturally transformable. These bacteria have developed highly specialized functions that will bind DNA fragments and transport them into the cell.

Griffith also showed that the transforming factor could be passed from the transformed cells to their progeny and thus had the characteristic of gene.

These mechanisms can be quite distinct. In the case of *Bacillus subtilis*, any DNA can be taken up.

- *Bacillus* and *Streptococcus* unwind the DNA and transport only a single strand.

- In contrast, *Haemophilus*, *Actinobacillus*, and *Neisseria* require a specific sequence to be present on the DNA fragments and transport double-stranded DNA fragments. Transformable organisms take up DNA when they are in a **competent** state.

- In *Bacillus*, this state is triggered by small diffusible molecules whose concentration indicates when the culture has reached a certain density.

- In *Haemophilus*, competence is induced by nutritional starvation. These signals somehow trigger the expression of proteins that enable the cells to bind and take up DNA.

- In nature, the DNA to be taken up is thought to be released into the environment by lysis of bacterial cells.

- Transformation is probably the least efficient mechanism of gene transfer because naked DNA is sensitive to nucleases in the environment.

- In the laboratory, mutant strains can be transformed to wild type by the addition of purified DNA extracted from a wild type strain. The process depends on the DNA and is sensitive to the addition of DNAse.

- The ability to introduce DNA into bacterial cells in the laboratory is the basis for "reverse genetics," in which a gene is first cloned, mutated *in vitro*, and reintroduced into the bacterial cell to study the resulting phenotype.

Natural Transformation

Cells that are in a state in which they can be transformed by DNA in their environment are said to be the competent. In significant number of bacteria, entry into the competent state is encoded by chromosal genes and signaled by certain environmental conditions. Such bacteria are now capable of undergoing natural transformation. For example, certain species of *Haemophilus*, *Bacillus*, *Actinobacillus* and *Neisseria*, have been found to be naturally transformable.

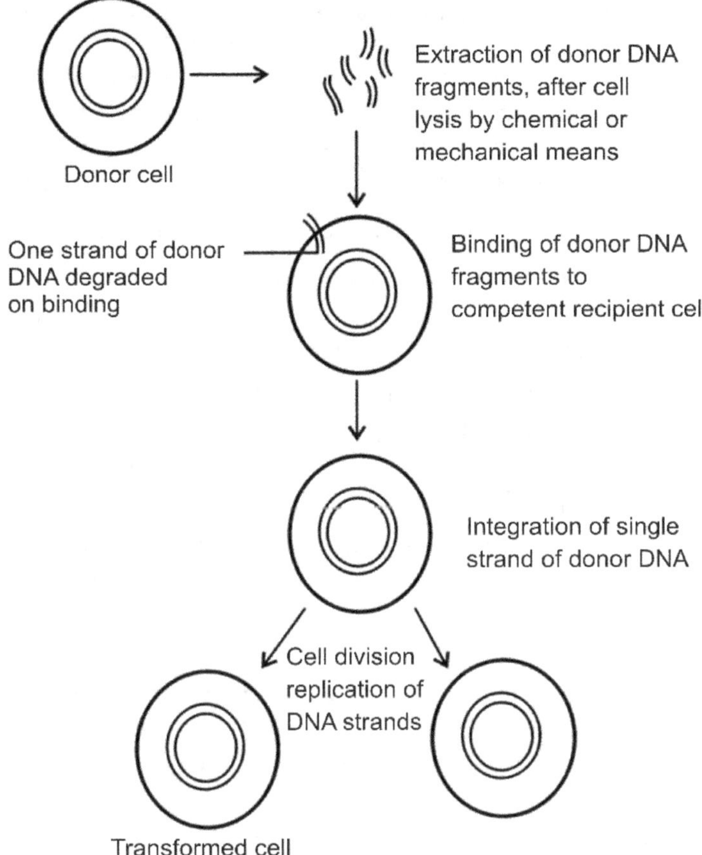

Fig. 4.10 Principle steps in bacterial transformation

Artificial Transformation

Bacteria which do not become competent under ordinary conditions of culture, they can made competent by artificial treatments such as exposure of cells to high concentrations of divalent cations like $CaCl_2$ such systems of transformations have been termed as artificial transformation. Some organisms that are not naturally transformable, like *E. coli*, can be made competent for transformation by treating the cells with CaCl2 or placing them in an electric field (electroporation).

Mechanism for Bacterial Recombination

Inside the recipient cell the donor DNA fragment is positioned alongside the recipient DNA in such a way that homologous genes are adjacent.

Enzymes act on the recipient DNA, causing nicks and excision of a fragment. Then the donor DNA is integrated into the recipient chromosome in place of the excised DNA. The recipient cell then becomes the recombinant cell because its chromosome contains DNA of both the donor and the recipient cell. (The excised DNA pieces from the recipient chromosome are probably broken down by specific enzymes.)

Generally the process of transformation involves the following stages:

1. Reversible binding of ds-DNA molecule to cell surface through receptor site.

2. Irreversible uptake of DNA of donor.

3. Conversion of ds-DNA of donor to SS-DNA by nucleolytic degradation of one strand.

4. Integration of a part of all single strands of donor DNA into the chromosome of recipient cell.

5. The segregation and phenotypic (a set of observable characteristics) expression of integrated donor gene or genes in the recombinant cell i.e., transformed cell.

Transformation process can be occurred without cell contact. It is DNAse sensitive recombination process. This process occurs in absence of DNAse in the medium. These two criteria helps in differentiating process from other two i.e., transduction and conjugation.

In bacterial recombination, cell do not fuse, and usually only a portion of the chromosome from the donor cell (male) is transferred to the recipient cell (female). The recipient cell thus becomes a merozygote, a zygote that is a partial diploid. Once merozygote transformation has occurred, recombination can take place.

Applications of transformation: The utilization of bacterial transformation in medicine, particularly in the pharmaceutical industry is an exciting development that has led to the fast and efficient production of many drugs needed by society. By placing certain suitable bacteria into a bath of calcium chloride, scientists have been able to artificially stimulate the bacteria to uptake certain chosen genes and then incorporate them into their genomes. This transgenic bacterium, if the process was successful, can then express the foreign genes by the production of proteins, and mass produce them because of their ability to speedily and exactly clone themselves. In one example, an E-coli bacterium was stimulated to uptake and incorporates into its genome the human gene for the production of insulin. So instead of painstakingly harvesting small amounts of insulin from hogs, insulin can now be mass produced by the transgenic bacterium. Other examples of important drugs that are produced utilizing the bacterial ability of transformation include human growth hormone, erythropoietin, a drug used to stimulate red blood cell production in people suffering from anemia, tissue plasminogen activator, which is used to dissolve blood clots, as well as several others.

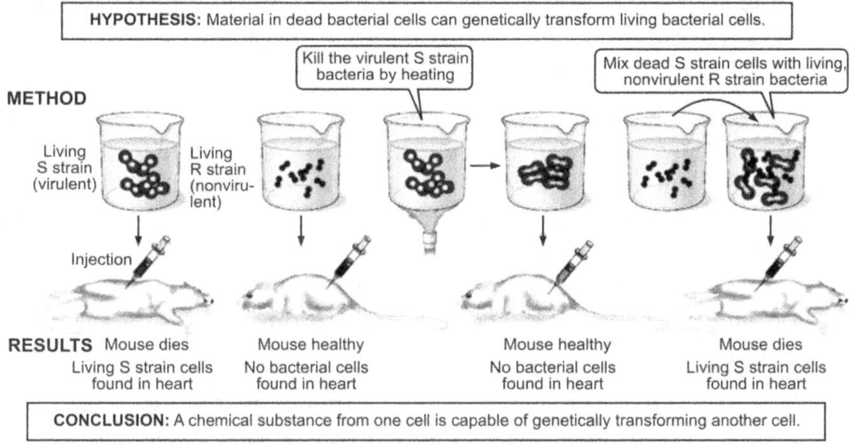

Fig. 4.11 Demonstration of genetic transformation

Pollution control is a major concern in the world today because of earth's limited resources. But there is an effective and natural way to help do away with pollution, and this process is called bioremediation. Bioremediation is the utilization of some types of transgenic bacteria, fungi, normal bacteria, and/or other microbes to decompose many forms of garbage and to break down petroleum products. An example of an instance where a transgenic bacterium was utilized in the fight against pollution is seen in the breakdown of naphthalene, an environmental pollutant found in many artificially created soils, by the genetically altered pseudomonas fluorescence. This bacterium was stimulated to uptake the gene for fluorescence so that as it broke down the naphthalene it would produce light in proportion to the amount of chemical it had broken down, thus allowing scientists to monitor the efficiency of the process. A more famous example (i) involving the use of transgenic bacteria genetically engineered for the breakdown of hydrocarbons in oil was seen in their use in the Exon-Valdez oil spill.

4.4.1.2   Bacterial Conjugation

Because lacking of knowledge of any mating system in bacteria, it was impossible to explore the system experimentally to Luria and Delbruck (1943) who had demonstrated that bacteria have a stable hereditary system. The first demonstrate of recombination in bacteria was achieved by Lederberg and Tatum in 1946 in a brilliant and remarkable experiment that opened the door to a whole new world of microbiology.

Conjugation in bacteria must be quite rare. Since it was not found by anybody (in spite of many attempts), so few possible recombinants were selected from a large population.

Two different auxotrophic (an organism having a growth requirement of specific nutrients not necessarily in the parental strain) strains of *E. coli* was combined and allowed to mate. Then combined cultures were plated on a minimal medium, which can grow only phototrophs (the organisms that can synthesize all their amino acid requirements). Phototrophic colonies were grown, then it was understood that growth of phototrophic bacteria is because of recombination between the auxotroph.

Polyauxotrophs (mutants with more than one nutritional requirement) were used so that back mutation or spontaneous reversion to the wild type would not occur to confuse the results. The photrophs which arose could not have arisen by the phenomenon of transformation. It is experimentally proved that bacterial recombination by conjugation is indeed a true sexual process. It is apparent that mating or conjugation in *E. coli* is radically different from sexual mating in higher organisms. It is not a reproductive process that occurs regularly at each generation. It does not involve meiosis since bacterial cells are haploid, or dies if it involves the fusion of gametes.

It involves the transfer of some DNA from one cell to another followed by separation of the mating pair of cells. In conjugation it is possible for large segments of the chromosome, and in special cases the entire chromosome is transferred.

Sex factors: There is a sexual differentiation in *E. coli*; in other words, different mating types of the bacterium exist. Male cells contain a small circular piece of DNA, which is in the cytoplasm and not part of the chromosome, called the sex factor or F factor (fertility factor).

These cells are referred to as F (+) and are donors in mating. Female cells lack this factor and are labeled F (-). They are recipient cells.

Crosses between two F (-) strains do not yield recombinants. However, in F (+) x F (-) crosses, the male replicates its sex factor, and one copy of it is almost always transferred to the female recipient. The F (-) cell is converted to an F (+) cell) (Fig. 4.12) and is itself capable of serving as a donor. So as long as the cell grows the conjugation process can continue in an infectious way with repeated transfer of the sex factor. The transfer of the factor is independent of the transfer of chromosomal genes.

F factor DNA is only sufficient to specify about 40 genes which control sex factor replication and synthesize sex pili. F factor DNA replicates independently of the F (+) donor cell's normal chromosome. The transfer of the F factor is also independent.

Sex pili seem to act to bind an F (-) cell to an F (+) cell, pulling the F (-) cell into close contact. Sex pili are tubules through which DNA passes from a F (+) to a Γ (-) cell during conjugation, although the DNA may be passed from one cell to another at sites of contact between them.

4.4.1.3   Extra Chromosomal Genetic Elements (Plasmids)

In addition to the normal DNA chromosome, extra chromosomal genetic elements are often found in bacteria. These elements are called plasmids and are capable of autonomous replication in the cytoplasm of the bacterial cell.

Plasmids are circular pieces of DNA that extra genes. Some plasmids are capable of either replicating autonomously or integrating into the bacterial DNA chromosome and are called episomes. Thus, the F factor of *E. coli* was called an episome because it can alternately exist in the F (+) of Hfr (high frequency recombination, or Hfr strains) state.

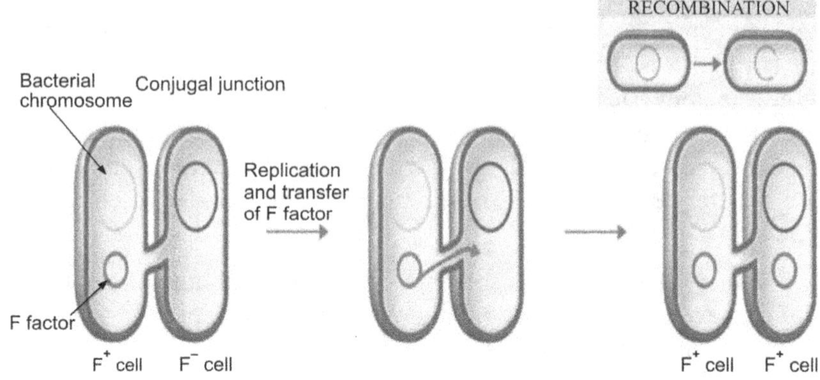

(a) When an F factor (a plasmid) is transferrred from a donor (F$^+$) to a recipient (F$^-$), the F$^-$ cell is converted to an F$^+$ cell.

Fig. 4.12 Bacterial conjugation

Applications of Bacterial Conjugation

Bacterial conjugation is a mechanism for horizontal DNA transfer with potential for universal DNA delivery. The conjugal machinery can be separated into three functional modules: the relaxosome, the coupling protein and a type IV protein secretion system. Module interchangeability among different conjugative systems opens up the possibility of "à la carte" engineering of DNA delivery into virtually any cell type.

4.4.1.4   Transduction

Bacteriophages have the ability to transfer genes from one bacterial cell to another, a process known as transduction.

Most bacteriophages, the virulent phages, undergo a rapid lytic growth cycle in their host cells. They inject their nucleic acid, usually DNA, into the bacterium, where it replicates rapidly and also directs the synthesis of new phage proteins. Within 10 to 20 min, the new DNA combines with the new proteins to make whole phage particles, which were released by destruction of the cell wall and lysis of the cell.

However, some bacterial viruses, the temperature phages, which ordinarily do not lyse the cell, carry DNA that can behave as a kind of episome in bacteria; like other episomes, such as the F factor, these viral genomes can become integrated into the bacterial genome; they are then known as prophages. Bacteria that carry prophages (lysogenic bacteria) can be induced with ultraviolet light and other agents to make the prophages start to replicate rapidly and go through a lytic growth cycle, resulting in lysis of the cell with release of new phage particles.

Phage's particles may become filled with cell chromosomal DNA or a mixture of chromosomal and phages DNA. Such aberrant phages can attach to other bacteria and introduce bacterial, rather just phage, DNA from one cell to another. Thus we can define bacterial transduction as the transfer by bacteriophages, serving as a vector, of a portion of DNA from one bacterium (a donor) to another (a recipient). There are two varieties of bacteriophage-mediated gene transfer: **generalized transduction** and **specialized transduction**.

Generalized transduction occurs as a result of the lytic cycle. In the process of packaging bacteriophage DNA, the head structures of some bacteriophages will package random fragments of the bacterial chromosome. Thus, the lysate contains two kinds of particles that differ only in the kind of DNA they contain. Most of the particles contain viral DNA. When these inject their DNA, the lytic cycle will repeat and new bacteriophage particles will be produced. A small fraction of the particles, possibly as high as 1%, contain fragments of the bacterial chromosome in place of the bacteriophage DNA. When one of these particles injects its DNA into the cell, the cell is not killed. The newly introduced DNA contains only bacterial genes and is free to recombine with the chromosome. Some transducing bacteriophages can introduce 100-200 kilobases of DNA. Because the bacterial fragments that are packaged are essentially random, virtually any bacterial gene of the bacterial chromosome can be transduced (hence, the term "generalized" transduction). Entire plasmids can be transduced by phages. Some plasmids, notably those encoding antibiotic resistance in *staphylococci* have evolved signals to allow efficient packaging by phage particles and subsequent transfer by transduction. Another element **pathogenicity island**, in the *Staphylococcus* chromosome which codes for toxic shock toxin senses the presence of an infecting phage, excises, replicates, and is efficiently packaged.

Transducing particles, like bacteriophage particles, are stable in the environment for long periods of time. Thus, bacterial genes can be stored in the environment and transduction of a bacterial cell may occur long after the original bacterial population was lysed by the bacteriophage infection. Studies on dissemination of antibiotic resistance have revealed generalized transduction to be a significant mechanism of gene transfer in nature.

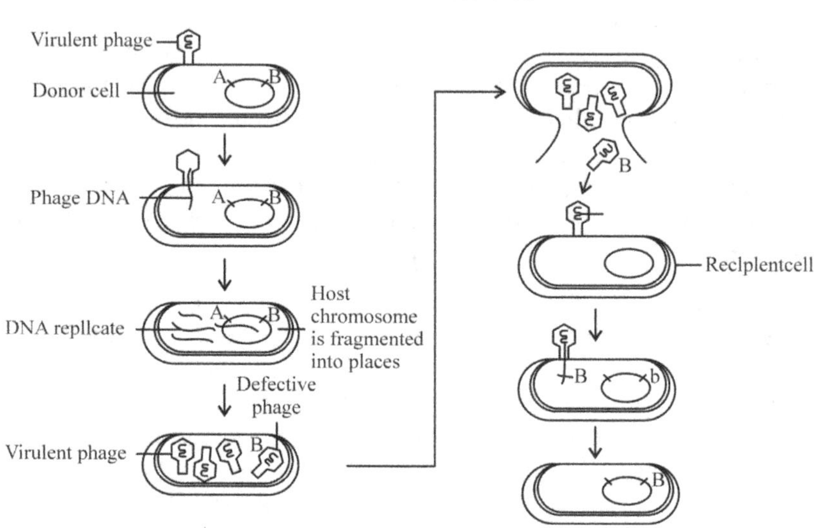

Fig. 4.13 Generalized transduction

Specialized transduction requires a temperate bacteriophage. In this class of transduction, a bacterial gene becomes associated with the bacteriophage genome (e.g. by recombination). When such a bacteriophage lysogenizes a new bacterial host, it brings with it the associated bacterial gene. Because it is a bacterial gene, its expression is not turned off by the bacteriophage repressor that inhibits expression of the lytic functions. A well known example is the b phage of *Corynebacterium diphtheriae*, which carries the gene for diphtheria toxin. Cells of *C. diphtheriae* that are non-lysogenic for the bacteriophage are incapable of causing diphtheria. *C. diphtheriae* cells that carry the b phage in the chromosome express the gene for diphtheria toxin and produce disease. Other examples include changes in the O-antigens of *Salmonella*, antibiotic resistance genes, erythrogenic toxin in *Streptococcus pyogenes*, the tissue destroying a-toxin of *Staphylococcus aureus*, enterotoxin of *E. coli*, cholera toxin of *Vibrio cholerae*, and neurotoxin by *Clostridium botulinum*. Such alterations of the properties of a bacterial cell by lysogeny with a temperate bacteriophage are known as lysogenic conversion shown in Fig. 4.14.

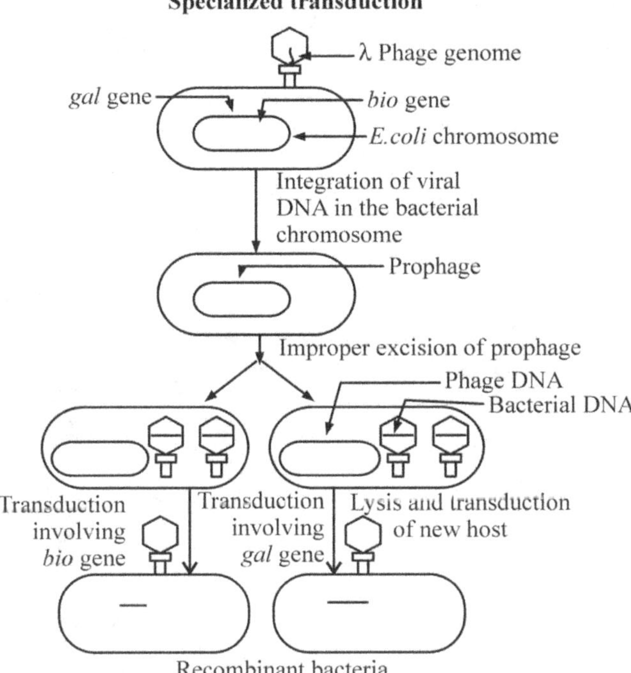

Fig. 4.14 Specialized transduction

4.4.1.5   Transduction - Uses in Research

Generalized transducing viruses are the most useful in mapping bacterial chromosomal genes. Since the amount of DNA that is packaged by the virus is determined by the size of the head of the virus, each viral particle holds the same amount of DNA. The initial cutting of the host chromosome is a random event, giving all genes approximately the same probability of being packaged and transferred. Each piece of DNA that is packaged will be the same length, meaning that the closer together two genes are, the higher the probability that the two genes will be present on the same fragment of packaged DNA. In other words, the closer together the genetic markers are, the higher the frequency of co-transduction. Therefore the distance between closely linked chromosomal genes can be calculated by measuring the frequency that two genes or genetic markers are co-transduced.

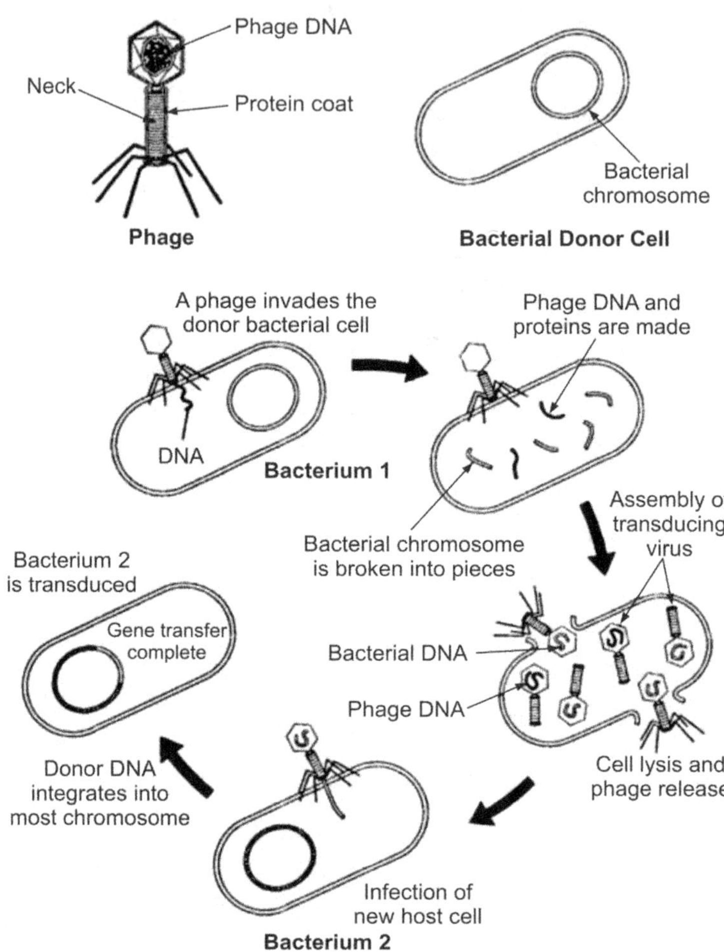

Fig. 4.15 Transduction

4.4.1.6 Microbial Biotransformation

- Microorganisms have the ability to enzymatically change a wide variety of chemical molecules.

- Biotransformation is defined as the transformation of a given molecule into a separate product with structural similarities using biological catalysts such as microorganisms.

- An enzyme, or a full, inactivated microbe that contains an enzyme or numerous enzymes synthesized in it, can be described as a biological catalyst. The distinction between a biotransformation and a bioconversion is minor.

- Because bioconversions rely on live organisms' catalytic activity, they can entail multiple chemical reaction stages.

- Bioconversions frequently require enzymes that are highly unstable for the substrates employed since a living microbe produces enzymes on a constant basis.

- Biotransformation and bioconversions have extremely similar features, and the terms are sometimes used interchangeably.

- Fermentation, on the other hand, is a branch of zymology that uses microorganisms; yeast has been known to convert sugar to alcohol since 1857, when French chemist Louis Pasteur discovered it.

- Biotransformation processes offer benefits in overcoming some of the inherent challenges, as well as examples of economically successful procedures.

- To put it another way, Biotransformation is the microbial (enzymatic) conversion of a substrate into a product using a small number of enzymatic processes (one or a few).

- Fermentation, on the other hand, includes a significant number of reactions (often complex in nature).

Biotransformation/Bioconversion Types

1) Biotransformation of microorganisms

2) Biotransformation of plant cell cultures

3) Biotransformation of animal cell cultures

Microbial transformation: When microorganisms carry out the transformation of organic substances, the process is known as microbial transformation.

Microorganisms are capable of chemically altering a wide range of organic substances.

During bioconversion, these bacteria produce enzymes that act on the organic component and convert it to other chemicals or change it.

Vinegar manufacturing, for example, is the oldest and most well-known transformation process.

Microbial cells, as opposed to other cells, are an excellent alternative for biotransformation for a variety of reasons, including:

1. **Surface-volume ratio:** The surface-volume ratio of microbial biotransformation is high.

2. **Microbial Cell Growth Rate:** A higher microbial cell growth rate minimizes the time required for biomass transformation.

3. **Metabolism Rate:** A faster rate of metabolism in microorganisms leads to more effective substrate transformation.

4. **Sterility:** Using microorganisms makes it easier to maintain sterile conditions.

Techniques for Biotransformation: A wide variety of biological catalysts can be utilized for biotransformation reactions.

Growing cells, resting cells, deceased cells, immobilized cells, cell-free extracts, enzymes, and immobilized enzymes are just some of the options.

Cells are cultured in a suitable medium to produce the required cells. The culture is supplemented with a concentrated substrate as the cells grow (6-24 hours).

In steroid biotransformation, emulsifiers such as Tween and organic solvents such as ethanol, acetone, dimethyl sulphoxide, and others may be required to solubilize substrates and/or products.

Spectroscopic or chromatographic techniques can be used to monitor the substrate conversion to product.

When the product formation is at its best, biotransformation can be stopped.

Non-proliferating cells

For the following reasons, non-growing cells are favoured for biotransformation reactions.

1. A very high substrate concentration can be employed (with high substrate concentration, growing cells stop their growth).

2. Cells can be cleansed and reused, ensuring that no contaminants are present.

3. The substrate to product conversion efficiency is good.

The process of biotransformation can be accelerated by establishing favourable environmental conditions (pH, temperature etc.).

1. Product isolation and recovery are straightforward.

➢ Cells that have become immobile

➢ Immobilized cells can be used to carry out continuous bio-transformations.

➢ Furthermore, the same cells can be reused multiple times.

➢ Immobilized cells are used in a variety of bioconversions with single or multistage reactions, such as the commercial synthesis of L-alanine and malic acid.

➢ enzymes that have been immobilized

➢ For bio-transformations, several immobilized enzyme systems have been developed, such as glucose isomerase and penicillin acylase.

Because of the following advantages, cell-free enzyme systems in the form of immobilized enzymes are the most widely utilized in bio-transformations.

1. There are no unfavourable side effects.

2. The required items are not deteriorated in any way.

3. There is no transport barrier across the cell membrane for the substrate or product.

4. Product isolation and recovery are simpler and easier.

Benefits of microbial biotransformation Biotransformation is also acknowledged to be in line with today's green chemistry strategy.

➢ Green chemistry is a term used to describe chemical industrial manufacturing processes that produce little waste and consume little energy.

➢ The process of microbial transformation can operate at near neutral pH, ambient temperatures, and atmospheric pressures, whereas chemistry frequently necessitates extremes of these conditions, which are not exactly environmentally friendly and industrially undesirable. Extreme pH, temperature, and pressure may cause harm to personnel performing harsh procedures, as well as the communities surrounding the areas.

➢ Regio specificity and stereo specificity of the microbial biotransformation process that permits racemic mixtures to be converted into chiral compounds.

➢ Microorganisms such as fungus and bacteria have the potential to produce vast amounts of biomass and a wide array of enzymes in a short period of time.

➢ Concerns about transmission of animal-based diseases such as bovine spongiform encephalopathy (BSE), scrapie, Kuru, and Creutzfeld-Jacob syndrome ex: growth hormone purified from cadaver pituitaries for dwarfism is now produced by a recombinant Escherichia coli Several individual reactions can be combined by a single microbial reaction

➢ Using a microbe to prepare an organic product is sometimes less expensive than synthesizing it chemically.

• Mammalian drug metabolism research can be supplemented with microbial biotransformation systems.

• Genetically modified microbes expressing human drug-metabolizing enzymes are increasingly more widely available.

• Instead of complicated chemical reactions, using microbes as metabolite factories is a viable strategy for biosynthesis of regioselective and stereospecific compounds.

Disadvantages

• Chemical processes are simpler to handle and require less complex equipment.

• Difficult Requires a specific organism

• Choosing an organism is a difficult task.

• Occasionally, the technique is not cost-effective.

• The amount of substrate added is restricted by several parameters.

4.4.1.6 Aspects of Microbial Biotransformations in Practice

1. Prerequisites

Microorganisms must meet two requirements:

➤ To obtain a specific product, the microorganism must possess the enzyme that causes the necessary transformation.

➤ It should be able to serve as a substrate for the beginning material.

➤ In the medium, organisms that can use the substrate flourish.

2. Organism selection

Organism selection is based on the following parameters:

- Microorganisms must be capable of producing the desired output

- Microorganism cultivation should be cost-effective.

- The reaction must be finished within a certain amount of time.

- Products should not be used to create microorganisms.

There are five basic approaches for organism selection.

1. Screening at random

2. System that runs in parallel

3. Disruption of normal metabolism

4. The technique of enrichment

5. There is a mixture of cultures.

➤ **Random screening:** The substrate is added to a large number of microorganisms, and the medium is evaluated for the presence of product after a certain amount of time

This method is presented for screening a large number of fungi for their spores' ability to carry out a specific steroid conversion.

The spores are spotted with the substrate on a glucose-treated TLC Plate, and the chromatogram is generated following incubation.

➤ **Parallel system:** A suitable organism is identified by a literature search for similar conversion and testing in the system under investigation.

➤ **Interfering with normal metabolism:** This strategy, which has proven successful in a number of circumstances, begins with the selection of an organism capable of converting the substrate into a product via the needed chemical.

The organism is then altered by mutation, or the conversion of the needed chemical is blocked.

- **Enrichment technique:** A considerable amount of substrate, along with water and supplementary nutrients, is introduced to soil samples.

The combination is placed aside for a period of time to allow those organisms capable of using this substrate to multiply.

Following that, the sample is examined for strains with the appropriate features.

For example, if a piece of paper is buried in soil, it will be covered by billions of individuals of the genus Cytophaga within a few days.

For the conversion of a certain substrate, it may be desirable to utilize a mixture of two or more microorganisms.

In most cases, the formation of such fermentation is too complicated to be useful. Enrichment technique: A considerable amount of substrate, along with water and supplementary nutrients, is introduced to soil samples.

The combination is placed aside for a period of time to allow those organisms capable of using this substrate to multiply.

Following that, the sample is examined for strains with the appropriate features.

For example, if a piece of paper is buried in soil, it will be covered by billions of individuals of the genus Cytophaga within a few days.

For the conversion of a certain substrate, it may be desirable to utilize a mixture of two or more microorganisms.

In most cases, the formation of such fermentation is too complicated to be useful.

Newer technologies are currently being used, such as Airlift fermentors and surface attached microorganism (biofilms) in a stationary fluidized bed reactor.

3. Diffusion: Within the cell, transformation occurs.

As a result, the rate limiting stage is achieving cell solubility of the substrate in medium and its rate of diffusion.

Emulsifiers such as Tween or low-toxicity water miscible solvents (ethanol, acetone, DMF, DMSO) may aid in the solubilization of poorly soluble substances.

4. **Side reactions are avoided by adjusting the temperature or pH of the medium.** Side reactions might yield undesired compounds and complicate the isolation process.

5. **Isolation and recovery of the end product:** The end product of transformation processes is usually extracellular and can be dissolved or suspended. Bacteria and yeast are not separated for further purification, as fungal mycelium is normally eliminated by filtration.

Because large amounts of the reaction product can be adsorbed on the cells, the separated cell must be washed frequently with water or organic solvents in all circumstances.

Depending on the product's solubility, recovery is accomplished through precipitation as calcium salt, adsorption or ion exchangers, extraction with appropriate solvents, or straight distillation from medium for volatile compounds.

4.4.1.8 Therapeutic Aspects of Microbial Transformation

A. Conversion of a rare substrate: To complete the conversion, energy is required.

This energy comes from the cell's reserve materials or the medium's components.

The presence of an enzyme that ordinarily catalysis the conversion of structurally comparable chemicals could explain the ability to convert specific drugs.

An alternative theory proposes that a mutation occurs somewhere in the organism's genealogy, allowing descendants to carry out the transition.

The enzyme has no function unless the substance (substrate) is present, and it only becomes visible when the substrate is present.

B. Interference with metabolic route: If the degradative pathway is impeded, any substance generated inside the cell can theoretically become a product.

The majority of organic compound breakdown is caused by oxidation and reduction.

This provides the cell with the energy it requires for production of cell constituents. The proper balance between biosynthesis and breakdown is maintained through mechanism control.

4.4.1.8.1   Microbial biotransformation Types

Hundreds of biotransformation's are known, but only a few of them are useful for the synthesis of commercially important chemicals.

When chemical techniques of producing a given substance are either difficult or expensive, bioconversion reactions become important.

Microbial transformations have several advantages over chemical transformations, such as reaction-specific processes, better stereo- and region-specificity, and softer reaction conditions, and are thus favoured in sectors that deal with preparative organic chemistry.

Oxidation/reduction, hydrolysis, condensation, and isomerization reactions are the most common microbial transformation reactions shown in Table 4.5

Table 4.5 Common Microbial Transformation Reactions

Type of reaction	Example	Commonly used microorganisms
Oxidation	Tryptophan $\rightarrow$ 5-Hydroxytryptophan Naphthalene $\rightarrow$ Salicylic acid	Bacillus subrins Coynebacterium sp
Reduction	Benzaldehyde $\rightarrow$ Benzyl alcohol Nitropentachlorobenzol $\rightarrow$ Pentachloaanaline	Saccaromyces cerevisdue Streptomyces aureolacents
Hydrolysis	Anhydrotetracycline $\rightarrow$ Tetracycine Menthyl laureate $\rightarrow$ Menthol	Streptomyces aureclacens Mycobacterium phie
Cendensation	Streptomycin $\rightarrow$ Steptomycin-phosphate	Streptomyces genesus

The following are some of the most important biotransformation reactions.

I. **The Oxidation Process:** Oxidation reactions are those that include the addition of oxygen and/or the removal of hydrogen.

The following reactions are included in it:

- **Hydroxylation (conversion efficiency of 100%):**

  Conversion of hydrogen to a hydroxyl group occurs in this sort of reaction R-H R-OH (hydroxylation)

  Bacillus subtilis, for example, hydroxylates tryptophan to 5-hydroxy tryptophan. At C-5, the hydroxylation takes place.

- **Epoxidation (about 25% conversion efficiency):**

This sort of conversion is nearly always associated with steroids.

Microorganisms that can do axial hydroxylation can likewise epoxidize a double bond at the same carbon atom.

For example, in the presence of Pseudomonas oleovorans, 1,7-octadiene is converted to 7,8-epoxy-1-octene.

Epoxidation happens at the C-7 and C-8 sites of 1,7-octadiene in this reaction.

- **Dehydrogenation (60% conversion efficiency):**

  In this reaction, conversion of a hydroxyl group to a carbonyl group takes place

  $$R\text{-}C\text{-}OH \Rightarrow R\text{-}C=O \text{ (dehydrogenation)}$$

  E.g., Gluacine is dehydrogenated to dehydrogluacine in presence of *Fusarium solani*

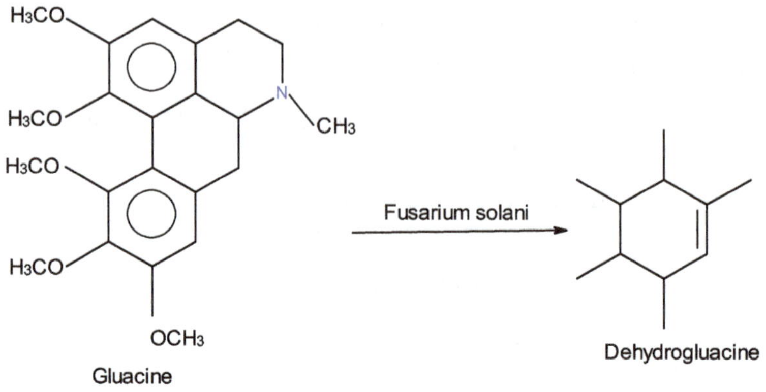

Fusarium solani

Gluacine

Dehydrogluacine

Oxidation of aliphatic side chains with the formation of aldehydes, ketones or carboxyl functions (80% conversion efficiency)

E.g., n-dodecylbenzene is oxidized to phenyl acetic acid in presence of *Nocardia sp.*

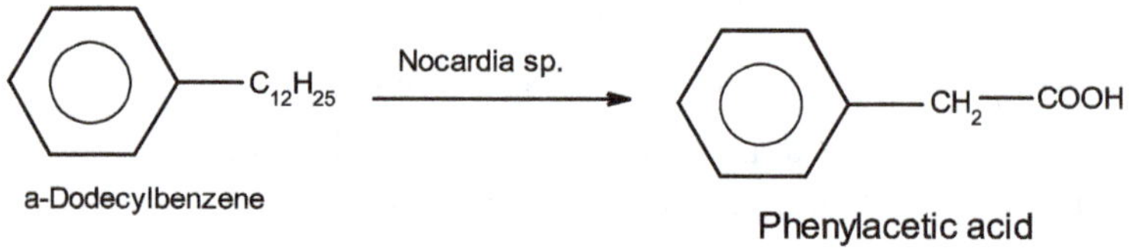

Nocardia sp.

a-Dodecylbenzene

Phenylacetic acid

Oxidative splitting of aromatic rings (70% conversion efficiency)

E.g., the conversion of naphthalene to salicylic acid by *Corynebacterium nov.sp.* In this reaction, one aromatic ring of naphthalene undergoes cleavage to form salicylic acid.

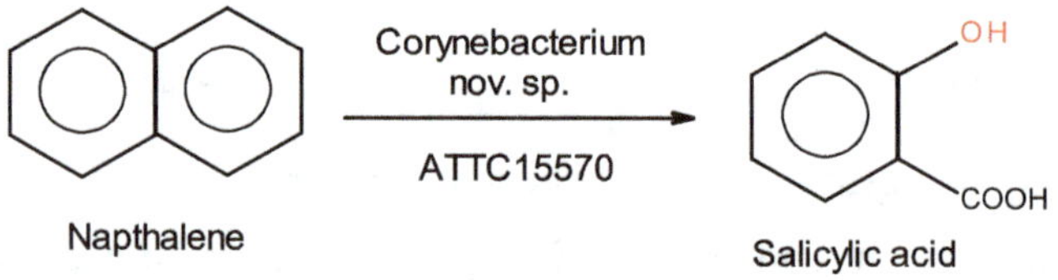

Corynebacterium nov. sp.

ATTC15570

Napthalene

Salicylic acid

Oxidation of heterofunctions: i.e., amino groups to nitro groups; formation of N-oxides and sulfoxides

E.g., the conversion of 2-amino-4-alkyl-imidazole to 2-nitro-4-alkyl-imidazole by *Streptomyces sp.*

2-Amino-4-alkyl-imidazole → Streptomyces sp. → 2-Nitro-4-alkyl-imidazole

where

$R_1 =$	$R_2 =$	Conversion efficiency (%)
H.	H.	
CH	H	50
OH	H	25
		36

Oxidative splitting of substituents i.e., oxidative deamination, N-CH 3 -demethylation, O-CH 3 -demethylation (100% conversion efficiency)

E.g., 10, 11-Dimethoxyaporphine conversion to Isoapocodeiene by *Cunnighamelle blaksleene*

10, 11-Dimethoxyaporphine → Cunnighamelle blakeclever ATCC 9245 → Isoapocodeine

II. Reduction reactions:

Reactions resulting in the addition of hydrogen and/or the removal of oxygen are reduction reactions. It includes following reactions.

Hydrogenation: Reduction   of   carbonyl   functions   i.e., R-C=O $\Rightarrow$ R-C-OH

E.g., Benzaldehyde is reduced to Benzyl alcohol by *Saccharomyces cerevisiae*

Reductive amination (also known as reductive alkylation) is a form of amination that involves the conversion of a carbonyl group to an amine via an intermediate imine. The carbonyl group is most commonly a ketone or an aldehyde

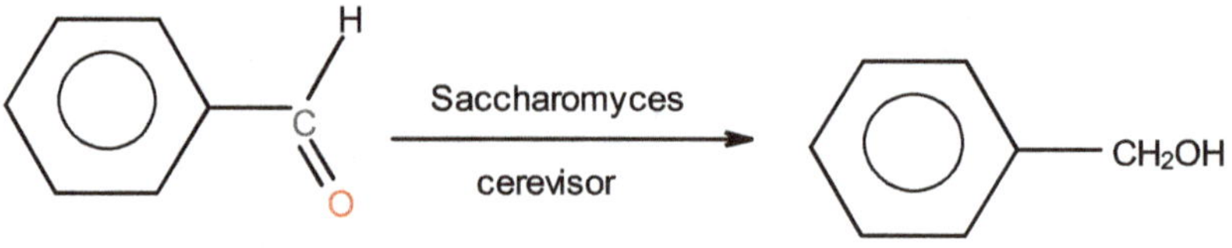

Benzaldehyde → (Saccharomyces cerevisor) → Benzyl alcohol

$$R-NO_2 \Rightarrow R-NH_2$$

$$R-NO_2 \Rightarrow R-NH_2$$

e.g., Nitropentachlorobenzene is converted to pentachloroaniline by *Streptomyces aurelociens*

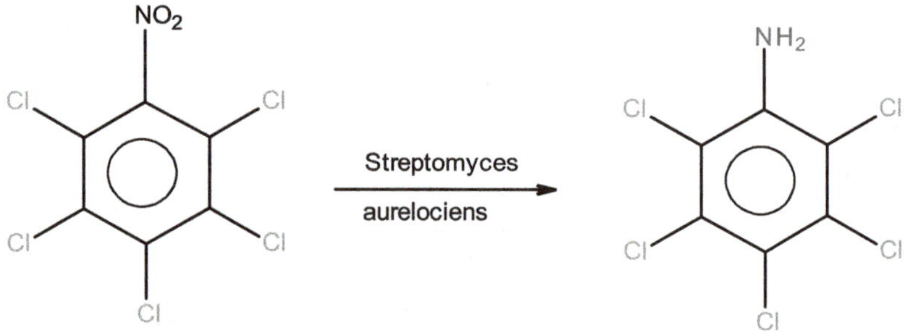

Nitropentachlorobenzene → (Streptomyces aurelociens) → Pentachloroaniline

III. Hydrolytic reactions:

A bond in a molecule is broken in a reaction with water, resulting in the formation of two compounds.

The water molecule splits in two at the same time, with hydrogen moving to one of the compounds and a hydroxide to the other.

$$R\text{-}COO\text{-}R' + H2O \quad R\text{-}COOH + R'\text{-}OH \quad R\text{-}COOH + R'\text{-}OH$$

$$R\text{-}COOH + R'\text{-}NH2 \quad R\text{-}COOH + R'\text{-}NH2 \quad R\text{-}COOH + R'\text{-}NH2 \quad R\text{-}COOH + R'\text{-}NH2 \quad R\text{-}COOH + R'\text{-}NH2 \quad R\text{-}COOH +$$

Hydration of carbon-carbon double bonds: For example, S. aureofaciens aids in the hydrolysis of anhydrotetracycline, allowing the C-C double bond between C-6 and C-5a to be broken and tetracycline to be obtained.

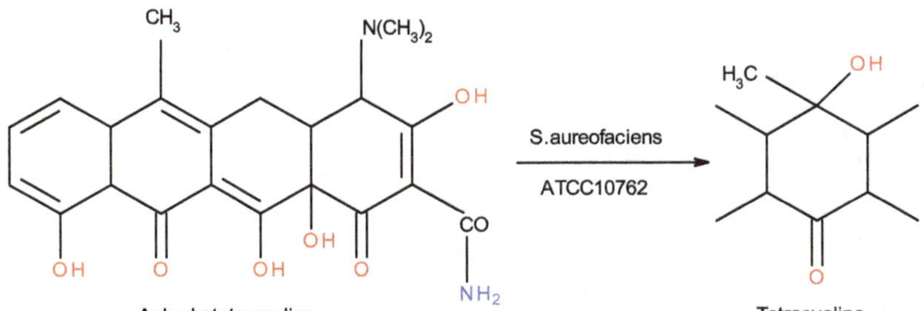

Anhydrotetracycline

S.aureofaciens
ATCC10762

Tetracycline

Hydrolysis of carboxylic acid esters:

E.g., Mycobacterium phlei aids in the hydrolysis of d,1-menthyl laureate into 1- menthol.

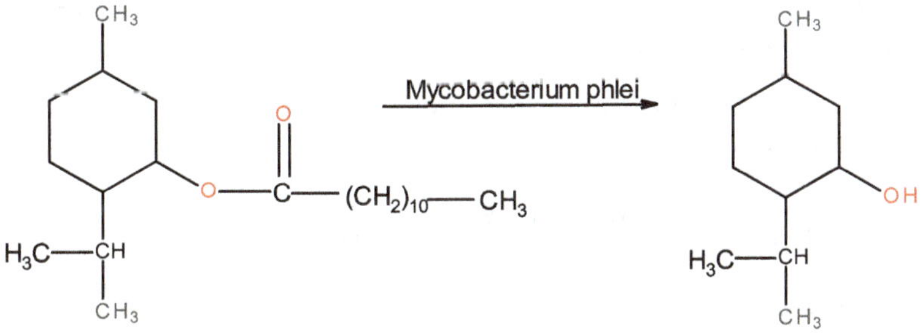

d,1-Menthyl laureate

Mycobacterium phlei

1-Menthol

Hydrolysis of N-derivatives:

E.g., Brevibacterium helps in the conversion of an alkyl nitrile to either an amide at pH 9 or a corresponding carboxylic acid.

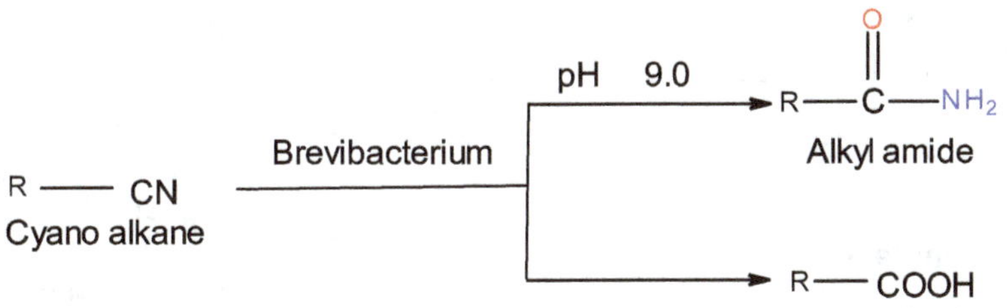

R —— CN
Cyano alkane

Brevibacterium

pH   9.0

$R—C(=O)—NH_2$
Alkyl amide

R—COOH
Carboxylic acid

Amination: Transformation of dihydroxyphenylpyruvic acid in to L-dopa can be performed by several micro-organisms using amination process

Dihydroxy phenyl pyruvic acid → (Cambacterium aurantiacun) → L-Dopa

IV. Condensation reactions:

When two or more molecules join to produce a bigger molecule, a minor molecule such as water or methanol is lost at the same time.

While this can happen in a variety of reactions, the term is mainly reserved for those that result in the formation of a new carbon-carbon bond.

Phosphorylation is the chemical process of adding a phosphoryl group (PO3-) to a molecule.

Streptomycin, for example, is phosphorylated by Streptomyces griseus to streptomycin-p.

$$\text{Streptomycin} \xrightarrow{\text{Streptomyces griseus}} \text{Streptomycin-P}$$

-N-Glycosidation:

E. coli helps in the N-glycosidation of 6-azauracil into 6-azauracil ribose due to the condensation reaction

6-azauracil → (E.coli ATCC 10798) → 6-Azauracil-riboside

O-glycosidation: Beauveria sulfurescens helps in the condensation of cyclofenil into methylglucopyranoside derivative.

4.4.1.7.2   The use of microbial biotransformation

Steroid biotransformation

- Steroids are a type of natural substance found in bile salts, adrenal-cortical and sex hormones, insect moulting hormones, sapogenins, alkaloids, and some antibiotics.

- The first microbial biotransformation of steroids took place in 1937.

- Corynebacterium sp. was used to make testosterone from dehydroepiandrosterone.

- Using Nocardia spp., cholesterol was synthesized from 4-dehydroeticholanic and 7-hydroxycholestrol.

The basic structure of all steroids is a cyclopentanoper-hydrophenanthrene, which is made up of four fused rings.

- Naturally occurring steroids, such as adrenal cortex hormones (cortisone, cortisol, corticosterone), progestational hormones (progesterone), androgens or male sex hormones (testosterone, dihydrotestosterone), and estrogens or female sex hormones (estradiol, estradiol, estradiol, estradiol, estradiol, estradiol, estradiol, estradiol.

- The biotransformation of steroids for the synthesis of steroid hormones is of major interest to the pharmaceutical sector.

- Steroid hormones and their derivatives have been utilized to treat a variety of ailments.

- Aside from their traditional uses as immunosuppressive, anti-inflammatory, anti-rheumatic, progestational, diurctic, sedative, anabolic, and contraceptive drugs, steroid compounds have recently been used to treat cancer, osteoporosis, HIV infections, and confirmed AIDS.

- Steroids are now one of the most important segments of the pharmaceutical industry, with global markets worth around $10 billion and annual production reaching 1,000000 tonnes.

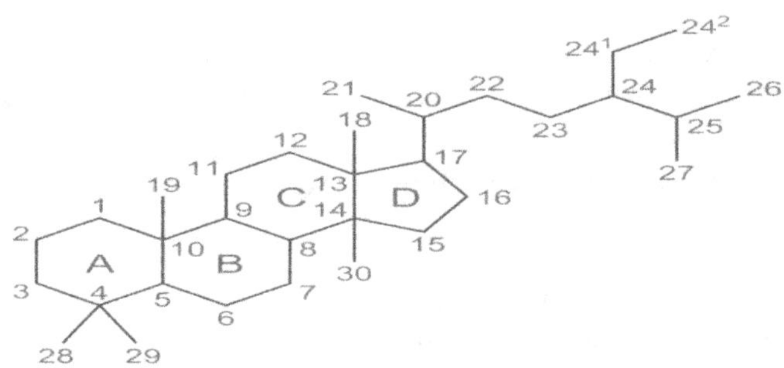

Fig. 4.16 Steroid structure

In the commercial manufacturing of testosterone and oestrogen, progesterone transformation of a C-19 steroid is used, and microbial dehydration of ring A is used in oestrogen production.

With the help of an enzyme called Arthrobacter simplex, the breakdown product 3-hydroxy-9,10-secoandrostatriene9,17-dione is formed from cholesterol via an opening of the B ring, with the formation of two important intermediate products, androstendione and androstadiendione.

4.4.2   Steroidal Transformation Types

I. REACTIONS TO OXIDATION:

- Hydroxylation is defined as the substitution of a hydroxyl group for a hydrogen atom at a specific position in a steroid, such as or, while maintaining the steroid's structure.

- The hydroxyl group gets its oxygen atom from molecular oxygen (gaseous), not from water. The stereochemical arrangement of the hydrogen atom that has been substituted is always retained by the hydroxyl group that is generated.

- For instance, certain microbes can attach hydroxyl groups to any of the steroid molecule's carbon atoms.

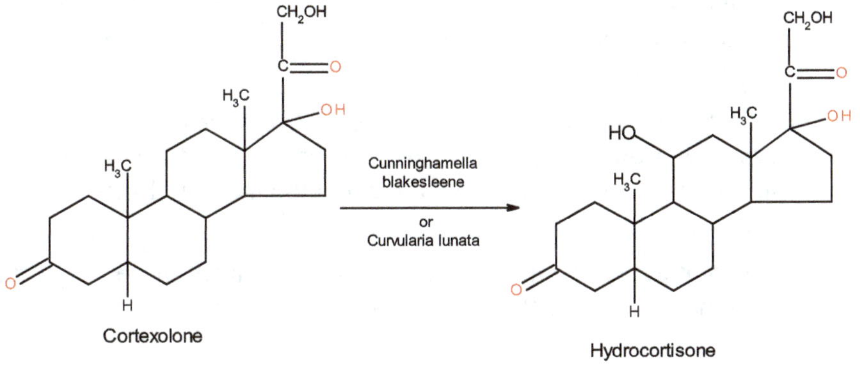

CH2OH
C
O
H3C
OH
H3C
O
H
Cortexolone
Cunninghamella
blakesleene
or
Curvularia lunata
HO
Hydrocortisone

- Fungi are the most active hydroxylating microorganisms, but some bacteria particularly the *Bacilli, Nocardia and Streptomyce*s show fair good activity.

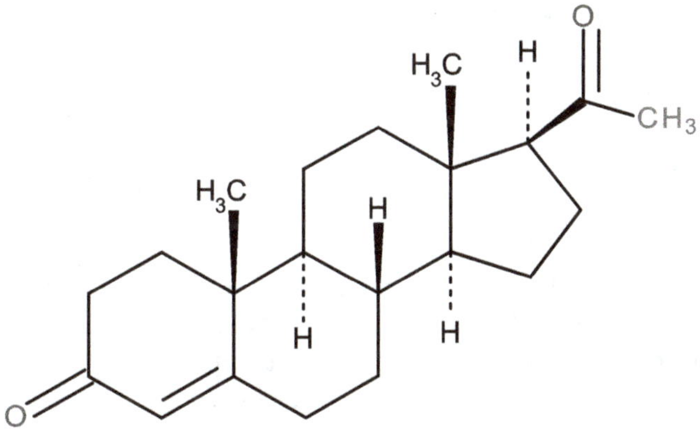

O
H3C
H
CH3
H

Progesterone

- Preliminary study on progesterone's 11 alpha-hydroxylation suggested that oxygen might be introduced into the steroid nucleus by bacteria in a site-specific and stereospecific manner without activation.
- These reactions were successful, allowing for the synthesis of cortisone at a low cost.

A. DEHYDROGENATION:

- All four rings of the steroid nucleus have been observed to dehydrate with the simultaneous insertion of a double bond, albeit the introduction of unsaturated bonds in Ring A is the only commercially important reaction.

- In 1955, Charney and colleagues discovered that inducing Corynebacterium simplex to dehydrogenate cortisol at the 1st position considerably enhanced the compound's anti-inflammatory capabilities.

- Prednisolone, the resulting chemical, was 3-5 times more active than the original drug and achieved similar *results*.

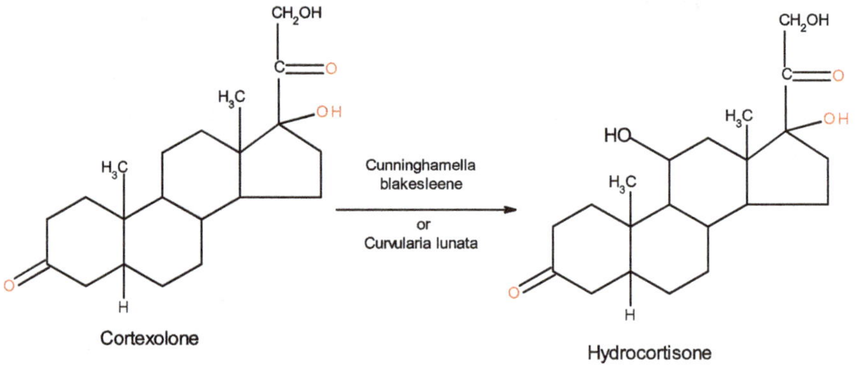

Cortexolone

Hydrocortisone

B. EPOXIDATION:

- The epoxidation of steroidal double bonds is a rare example of biological epoxidation. The 9, 11- epoxidation of 9(11)-dehydro-compounds, and the 14, 15-epoxidation of 14(15)-dehydrocompounds, using *Curvalaria lunata*.

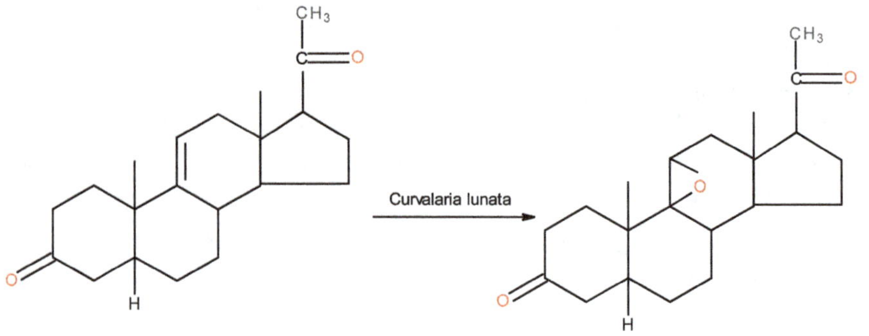

- Ring A Aromatization: Microbial aromatization of suitable steroid substrates can result in ring A aromatic compounds, particularly estrogens, which are an important component of oral contraceptives and play a key role in menopausal replacement therapy. With modest amounts of estradiol-17, cell free extracts of Pseudomonas testosterone may convert 19-nor-testosterone to estrone.

C. STEROID NUCLEUS DEGRADATION

- The aliphatic side chain of steroids is selectively removed during side chain degradation, leaving the steroidal nucleus intact.

- The enzyme responsible for the conversion is specifically blocked.

- Several organisms can break down the side chain to produce C-17 keto steroids, as shown below.

Side chain cleavage of cholesterol

D. STEROIDAL RING DEGRADATION

- The degradative product 3-hydroxy-9, 10-secondrosta-1,3,5(10) triene-9,17-dione is produced from cholesterol via a strategical cleavage of the ring B in the steroid nucleus, and generates androstendione and androstadiendione as intermediate products.

- Degradation of cholesterol by *Mycobacterium species* is restricted to side chain only when Ni^{2+} or Co^{2+} ions are added to the growth medium.

- *Aspergillus orchraceus* convert progesterone to 11- α - hydroxyprogesterone and this is further converted to 6- β -11- α - dihydroxy progesterone in the presence of Zn^{2+}. In the absence of Zn^{2+} only 11- α -hydroxyprogesterone is formed.

II. REDUCTION REACTIONS:

E.g., Reduction of aldehydes and ketones to alcohols

- Estrone is converted by *Streptomyces* to estradiol

A. Hydrolysis reactions:

E.g., Hydrolysis of esters- *Flavobacterium dehydrogenans* contain a specific enzyme acetolase which hydrolyses the steroidal acetates

1. Esterification:

- It usually involves acetylation process

  E.g., Androstenedione is esterified to testosterone acetate in the presence of *Sacromyces fragilis*

2. Prostaglandins undergo microbial transformation.

- These are hormones made up of C-20 unsaturated fatty acids.

- These include PGE-2, which is used as a contraceptive, PEG-2, which is used to relieve childbirth pain, PEG-1, which is used to treat congenital heart failure, and PEG-2, which is used to treat digestive problems.

- Microbial transformation with pathogenic fungus like Cryptococcus neoformans can create these prostaglandins from unsaturated fatty acids.

3. L-Ascorbic acid transformation by bacteria (vitamin C)

- Reichstein-Grussner synthesis is the name of the method that produces L-ascorbic acid.

- This multi-step microbial conversion process produces L-ascorbic acid, which is employed in vitamin manufacturing and as an antioxidant in food production.

- Acetobacter suboxydans performs the oxidation of D-sorbitol to L-sorbose in a submerged process at 30-35°C with vigorous stirring and aeration.

- The first phase involves Erwinia species oxidizing glucose to 2,5-diketo-D-gluconic acid via D-gluconic acid and 2-keto-D-gluconic acid;

- the second step involves Erwinia species oxidizing glucose to 2,5-diketo-D-gluconic acid via D-gluconic acid and 2-keto-D-gluconic acid.

- A Corynebacterium species catalyses the reduction of 2,5-DKG to 2-keto-1-gulonic acid in the second step.

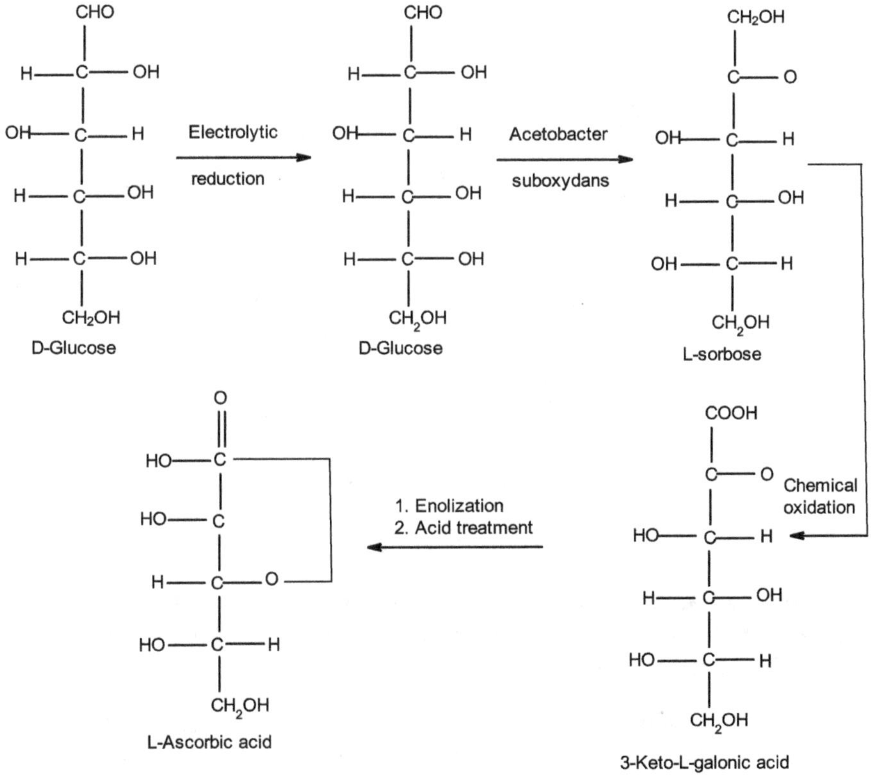

D-Glucose → (Electrolytic reduction) → D-Glucose → (Acetobacter suboxydans) → L-sorbose → (Chemical oxidation) → 3-Keto-L-galonic acid → (1. Enolization 2. Acid treatment) → L-Ascorbic acid

4. Antibiotic Microbial Transformation:

- The goal of microbial transformation of existing antibiotics is to generate novel, modified, and better antibiotics with properties such as lower toxicity, a broad antibacterial range, improved oral adsorption, and less resistant/allergic effects.

- Microorganisms can phosphorylate erythromycin, rendering it inactive.

- Streptomyces vendargensis glycolates and inactivates erythromycin, the final product of which is 2'-(0-[D-glucopyranosyl]) erythromycin A).

- A glycosylation system like this could safeguard macrolide-producing microorganisms during antibiotic production or serve as a method for pathogens to develop macrolide resistance.

1. Structures of compounds 1 (R - H) and 2 (R - glucose)

In most cases, any transformation step causes a partial or complete inactivation of antibiotic. Several typical examples of the many possible reactions are given here,

- Indirect transformation: Affected antibiotics are generated in the presence of inhibitors or changed precursors in the media during regulated biosynthesis.

- Streptomyces parvulus, for example, creates two novel actinomycin's that contain cis-4-methylproline instead of proline.

- When mutations that prevent the manufacturing of a certain antibiotic were utilized, new compounds were discovered.

- Only a few better antibiotics, such as 5-epi-sisomicin, have been developed using mutational synthesis and are currently being tested in clinical studies.

Direct transformation: The antibiotics were inactivated by hydrolysis of the functional groups.

However, in the instance of lankacidin-C-14-butyrate, a bioconversion product generated by Bacillus megaterium IFO 12108 from lankacidin C and methyl-butyrate, increased antibacterial activity was found with lesser toxicity.

5. Glycoside transformation by bacteria:

- For example, Eubacterium lentum Cultures Reductively Inactivate Digitoxin.

- By reducing the double bond in the lactone ring, the anaerobe Eubacterium lentum inactivates the cardiac glycoside digitoxin.

- When the substrate was incubated at a concentration of 10 mcg/ml, the conversion was quantitative.

- **On the biotransformation of phenol and monofluorophenols by the cultured cells of *Eucalyptus perriniana*, phenyl and fluorophenyl β -D-glucosides were isolated after a 1-h incubation.**

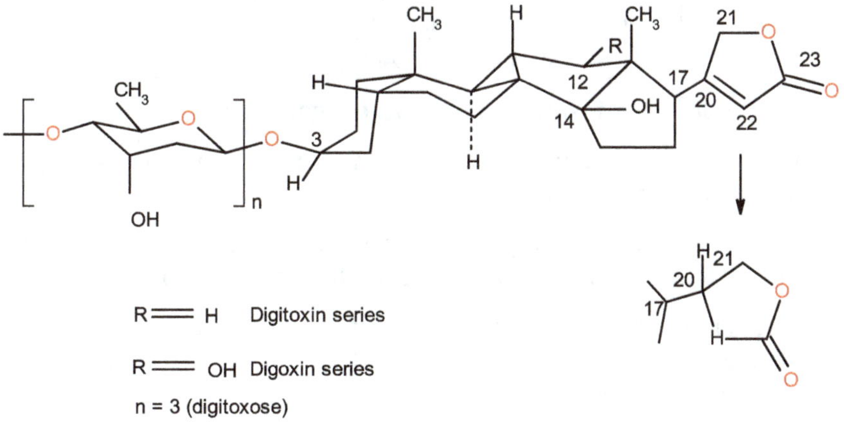

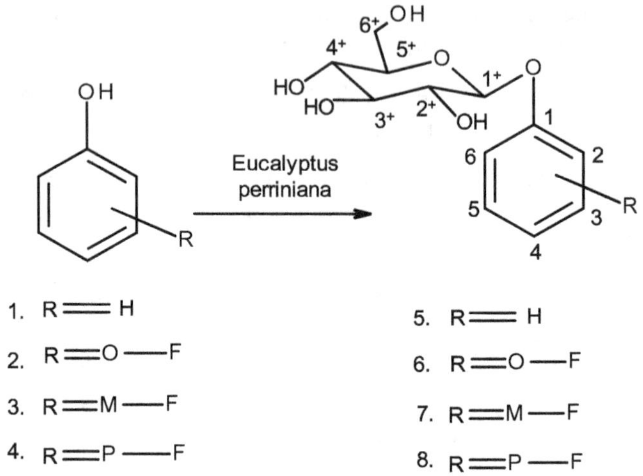

Fig. 4.17 diagram — Eucalyptus perriniana biotransformation

Fig. 4.17 Biotransformation of 1-4 by the cultured cells of E. Perriniana. 1. Phenol, 2. 2-fluorophenol, 3. 3-fluorophenol, 4. 4-fluorophenol, 5. Phenyl β-D-glucoside, 6. 2-fluorophenyl β-D-glucoside, 7. 3-fluorophenyl β -D-glucoside, 8. 4-fluorophenyl β-D-glucoside

Table 4.6 The glucosylation of 1-4 by the cultured cells of E.perriniana

	Product	Yield (%)*
1	Phenyl-1-β-D-glucoside (5)	17.2
2	2-Fluorophenyl-β-D-glucoside (6)	49.2
3	3-Fluorophenyl β-D-glucoside (7)	19.6
4	4-Fluorophenyl β-D-glucoside (8)	28.0

6. Pesticide Transformation by Microorganisms:

- Plant disease and pest control agents are essential for the world's population's existence.

- High compound stability is necessary for vector control systems, yet this stability has a negative impact on the environment.

- Microbial transformation is of interest in this regard, not for the generation of new active agents, but for the maximum feasible environmental detoxification.

- This entails xenobiotic enzymatic transformations.

- Xenobiotics can be removed from the ecosystem using a variety of methods.

Metabolism: Xenobiotics can be used as microbial growth and energy production substrates.

- Some substrates are completely broken down into carbon dioxide and water.

- Arthrobacter species, for example, transform the herbicide dalapon (a chlorinated fatty acid) into pyruvate. Co-metabolism: Co-metabolism usually results in a simple change of molecules, which can lead to a decrease or increase in toxicity.

- The microorganisms involved do not acquire energy from the transformation reaction and must thrive on a different substrate.

- The combined action of various organisms can result in the complete disintegration of a chemical.

- Dehalogenation events, for example, are key cometabolism reactions that may allow pesticide molecules to be broken down further.

- Because of their intricate structure and high degree of halogenation, some chemicals, such as chlordecone, a hexachlorocyclopentadiene derivative with outstanding insecticide properties, are difficult for microbes to attack.

7. Pollutant Transformation by Microbes

- In recent years, there has been a lot of interest in employing microorganisms to biotransform various toxins in order to clean up the polluted environment.

- A wide range of chemicals, including polyaromatic hydrocarbons (PAHs), pharmaceuticals, radionuclides, hydrocarbons (e.g., oil), and polychlorinated biphenyls, have been bioremediated using the catabolic diversity of bacteria (PCBs).

- The biotransformation of a wide spectrum of xenobiotic compounds has been linked to both aerobic and anaerobic bacterium species discovered.

- Aerobic genera include Bacillus, Pseudomonas, Escherichia, Rhodococcus, Gordonia, Moraxella, Micrococcus, and Methanospirillum, Pelatomaculum, Syntrophobacter, Desulfotomaculum, Syntrophus, Desulfovibrio, and Methanosaeta, while anaerobic genera include Methanospirillum, Pelatomaculum, Syntropho

- Acetone, cyclohexane, styrene, benzene, ethylbenzene, propylbenzene, dioxane, and 1,2-dichloroethylene have all been catabolized by Mycobacterium vaccae. PCB (Polychlorinated Biphenyls) are known to be easily degraded by Pseudomonas and Bacillus.

- Pseudomonas, Acetobacter, and Klebsiella bacteria have also been found to be capable of bio-fixing carcinogenic azo-compounds.

- Pseudomonas BCb12/1 and BCb12/3 have been discovered to have outstanding low ethoxylated NPnEO degrading abilities (Non phenol Polyethoxylates).

- The breakdown of Phthalate molecule is primarily carried out by anaerobic methanogens (Methanospirillum hungatei, Methanosaeta concilii, Syntrophobacter fumaroxidans).

- Cunninghamella elegans, Pseudomonas knackmussii, and Pseudomonas pseudoalcaligenes KF707 have recently been found to be capable of biotransforming potential contaminants containing the pentafluorosulfanyl (SF5-) functional group.

Biotransformation of petroleum:

- Hydrocarbons derived from petroleum are the lifeblood of our industries and daily lives.

- However, one of the most pressing concerns of days is the hydrocarbon contamination caused by petrochemical industry activities.

- Many aquatic and marine microflora have been shown to play an essential part in oil spill biodegradation by breaking down oil pollutants into harmless forms.

- Bacteria, yeast, and fungi are the primary biotransformers of petroleum hydrocarbons.

- Bacterial taxa include Rhodococcus, Pseudomonas, Arthrobacter, and Mycobacterium are active degraders of petroleum hydrocarbons by alkylaromatic degradation.

- Gordonia, Brevibacterium, Corynebacterium sp., Flavobacterium sp., Pseudomonas fluorescens, Pseudomonas aeruginosa, Actinocorallia,

Klebsiella, Rhizobium, Bacillus sp., and Alcaligenes sp., Aeromicrobium, Dietzia, Burkholderia, and

- sAspergillus, Penicillium, Talaromyces, Amorphoteca, Neosartorya, and Cephalosporium have all been isolated from petroleum sites and have been shown to play a vital role.

4.5   Mutagenesis and its Types

Genetics includes the study of the inheritance (heredity) and the variability of the characteristics of an organism. Inheritance is based on genes that are faithfully transmitted from parents to offspring during reproduction. Nevertheless, "mistakes" the changes in the genetic material do occur. Such sudden, heritable change in the genetic material are called mutations.

In 1880s, for the first time Hugo de Vries (1848-1935), a Dutch botanist, one of the independent rediscoveries of Mendelism, put forward his views regarding the formation of new species in 1901. He used the term mutation to describe the phenotypic changes in evening primrose, *Oenothera lamarckiana*.

The term mutation is derived from the Latin word *mutare* means to change.

Mutation refers to any heritable change in nucleotide sequence of a gene of the organisms irrespective of altered phenotypic expression of characters of the organisms.

When a bacterial cell divides, the two daughter cells are generally indistinguishable. Thus, a single bacterial cell can produce a large population of identical cells or clone. On solid medium, a clone is manifested as an easily isolated colony. Occasionally, a spontaneous genetic change occurs in one of the cells. This change (**mutation**) is heritable and passed on to the progeny of the variant cell to produce a **subclone** with characteristics different from the original (**wild type**) parent. This is termed **vertical inheritance**. If the change is detrimental to the growth of the cell, the subclone will quickly be overrun by the healthy, wild type population. However, if the change is beneficial, the subclone may overtake the wild type population. This is an example of how evolution is directed by **natural selection**.

The term mutation refers both to the change in the genetic material and to the process by which the change occurs. These changes are associated with the two fundamental properties of the cell (or) organism, namely the genotype and the phenotype.

The genotype refers to the genetic constitution of the cell. The phenotype is the expression of the genotype in observable properties characteristics of the cell (or) organism. The genotype of a culture of cells remains relatively constant during the growth. However, it can change by mutation. This change can result in an alteration in the observable properties (or) phenotype of the cells.

Spontaneous Mutations occurs without known cause, they are resulting from an inherent low level of metabolic errors that is mistakes during DNA replication. Induced mutations are resulting from exposure of organisms to mutagenic agents such as ionizing radiations and various chemicals that react with DNA. Spontaneous mutations occur infrequently, although the observed frequencies vary from gene to gene and from organism. Treatment with mutagenic agents can increase mutation frequencies by orders of magnitude.

Mutagens: Mutagens are chemical (or) physical agents that increase the frequency at which mutations occur during the growth of culture.

Mutation that occurs due to physical agents is called physical mutagenesis, if it is due to chemical agents then it is referred as chemical mutagenesis. These mutagens act in one (or) the other of two quite different ways.

1. Some Chemical mutagens become associated with the DNA that are called intercalating agents (or) some incorporated into it called base analogues.

2. A large variety of other mutagens are reacting mutagens which react chemically with DNA – usually with one of its purine (or) pyrimidine bases.

4.5.1   Chemical Mutagens

Table 4.7 Chemical Mutagens

Class	Example
Aziridines	Ethyleneimine
Mustard-Ist mutations identified	N$_2$ mustard, sulphur mustard
Epoxides	Ethyleneoxide, diepoxybutane
Miscellaneous	Hydroxylamine

DNA repair mechanisms: DNA damage can occur by UV radiation, x-rays and certain chemicals. Cells contain specific enzymes which can repair damaged DNA.

♦ Many kinds of bacterial cells and yeasts have been shown to possess an efficient photo reactivating mechanism for repairing damages caused by UV radiation.

♦ Photoreactivation occurs when cells exposed to lethal doses of UV light are immediately exposed to visible light. A special enzyme designated PRE, induced by visible light, splits or unlinks the dimers formed because of exposure to UV light and restores the DNA to its original state.

Excision repair: Some bacteria have enzymes called endonucleas and exonucleases that excise or cut out a damaged segment of DNA.

♦ Enzymes such as polymerases and ligases, repair the resulting break by filling in the gap and joining the fragments together. This mechanism is termed as excision repair.

SOS repair: SOS (save our soul) repair is a by-pass repair system. It is also called emergency repair. The process by which *E.coil* repairs large amounts of DNA damage is called inducible or SOS repair. This process is not a single discrete mechanism but includes diverse responses such as the ability to repair pyrimidine dimers, to induce various prophages, to shut off respiration, and to delay septum formation during cell division. The process is a very efficient one; however, it tends to insert mismatched bases and thus is error prone and introduces additional mutation.

Intercalating agents: These are planar molecule and can insert between the stacked pairs of bases in the core of DNA molecule. Such incorporation distorts the backbone of the double helix results in frame – shift mutations when the distorted helix is replicated.

Base analogues: Mechanism of mutagenic action of base analogues can be illustrated by considering example of 2-aminopurine which is commonly used mutagen. In its usual amino form it pairs with thyme and in imino form it pairs with cytosine. Thus it usually has paring properties like adenine, but the probability of its being in the imino form is greater.

4.5.2   Physical Mutagens

Mutations also results from ionizing and non-inoizing radiations. H. J. Muller was the person who first demonstrated that mutation could be induced by an external factor. Examples for ionizing radiations are penetration into living tissues. The high energy rays collide with the atoms and cause the release of electrons, leaving positively changed free radicals (or) ions. These ions in turn collide with other molecules, causing the release of further electrons. The net result is that a "core" of ions is formed. This process of ionization is induced by X-rays, protons and neutrons as well as alpha, beta and gamma rays replaced by radioactive isotopes of the elements ^{32}P, ^{35}S and cobalt-90.

Mechanism of X-rays (Ionizing radiations)

These ionizing radiations produce gross changes in structure of the chromosome. These changes in chromosome structure result from breaks in chromosome caused by ionizing radiations. For example X-rays causes breakage of covalent bonding.

Ultra-Violet Radiations

In contrast to X-rays, they do not pocess sufficient energy to induce ionization. However they are readily absorbed by purines and pyrimidines which then enter a more reactive (or) excited state. Because of their lower energy they penetrate tissues slightly, only the surface layers of cells in muticellular organisms.

The maximum absorption of UV by DNA is at wavelength of 254 nm. The principal damage caused by UV light is the formation of pyrimidine dimers, the most common being thymine dimers between adjacent bases which causes a distortion of DNA helix.

4.5.3 Occurrence of Mutations

Mutations most commonly occur during DNA replication. The occurrence of mutation may be spontaneous or induced.

Spontaneous mutations: This type of mutation is commonly referred as Naturally occurring mutation. The best example for spontaneous mutation is Tautomerism (changing from one form to another, keto – enol and vice versa).

Induced mutations: Any agent that increases the mutation rate is called as mutagen. Mutations obtained by the use of a mutagen are said to be induced.

◆ The major effect of UV light is to cause the formation of dimers by cross linking between adjacent pyrimidine, especially thymine, residues in DNA. These cross linked residues disrupt the normal process of replication.

◆ When X rays interact with DNA, the result is usually a break in the phosphodiester backbone of the nucleic acid.

4.5.4 Features of Spontaneous Mutations

Mutations can arise for number of reasons

1. Errors in DNA replication

2. Physical damage of DNA

3. Chemical damage

4. Recombination and transposition.

One main cause of spontaneous mutations results from the fact that bases can exist as different forms called tautomers, which are capable of forming different base pairs. During replication, adenine, which normally base-pairs with thymine in its normal amino form, switches to its rate imino form (tautomerism) and base pairs with cytosine instead of thymine. If this error is not repaired before the next round of replication the A-T base pair will change to a G-C base pair.

Adenine Base Tautomerization Adenine (aminoform) (iminoform)

Base-pairs with thymine Base-pairs with cytosine

Adenine changes from amino to imino form reverts to aminoform

Fig: Spontaneous mutations of as A-T base pair to G-C as result of adenine base tautomerization.

4.5.5   DNA Repair Mechanisms

Damaged DNA resulted due to the mutations can be repaired by three mechanisms.

1. Photoreactivation (PR)

2. Excision repair

3. Post replication recombination repair

1. Photo reactivation mechanism used in breaking of thymine dimers resulted from UV induced mutions. PR involves an enzyme that splits the thymine dimers by binding in the presence of visible light, specifically light within the blue region of the spectrum.

2. Endonuclease catalyses the first step, they recognizes the thymine dimers & cleaves the posphodiester backbone of the DNA strand containing the dimmer at a site near the damage. An Exo-nuclease then removes a segment of strand adjacent to the Endo-nuclease including dimmer. A DNA polymerase (DNA poly I) then fills the gap using complementary strand as a template. At last DNA ligase then catalyzes closer of final phosphor-diester linkage between adjacent nucleotides.

3. The third type of dark repair of UV damage involves both replication and recombination, that is why it is called a post replication recombination repair. When DNA molecules containing thymine dimers are replicated, gaps are formed in the nascent complementary strands opposite the dimers because DNA polymerases cannot use the distorted strands of a template. After a lag due to the thymine dimmer blockage replication is reinitiated at secondary initiation sites beyond the dimmer. This results in progeny double helices with thymine dimers in one strand and gaps in the complementary strand. If these two "sister" chromosomes recombine such that the dimers and gaps end up in one chromosome and the intact undamaged segments end up in the other chromosome, the latter will be functional and produce viable cell.

4.5.6   Types of Mutations

Two common types of mutations (Fig 4.18) are point mutations and frameshift mutations.

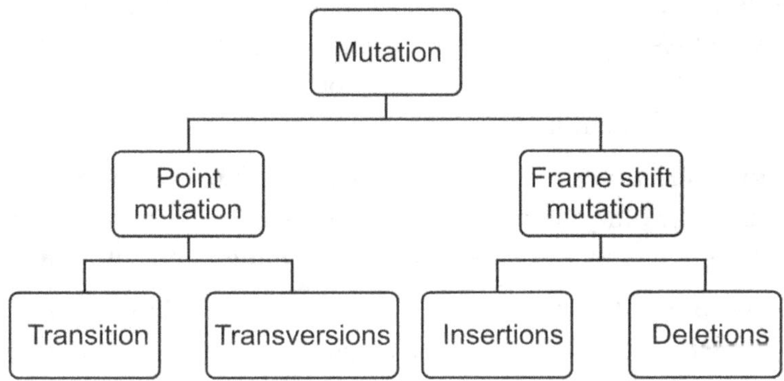

Fig. 4.18 Classification of mutations

1. **Point Mutations:** Point mutations occur as a result of the substitution of one nucleotide for another in the specific nucleotide sequence of a gene.

   Transition: Mutations resulting from tautomeric shifts in the bases of DNA involve the replacement of purine in one strand of DNA with the purine and the replacement of pyrimidine in the complementary strands with other pyrimidine. Such base pair substitutions are called transitions. The substitution of one purine for another purine or one pyrimidine for another pyrimidine is termed as Transition.

   Transversion: The replacement of a purine by a pyrimidine, or vice versa is termed as Transversion.

   This base-pair substitution may result in one of three kinds of mutations affecting the translation process.

   (i)   Missense mutation

   (ii) Nonsense mutation

   (iii) Neutral mutation

Missense mutation: The altered gene triplet produces a codon in the mRNA which specifies an aminoacid different from the one present in the normal protein. This mutation is called as missense mutation. *Ex:* Sickle cell anaemia.

Nonsense mutation: This type of mutation occurs due to incomplete protein synthesis i.e., premature termination of protein formation during translation. As a result of this mutation an incomplete polypeptide is formed which is nonfunctional.

Neutral mutation: The altered gene triplet produces a mRNA codon which specifies the same amino acid because the codon resulting from mutation is a synonym for the original codon this is a neutral mutation.

2. **Frameshift Mutations:** They involve the addition (or) deletion of one (or) few base pairs. Base pair additions and deletions are combinedly referred to as frameshift mutations. These mutations alter the reading frame of all base-pair triplets in the gene.

In prokaryotes large proportions of spontaneous mutations are occurring and they are found to be single base pair insertions (additions) and deletions rather than base-pair substitutions.

These mutations result from an addition or loss of one or more nucleotide in a gene and are termed insertion or deletion mutation respectively. This results in a shift of the reading frame.

♦ Frame shift mutations generally lead to nonfunctional proteins, because, entirely new sequence of amino acids is synthesized from a frame shift reading of the nucleotide sequences of mRNA shown in Fig. 4.18.

4.5.7   Detection and Isolation of Mutants

Mutation occurring in micro-organisms can be detected and efficiently isolated from the parent organisms of other mutants. Awareness of wild type characters of an organism is essential for studying mutation so that mutants can easily be detected. Since, mutations are rare about one per 10^7 to 10^{11} cells, it is very important to have a very sensitive detection system so that the rare mutant may not be missed from detection.

Some of the methods of detection have been described as below.

4.5.8   Replica Plating Technique

This technique is used to detect auxotrophic mutants which differentiates between mutants and wild type strains on the basis of ability to grow in the absence of an amino acid. Isolation of a leucine auxotroph through replica plating follows the following steps

(i)   Generates the mutants by treating a culture with a mutagen.

   e.g., nitrosoguanidine

(ii)   Inoculate a plate containing complete growth medium and incubate it at proper temperature. Both wild type and mutant survivors will form colonies on the complete medium. This plate containing complete medium is called masterplate.

(iii)   Prepare a piece of sterile velvet (Fig. 4.19) and gently press on upper surface of master plate to pick up bacterial cells from each colony. As pressed on master plate, again gently press the velvet on replica plates containing complete medium in one set and lacking only leucine in the other set. Thus, the bacterial cells are transferred in replica plates in the same position as in master plate.

(iv)   Incubate the plates and compare the replica plates with master plate for the bacterial colony not growing on replica plate. The leucine auxotrophs (Leu⁻) will not grow on replica plates devoid of leucine. Isolate and culture Leu⁻ cells growing on complete medium.

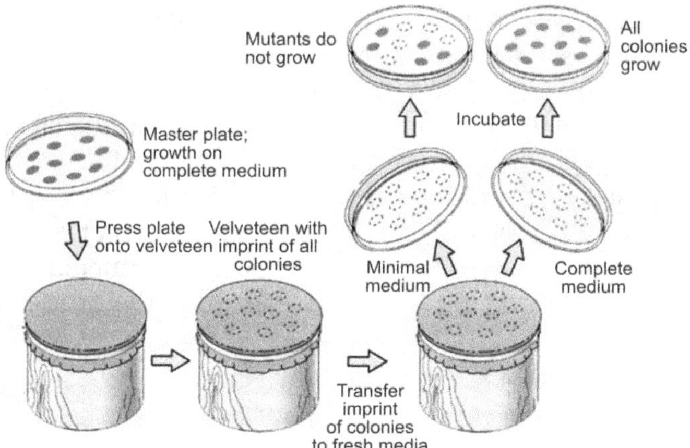

Fig. 4.19 Replice plating technique for isolation of mutants

Replica plating can also be used to isolate the temperature sensitive mutants. It involves by forming colonies at 30 °C and then transferring these colonies on two plates, one incubated at 30 °C and the other at 42 °C. The colony which grow at 30 °C and absent at 42 °C certainly consist of temperature sensitive mutant.

4.5.9   Resistance Selection Method

It is the other approach for isolation of mutants. Generally the wild type cells are not resistant either to antibiotics or bacteriophages. Therefore, it is possible to grow the bacterium in the presence of the agent (antibiotics or bacteriophage and 100k for survivors). This method is applied for islolation of mutants resistant to any chemical compounds that can be amended in agar, phage resistant mutants.

4.5.10   Substrate Utilization Method

This method is employed in the selection of bacteria. Several bacteria utilize only a few primary carbon sources. The cultures are plated onto a medium containing an alternate carbon sources. Any colony that grows on medium can use the substrate and are possibly mutants. These can be isolated.

Sugar utilization mutants are also isolated by means of colour indicator plates. A popular medium (EMB agar) is used for this purpose. EMB agar contains two dyes eosin and methylene blue in the medium. Colour of these dyes is sensitive to pH. This medium also contain lactose sugar as carbon source and complete mixture of aminoacids. Therefore, both lactose wild type (Lac^+) and lactose mutant (Lac^-) cells can grow and form colonies on EMB agar plates. The Lac^+ cells catabolize lactose and secrete acids, therefore, local pH of the medium decreases. This results in staining of colony to dark purple. On the other hand, Lac^- cells are unable to utilize lactose and use some of the aminoacids as carbon source. After utilization of aminoacid, possibly ammonia is produced that increases the local p^H and decolourizes the dye resulting in white colony.

4.5.11   Carcinogenicity Test

This method is based on detecting potential of carcinogens and testing for mutagenicity in bacteria. Ames et al. (1973) developed a method for deletion of mutagenicity of carcinogens which is commonly known as Ames test. It is widely used to detect the carcinogens. The Ames test is a mutational reversion assay in which several special strains of *salmonella typhimurium* are employed. Each strain contains a different mutation in the operon of histidine biosynthesis.

The Ames test employs the following steps:

(i)   Prepare the culture of *salmonella* histindine auxotrophs (His⁻)

(ii)   Mix the bacterial cells and test substance (mutagen) in dilute; molten the top agar with a small amount of histidine in one set, and control with complete medium plus large amount of histidine.

(iii)   Pour the molten mix on the top of minimal agar plates and incubate at 37°C for 2-3 days. Until histidine is depleted all the His⁻ cells will grow in the presence of test mutagens. When histidine is completely the original wild type characters) will grow on agar plate. The number of spontaneous reverants is low, whereas the number of reverants induced by the test mutagen is quite high. To estimate the relative mutagenicity of the mutagenic substance the visible colonies are counted and compared with control. The high number of colonies represents the greater mutagenicity.

A mammalian liver extract is added to the above molten top agar before plating. The extract converts the carcinogens into electrophilic derivatives which will soon react with DNA molecule. In natural way this process occurs in mammalian system when foreign substances are metabolized in the liver does, therefore, the liver extract is added to this test, just to promote the transformation shown in Fig. 4.20.

The Ames test has now been used with thousands of substances and mixtures such as the industrial chemicals, food additives, pesticides, hair dyes and cosmetics.

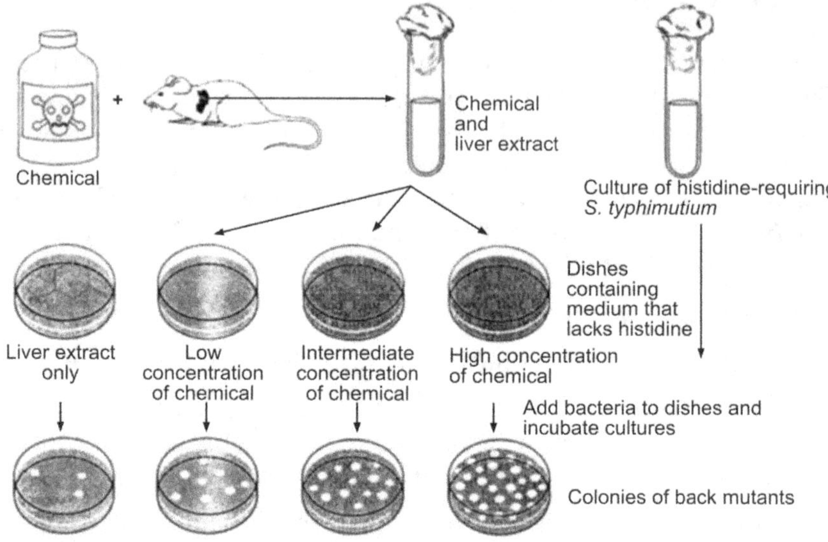

Fig. 4.20 The Ames test

4.6   DNA Replication

Bacteria are almost always haploid, which means that their chromosomes are unpaired. In contrast, most eukaryotic cells are diploid, they have paired homologous chromosomes which may be heterozygous (carry different alleles or genus occupying the same relative locus on homologous chromosomes) shown in Fig. 4.19.

♦ All bacteria have their genetic loci in a single linkage group; that is, they have a single chromosome per genome.

♦ The chromosome of a typical bacterium is a circular double stranded DNA molecule; that is, the double helix for a complete genome has no free ends.

♦ The circular chromosome is further twisted on itself in the bacterial cell to form a supercoil.

♦ It has an approximate molecular weight of 2.5×10^9 Daltons and has about 4×10^6 base pairs.

There are three general methods of replication of the DNA molecule.

Theta mode: The replication of a circular DNA molecule is initiated at a certain point called the origin, which is specific for each bacterial species.

♦ Replication proceeds in two directions around the chromosome, leading to the formation of a "bubble" which increases in size as replication proceeds. This mode is called theta because intermediate structures resemble the Greek letter θ.

♦ In this process, a circular parental chromosome is replicated to two circular daughter chromosomes, in each of which one strand of the parental DNA molecule is conserved and a complementary strand is newly synthesized.

Sigma (σ) or "Rolling circle" mode: Replication begins with the cleavage of phosphodiester bond in one strand of the circular DNA molecule to produce a nick with $3' - OH$ and $5' - po_4$ ends on that strand.

♦ The complimentary circular strand then serves as template for the synthesis of a new strand. As this strand grows at the $3' - OH$ end, the $5' - po_4$ end of the some strand is displaced to form a "tail" on the circle.

♦ As the replication proceeds, a circular parental molecule is converted to two daughter molecules, one circular and the other linear. This mode is called sigma because intermediate structures have the Greek letter σ conformation.

♦ The sigma mode of DNA molecule replication is carried out by some bacteriophages, such as λ and $\phi \times 174$ whose progeny viral DNA is linear.

Linear mode: All eukaryotic organisms and some viruses have linear DNA molecules. Replication of these chromosomes is initiated at specific sites by the formation of replication bubbles.

♦ Small viral linear DNA molecules may have only one point of initiation points per molecule.

♦ Large DNA molecules of eukaryotes may have hundreds of initiation points per molecule.

♦ A replication bubble grows in size as DNA replication (Fig. 4.22) proceeds from the point of initiation. Adjacent bubbles fuse to form larger ones as replication proceeds.

- Upon completion of replication, two linear double-helical daughter molecules are formed from one linear parental molecule.

- Prokaryotes replicate their DNA from one origin or growing point per molecule while eukaryotes replicate from many origins per molecule.

- Replication may occur in either a unidirectional or bidirectional manner from each origin.

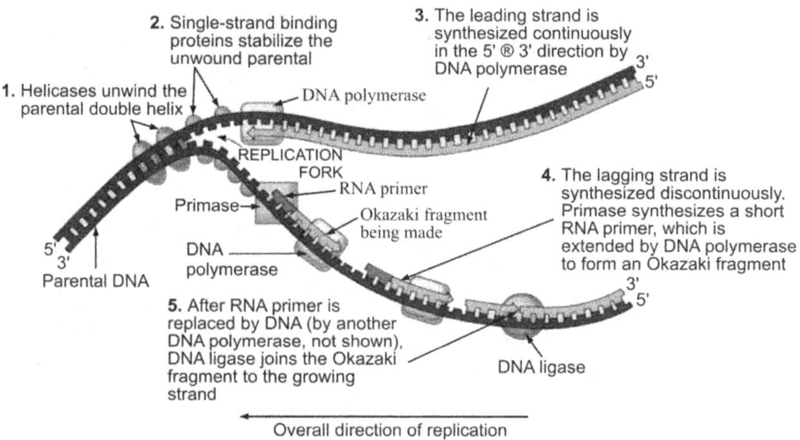

Fig. 4.21 A Summary of DNA replication

Events at the growing point (Replication Fork)

- At the growing point both DNA strands are duplicated.

- Prokaryotic DNA strands are synthesized at the rate of about 1000 nucleotides per second, at a replication fork.

- Eukaryotic DNA strands are synthesized more slowly at about 100 nucleotides per second.

- Many enzymes are involved in this synthesis; they are helix-unwinding protein (ATP-dependent), a helix-destabilizing protein, and a helix-relaxing protein (DNA gyrase). These enzymes participate on opening the parental DNA helix, a head of the replication fork.

- DNA replication is discontinuous, that is, the strands are replicated in small fragments called "Okazaki" fragments, in the 5'-3' direction.

- Initiation of DNA replication requires a primer, a short sequence of RNA that is synthesized by RNA polymerase and is complementary to the DNA which serves as a template.

4.7   Transcription (RNA Synthesis)

DNA itself cannot directly order for the synthesis of aminoacids but forms its transcripts first which is then translated into protein. For the first time in 1958 F. crick suggested that there is unidirectional flow of information from DNA to RNA to protein.

This sequential transfer of information from DNA to protein via RNA is known as central dogma.

♦ The tRNA, mRNA and rRNA are involved in the process of transcription. However an enzyme transcriptase i.e. DNA-dependent RNA polymerase is required for the synthesis of RNA by using ribonucleotide triphosphates i.e., ATP, GTP, CTP and UTP.

♦ The synthesis of RNA is different from that of DNA in the following features.

(i)   Only one of the two strands of any given segment of DNA serves as the template.

(ii) Only specific, relatively short lengths of DNA are transcribed i.e., and RNA chain is a transcript of a short section of DNA.

♦ Transcription is the first step in gene expression. The process involves separation of the two DNA strands, one of which serves as a template for the synthesis of a complementary strand of mRNA by DNA-dependent RNA polymerse.

Transcription stages: Transcription involves 3 steps shown in Fig. 4.23.

1. Initiation
2. Elongation
3. Termination

Initiation: The enzyme RNA polymerase plays a key role in recognition and binding of initiation site. Transcription initiated at specific sites on the bacterial chromosome that are defined by short sequences of bases of DNA called promoters. RNA polymerase binds to the promoter over a relatively long region intending from approximately 45 base pairs upstream from the point at which transcription is transcription/mRNA synthesis.

Elongation: once initiated σ factor is released and binds to another core enzyme.

♦ When both core enzyme and sigma particle are combined there it is called as holoenzyme.

Termination: Termination of mRNA synthesis is also at specific regulatory sequences of DNA nucleotides along the DNA molecule which are recognized by the RNA polymerase. Furthermore, a tetrameric protein factor called the rhofactor binds to RNA polymerase and promotes its termination.

There are two types of mechanisms that brings about termination.

(i)   Rho-independent termination

(ii) Rho-dependent termination.

Rho-independent termination: The Rho-independent signal for termination is recognized by DNA itself. RNA forms a hair pin loop like structure.

Rho-dependent termination: This termination requires the Rho protein encode by rhogene. The Rho factor is a hexamer. Rho factor moves along RNA from its binding site to the enzyme RNA polymerase. The movement is facilitated by the hydrolysis of ATP that provides energy, which is required for the separation of core enzyme, RNA.

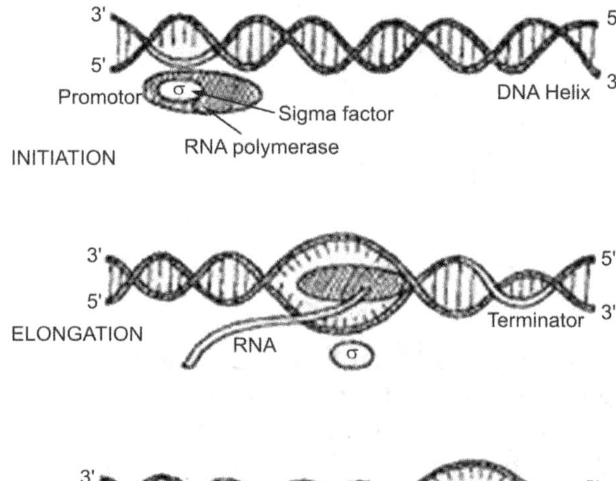

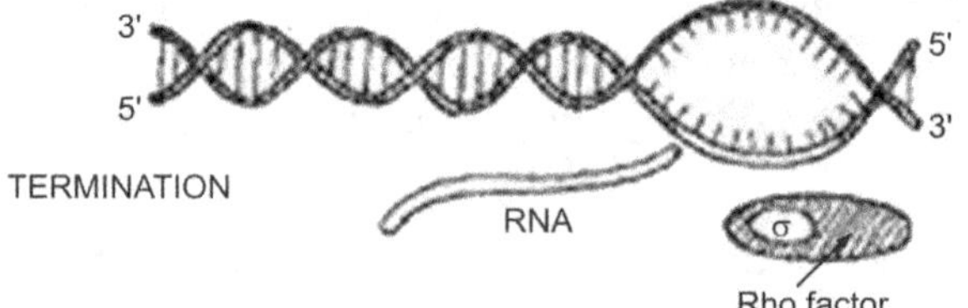

Fig. 4.22 Summary of RNA synthesis

4.8   Translation

Translation is the process in which the genetic information present in the mRNA molecule directs protein synthesis. mRNA has codons, capable of specifying a particular aminoacid. All the three types of RNAs are involved in protein synthesis in the following main steps:

(i)   Activation of aminoacids

(ii)   Transfer of aminoacid to tRNA

(iii)   Assembly of the protein chain on the Ribosome.

(i)   **Activation of aminoacids:** In protein synthesis only L-aminoacids take part. The D-aminoacids are screened from the all 20 aminoacids. Each aminoacid has a specific aminoacyl tRNA synthetase and a specific tRNA. The aminoacids are activated by aminoacyl-tRNA synthetase. This activation reaction requires energy in the form of ATP.

The activated aminoacid remains tightly bound to the enzyme after activation.

(iv)   **Transfer of aminoacid to tRNA:** The process of transfer of activated aminoacids to tRNA is called charging of tRNA. This reaction is catalyzed by the enzyme that was originally bound to the aminoacid.

The tRNA function in protein synthesis is to carry aminoacids and recognize codons in mRNA.

Clover leaf model of t-RNA

♦   Ist arm called acceptor arm. It accepts the aminoacids.

♦   IInd called D arm/DHU arm (digydroxy uridine)

♦   IIIrd arm called anticodon arm which specifically recognizes the complementary codon in mRNA for a specific aminoacid.

♦   IVth arm called variable arm. It has no particular shape and function.

♦   Vth arm is called Tpc (Thymine, pseudouridine and cytosine). Thymine is an exception because RNA has oracil in the place of Thymine.

(iii)   **Assembly of the protein chain on the ribosome:** The ribosome is the site of protein synthesis. Its rRNA is transcribed from certain portions of DNA by the same energy requiring process used for synthesis of mRNA and tRNA.

The ribosomes of E.coil have been studied extensively and have been found to consist of two subunits, which are identified by a sedimentation constant (s) and determined by ultracentrifugation studies. The larger subunit is a 50s particle, while the smaller unit is a 30s particle. Ribosomal subunits may associate or dissociate with each other. The association of 30s and 50s submit to form a 70s ribosome shows that the sedimentation behavior of the 70s ribosomes is not a simple addition of the units of the smaller particles. Each subunit is made up of ribosomal RNA molecule and numerous proteins.

4.8.1   Steps of the Synthesis of a Protein Chain on a Ribosome

Step 1: A ribosome binds to one end of a mRNA molecule at a specific site.

Step 2: A charged tRNA carrying the first aminoacid molecule then attaches to the chain-initiating codon(x) of the mRNA.

Step 3: Another tRNA carrying the second aminoacid binds at the next codon(y).

Step 4: The amino group of the aminoacid on the second tRNA reacts with the active terminal carboxyl group on the aminoacid of the first tRNA is then to form a dipleptide; the first tRNA is then released. The mRNA is moved along the ribosome to position the next codon(z) in readiness for the tRNA carrying the third aminoacid.

A single molecule of mRNA is long enough for several ribosomes to read the molecule at the same time. When a number of 70s ribosomes are actively engaged in protein synthesis on a strand of mRNA, this is called polysome.

4.9   Gene Regulation

The DNA of a microbial cell consists of genes, a few to thousands, which do not express at the same time. At a particular time only a few genes express and synthesize the desired protein. The other genes remain silent at this moment and express when required.

♦ Requirement of gene expression is governed by the environment in which they grow. This shows that the genes have a property to switch on and switch off.

♦ 20 different aminoacids constitute different proteins. All are synthesized by codons. Therefore, synthesis of all the aminoacids requires energy which is useless because all the aminoacids constituting proteins are not needed at a time. Hence, there is need to control the synthesis of those aminoacids which are not required. Therefore, a control system is operative which is known as "Gene regulation".

♦ There are certain substrates called inducers that induce the enzyme synthesis.

For example, if yeast cells are grown in medium containing lactose, an enzyme lactase, is formed. Lactase hydrolyses the lactose into glucose and galactose. In the absence of lactose, lactase synthesis does not occur. This shows that lactose induces the enzymes lactase. Therefore, lactase is known as inducible enzyme.

4.9.1 The Lac Operon

For the first time Jacob and Monod (1961) gave the concept of operon model to explain the regulation of gene action.

An operon is defined as several distinct genes situated in tandem (an arrangement in which a team of machines, are lined up one behind another, all facing in the same direction) all controlled by a common regulatory region. Commonly an operon consists of repressor, promoter, operator and structural gens. The message produced by an operon is polycistronic because the information of all structural genes resides on a single molecule of mRNA.

♦ The lactose utilizing system (Fig. 4.22) consists of two types of components; the structural genus (lac z, lac y and lac A) the products of which are required for transport and metabolism of lactose and the regulatory genes (lac I, lac O, lac P). These two components together comprises of the lacoperon.

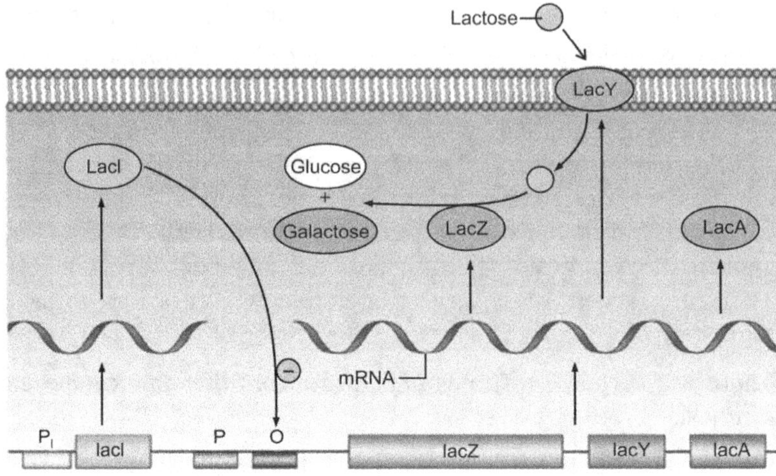

Fig. 4.23 Gene regulation by lac operon

The regulation of lacoperon of E.coil has the following:

(i) **Structural genes:** The lactose operon of *E.coil* is composed of three structural z, y and A. 'Z' gene transcribes mRNA for a single long polypeptide chain to form the enzyme b-glactosidase. This enzyme catalyses the hydrolysis of lactose in glucose and galctose. 'y' gene transcribes the mRNA that translates the permease protein. The enzyme permease facilitates the lactose to enter inside the bacterium.

'A' gene specifies the enzyme transcetylase.

(ii) **Operator gene:** Operator lies immediately left to the structural gene. When the operator is 'on', the structural gens can't function. Operator is the target for the attachment of repressor protein produced by the regulator gene. The base pairs in the operator region are palindrome i.e., show two fold symmetry from a point. The repressor proteins bind to the operator and form an operator-repressor complex which in turn physically blocks the transcription of z, y and A genes by preventing the release of RNA polymerase to begin transcription.

(iii) **The promoter gene:** The actual site of transcription initiation is known as promoter region. It is left the operator region. mRNA transcription by the RNA polymerase. This enzyme first along the operator region and structural genes, like operators the promoter region consists of palindromic sequence of nucleotides.

(iv) The repressor (Regulator) gene: The regulator gene transcribes the mRNA for the protein called repressor. This lac repressor regulates the expression of structural genes by binding the operator region. In the absence of lactose, repressor binds to the operator and blocks the path of RNA polymerase and presents the expression of structural genes.

4.9.2   Positive Regulation of the Lac Operon-Catabolic Control

Positive control of enzyme synthesis is said to occur when an association between a protein and a part of the regulatory region of an operon is essential for expression of related structural genes in the operon. Expression of the lac operon is inhibited when a more efficient source of energy, such as glucoses is present in the medium. The presence of glucose results in a decreased concentration of intracellular cyclic Amp. Cyclic Amp is necessary for the efficient expression of the lac operon since it activates the catabolite gene activator protein (Cap), which in turn activates transcription of lac mRNA by RNA polymerase at the promoter site.

Phenotypic Changes due to Environmental Alterations

Bacteria, like the cells of higher organisms, carry more genetic information-their genotype-than is utilized or expressed at any one time. The extent to which this information is expressed depends on the environment. A facultative anaerobic bacterium will produce different end products of metabolism, depending on the presence or absence of oxygen during growth. The presence or absence of oxygen determines which enzymes function and which donot. The outstanding feature of a phenotypic change due to environment is that it involves most of the cells in the culture. A phenotypic change of this type is not inherited: rather, it occurs when some condition of the environment changes. A return to the original phenotype occurs when the original environmental conditions are restored.

Genotypic changes: The genotype of a cell is determined by the genetic information contained in its chromosome. The chromosome is divided into genes.

♦ A gene is a functional unit of inheritance. It specifies the information of a particular polypeptide as well as various type of RNA.

♦ Each gene consists of hundreds of nucleotide pairs.

♦ Any gene is capable of changing or mutating to a different form so that it specifies information of an altered or new protein which may in turn change the characteristics of the cell.

For example, the substitution of even one aminoacid among several hundred in a polypeptide chain may cause the protein to be non functional.

♦ A mutation is a change in the nucleotide sequence of a gene. This gives rise to a new genetic trait, or a changed genotype.

♦ A cell or an organism which shows the effects of a mutation is called a mutant. Thus we occasionally see sudden changes in familiar plants and animals.

♦ In nature, mutations are rare events which occur at random and arise spontaneously with no regard to environmental conditions.

4.9.3   Tryptophan Operon

Operon is the coordinated unit of genetic expression in bacteria. The *trp* operon is an operon a group of genes that are used, or transcribed, together that codes for the components for production of tryptophan. The *trp* operon is present in many bacteria, but was first characterized in *Escherichia coli*. The operon is regulated so that when tryptophan is present in the environment, the genes for tryptophan synthesis are not expressed. It was an important experimental system for learning about gene regulation, and is commonly used to teach gene regulation.

♦ Tryptophan is an aromatic amino acid and is required for the synthesis of all proteins that contain tryptophan.

♦ The 20 common amino acids are required in large amounts for protein synthesis, and E.coil can synthesize all of them.

♦ The genes for the enzymes needed to synthesize a given amino acid are generally clustered in an operon and are expressed whenever existing supplies of that amino acid are inadequate for cellular requirements.

♦ When the amino acid is abundant, the biosynthetic enzymes are not needed and the operon is repressed.

♦ The *E.coil* tryptophan (trp) operon includes five genes for the enzymes required to convert chorismate to tryptophan.

♦ The five structural genes are [trp E, trp D, trp C, trp B, trp A] and the regulatory elements – primary promoter (trp p), operator (trp O), attenuator (trp a), secondary internal promoter (trp P_2) and terminator (trp t)

♦ The five structural genes of tryptophan operon code for three enzymes (two enzymes contain two different subunits) required for the synthesis of tryptophan from chorismate.

♦ The mRNA from the trp operon has a half-life of only about 3 min, allowing the cell to respond rapidly to changing needs for this amino acid.

4.9.3.1   Tryptophan Operon Regulation by a Repressor

♦ The trp repressor is a homo dimer, each subunit containing 107 amino acid residues.

♦ When tryptophan is abundant it binds to the Trp repressor, causing a conformational change that permits the repressor to bind to the trp operator and inhibit expression of the trp operon.

♦ The trp operator site overlaps the promoter, so binding of the repressor blocks binding of RNA polymerase.

♦ Once again, this simple on/off circuit mediated by a repressor is not the entire regulatory story. Different cellular concentrations of tryptophan can vary the rate of synthesis of the biosynthetic enzymes over a 700-fold range.

Attenuator as the second control site for tryptophan operon (Fig.4.25)

♦ The trp operon attenuation mechanism uses signals encoded in four sequences within a 162 nucleotide leader region at the 5' end of the mRNA, preceding the initiation codon of the first gene.

♦ Within the leader lies a region known as the attenuator, made up of sequences 3 and 4. These sequences base-pair to form a $G \equiv C$-rich stem-and-loop structure closely followed by a series of U residues.

♦ The Attenuator structure acts as transcription terminator.

♦ Sequence 2 is an alternative complement for sequence 3.

- If sequence 2 and 3 base pair, the attenuator structure cannot form and transcription continues into the trp biosynthetic genes, the loop formed by the pairing of sequences 2 and 3 does not obstruct transcription.

- Regulatory sequence 1 is crucial for the tryptophan sensitive mechanism that determines whether sequence 3 pairs with sequence 2 (allowing transcription to continue) or with sequence 4 (attenuating transcription).

- Formation of the attenuator stem-and loop structure depends on events that occur during translation of regulatory sequence 1, which encodes a leader peptide (so called because it is encoded by the leader region of the mRNA) of 14 amino acids, two of which are Trp residues.

- When Tryptophan concentrations are high, concentrations translation to proceed rapidly past the two Trp codons of sequence 1 and into sequence 2, before sequence 3 is synthesized by RNA polymerase.

- In this situation sequence 2 is covered by the ribosome and unavailable for pairing to sequence 3 when sequence 3 is synthesized; the attenuator structure (sequence 3 and 4) forms and transcription halts.

- When tryptophan concentrations are low, however, the ribosome stalls at the two Trp codons in sequence 1, because charged tRNA Trp is less available. Sequence 2 remains free while the sequence 3 is synthesized, allowing these two sequences to base-pair and permitting transcription to proceed.

- When tryptophan levels are high, the ribosome quickly translates sequence 1 (open reading frame encoding leader peptide) and blocks sequence 2 before sequence 3 is transcribed. Continued transcription leads to attenuation at the terminator-like-structure formed by sequences 3 and 4 incomplete.

When tryptophan levels are low, the ribosome pauses at the Trp codons in sequence 1. Formation of paired structure between sequences 2 and 3 prevents attenuation, because sequence 3 is no longer available to form the attenuator structure with sequence 4.

- Two polycistronic mRNAs are produced from tryptophan operon one derived from all the five structural genes and the other obtained from the last three genes.

♦ Besides acting as a core pressor to regulate trp operon, tryptophan can inhibit the activity of the enzyme anthranilate synthetase.

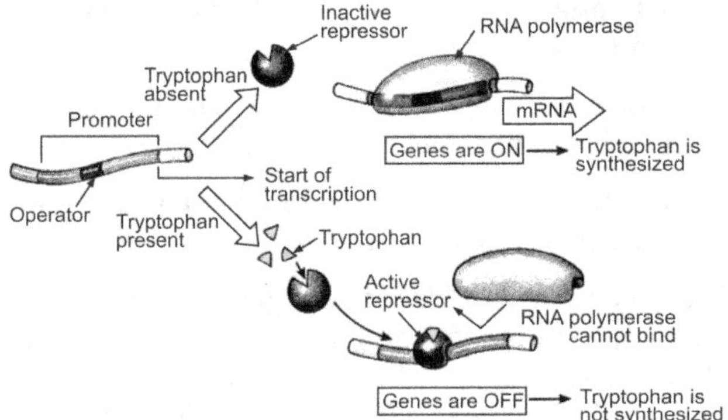

Fig. 4.24 Gene regulation by tryptophan operon

4.10 Phase Variation

• Phase variation is defined as the random switching of phenotype at frequencies that are much higher (sometimes >1%) than classical mutation rates.

• Phase variation contributes to virulence by generating heterogeneity; certain environmental or host pressures select those bacteria that express the best adapted phenotype

• Phase variation is a method for dealing with rapidly varying environments without requiring random mutation employed by various types of bacteria, including *Salmonella* species.

• It involves the variation of protein expression, frequently in an on-off fashion, within different parts of a bacterial population.

• Although it has been most commonly studied in the context of immune evasion, it is observed in many other areas as well.

• *Salmonella* use this technique to switch between different types of the protein flagellin. As a result, flagella with different structures are assembled.

• Once an adaptive response has been mounted against one type of flagellin, or if a previous encounter has left the adaptive immune system ready to deal with one type of flagellin, switching types renders previously high affinity antibodies, TCRs and BCRs ineffective against the flagella.

- The flagellar antigens of most ***salmonellae*** exist in one of two phases, phase 1 and phase 2.

- Phase 1 antigen is more specific and is shared by a few species only and designated as a, b, c, d etc., upto z, and after z as z_1 z_2 z_3 up to z_{14}.

- Phase 2 antigen is nonspecific or group phase and is shared by several unrelated species of *salmonellae*.

- It is always necessary to identify antigenic factor of flagella in phase 1 and sometimes in phase 2 and for which a culture in the alternative phase has to be produced. This is done by passing the bacteria through a Craigie's tube, containing homologous phase antiserum incorporated in agar.

V → w Variation

♦ The virulence of *Salmonella typhi* is associated with the presence of the Vi antigen

Fresh isolates of *S.typhi* with Vi antigen are generally inaggulutinable by O – antiserum because Vi antigen completely masks the O antigen (**O antigen** (Ger. *ohne Hauch,* without film), the antigen that occurs in the bodies of bacteria).

♦ These are called v forms.

♦ The V forms are only agglutinable by Vi antiserum.

♦ Organisms lose their Vi antigen either partially or completely after repeated   subculture in the laboratory.

♦ With partial loss of Vi antigen, *S .typhi* are agglutinable by both O and Vi antisera and these intermediate forms are called Vw forms.

♦ When there is complete loss of Vi antigen, the strain is agglutinable only by O – antiserum. These are called w form.

The Vi antigen of *S. paratyphi* and *S. Dublin* generally cannot completely mask the O antigen.

S-R Variation

The smooth to rough variation occurs due to mutation and is associated with

(a) Change of colonial morphology from smooth to rough.

(b) Loss of O antigen and virulence of the strain. It can be avoided by maintaining laboratory cultures in Dorset's egg medium or by lyophilisation.

♦ Only *Rickettsiae* show phase variation.

♦ The freshly isolated organisms are in phase I and on repeated passage on yolk sac they attain phase II.

Unlike other *Rickettsial* spescies, *Coxiella burnetii* contain two distinct plasmids.

Questions

1. Describe immunoblotting procedures in detail (ELISA, Western and Southern Blotting techniques).

2. Describe the genetic organization of Eukaryotes and Prokaryotes in detail.

3. Have a conversation about microbial genetics.

4. Discuss microbial biotransformation and its applications.

5. Define the term "mutation." Make a list of the different types of mutants.

5 FERMENTATION AND FERMENTATION PRODUCTS

5.1 History and Design of Fermenters

What is Fermentation? Fermentation is the chemical transformation of organic substances into simpler compounds by the action of enzymes, complex organic catalysts, which are produced by micro-organisms such as molds, yeasts, or bacteria. Enzymes act by hydrolysis, a process of breaking down or predigesting complex organic molecules to form smaller (and in the case of foods, more easily digestible) compounds and nutrients. The word "fermentation" is derived from the Latin meaning "to boil," since the bubbling and foaming of early fermenting beverages seemed closely akin to boiling. This concept is also known as zymosis.

For the first time, large scale aerobic fermenters were used in central Europe in the year 1930's for the production of compressed yeast.

♦ The fermenter consisted of a large cylindrical tank with air introduced at the base via network of perforated pipes

♦ Mechanical impellers were used to increase the rate of mixing and to break up and disperse the air bubbles

♦ Baffles on the walls of the vessels prevented a vortex forming in the liquid

Basic functions of fermenters: The main function of a fermenter is to provide a controlled environment for growth of a micro-organism;

♦ The vessel should be capable of being operated aseptically for a number of days and should be reliable for long term operation.

♦ Adequate aeration and agitation should be provided

♦ The power consumption should be low

5.2   Types of Fermenter

(i)   Fluidized bioreactor

(ii)   Loop or Air lift bioreactor

(iii)   Membrane bioreactor

(iv)   Pulsed column bioreactor

(v)   Bubble column bioreactor

(vi)   Photo bioreactor

(vii)   Packed tower bioreactor

Construction of Fermenters: The materials used for the construction of a fermenter should be

1.   The materials that have no effect of sterilization

2.   Its smooth internal finish. There are two types of such materials
    (i)   stainless steel
    (ii)   glass

♦ Control of temperature is essential

♦ Aeration and Agitation required to meet the metabolic requirements of the microbes

♦ The agitator (impeller) is required

♦ Stirrer gland and bearing

♦ Baffles to prevent vortex formation

♦ Sparger to supply sterile oxygen

Design and operation: These are designed to provide support to the best possible growth and biosynthesis for industrially important cultures. These vessels must be strong enough to resist the pressure of large volume of agitating medium.

The achievement and maintenance of Aseptic Conditions: The following operations may have to be performed to achieve and maintain aseptic conditions during fermentation:

(i)   sterilization of the fermenter

(ii) sterilization of the air supply

(iii) aeration and agitation

(iv) the addition of inoculum, nutrients and other supplements

(v)   sampling

(vi) foam control

(vii) monitoring and control of various parameters

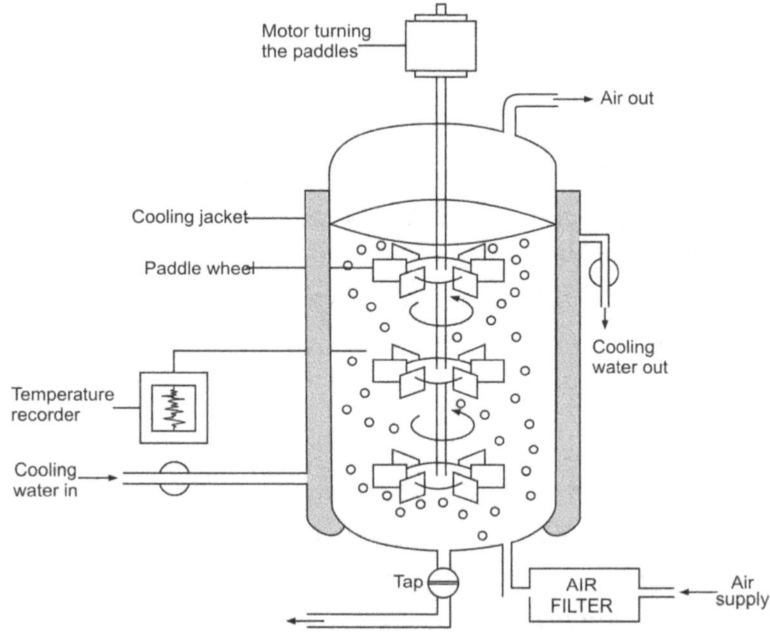

Fig. 5.1 Fermenter

Batch fermentation: Batch fermentation is a process in which a large volume of nutrient medium is inoculated to proceed for the harvest and recovery of the product. This ends the batch fermentation as the vessel is cleansed and desterilized for subsequent batches.

Fed-batch fermentation: In fed-batch fermentation, substrate is added in increments as the fermentation progresses.

Continuous fermentation: During continuous fermentation, some parts of the components (media and inoculums) of upstream process are withdrawn intermittently and replacement or withdrawn substances are made by adding the fresh medium or nutrients.

Scale-up fermentations: The determination of the proper incubation conditions to be employed with large scale production tanks as based on information obtained with various sized smaller tanks is called "scale up". This process allows to carryout laboratory procedure at industrial scale.

Culture preservation

1. *Methods of preservations*

    (a)   Agar slant culture

    (b)   Agar slant culture covered with oil

    (c)   Saline suspension

    (d)   Preservation at very low temperature

    (e)   Preservation by drying in vacuum

    (f)   Lyophilization or freeze drying

2. *Stock culture collection centers*

    (a)   American type culture collection, Rockville, Maryland, USA

    (b)   Indian collection of industrial micro-organisms, National chemical laboratory, Pune

    (c)   Institute of Pasteur, Paris (France)

    (d)   Institute of microbial technology, Chandigarh

Criteria used for the Selection of Micro-organisms for Fermentation

The microbes should have following attributes:

(i)   The strain must be genetically stable

(ii)   The strain should be readily maintained for reasonably long period of time

(iii)   The strain must readily produce many vegetative cells, spores or other structures

(iv)   The strains should be able to protect themselves from contamination

1. *Methods of culture maintenance*: There are three methods for culture maintenance:

(a) drying organisms on soil or some other solid

(b) storing organisms on agar slants and

(c) removing the water from the cells or spores by lyophilization and storage of dried product.

5.3   Fermentation Methods

1)   Solid state fermentation

Microbial growth and product conformation occur at the surface of solid substrates in this type of fermentation. Mushroom cultivation, mold-ripened cheeses, and start cultures are all examples of this type of fermentation. Extracellular enzymes, certain important chemicals, fungual poisons, and fungal spores have all been produced using this method. Traditional substrates include rice, maize, soyabean, and other agricultural items. The substrate contains a diverse range of nutrients that may or may not require supplementation. Such a substrate favours mycelia organisms, which can thrive in high-nutrient environments and produce a wide range of extracellular enzymes.

Solid-state fermentation is separated into two categories:

i) Fermentation of low moisture solids without or with intermittent/continuous agitation

ii) Suspended solid fermented in a closed container columns through which liquid is circulated. The fungi i.e., obligate aerobes are used shown in Table 5.1

Examples of solid-state fermentation

Table 5.1 Examples of solid-state fermentation

PRODUCT	SUBSTRATE	PRIM GENUS	PRODUCT USED AS
Soy sauce	Soybean, wheat	*Aspergillus soyeae*	Food
Hamanatto	Soyabean, wheat	*Aspergillus sp.*	Food
Sufu	Tofu	*Actinomucor sp.*	Food
Cellulase	Wheat bran	*Trichoderma reesei*	Enzymes
Amylase	Rice	*A.oryzae*	Enzyme

2) submerged fermentation

i) ***Batch culture:*** It is a closed culture system in which only a small amount of nutrient media is present. After inoculation, the culture enters a lag period, during which the cell size expands but not their numbness. The culture enters the lag phase, or exponential growth phase, in which cells proliferate at their fastest pace and their formation time is at its shortest. A rise in nutrients occurs, as well as the accumulation of inhibitory end products in the media.

Increase in cell number at different intervals of time is collected to create a typical growth curve.

ii) ***fed-batch culture:*** Fed-batch culture occurs when a batch culture is fed with fresh nutritional media without removing the raising microbial culture. Supplementation is possible with fed-batch culture.

iii) ***Continuous culture:*** contrary to batch culture where the exponential growth of microbial population is confined only for many generations, it's frequently desirable to maintain prolonged exponential growth of microbial population in artificial operations.

3) Anaerobic fermentation

A provision for aeration is usually not required in anaerobic fermentation. However, in rare circumstances, aeration may be required prior to the inoculum being mixed. When the fermentation process starts, the gas created by the process creates enough mixing. Carbon dioxide, hydrogen, ammonia gas, or an appropriate blend of these should be used to replace the air in the fermentor's headspace. Oxygen-freeze sterile carbon dioxide or other gases are bubbled through the media in the case of acetogens and other gas utilises back. Acetogens were cultivated in 400 fermenters using sterile carbon dioxide, with each run yielding 3kg of cells.

4) Aerobic fermentation

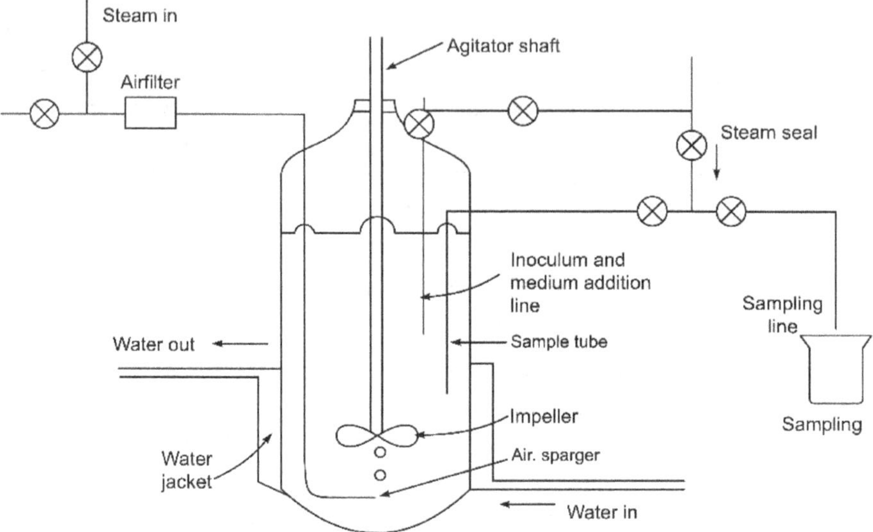

Fig. 5.2 Schematic representation of Aerobic fermentation

The supply for sufficient aeration is the main feature of aerobic fermentation; in some situations, the amount of air required per hour is around 60 times the medium volume. As a result, bioreactors used for aerobic turmoil contain a provision for a safe amount of sterile air, which is usually sprayed into the medium. This fermentor may have a media for moving and miming the medium and cell in the medium. Aerobic fermenters come in a variety of shapes and sizes:

i)   stirred-tank type, which includes mechanical motor-driven stirrers.

ii) Air-lift type: No mechanical stirrers are utilised, and agitation is achieved by air bubbles formed by the air supply shown in Fig 5.2.

5) Immobilized cell bioreactors

Cell immobilized is advantageous when

i)   the enzyme of interest is intercellular and

ii) the enzymes are unstable after extraction, cell immobilisation is helpful.

iii) Interfering enzymes are not present in the cell, or they are easily inactivated or eliminated.

iv) Products are molecules with a low molecular weight that have been discharged into the medium.

E.coli cells entrapped in polyacrylamide gel for the manufacture of L-aspartic acid are an example of cell immobilisation in commercial amino acid production.

5.4   Fermentation Media

All microorganisms need for their microbial activity the presence of several nutrients.

Carbohydrates

Carbohydrates can be utilised by any microbes, however this group of organic substances is not required in any way. Glucose is the sugar that is most easily digested. Disaccharides are used by the majority of fungus.

Lipids

The following is a summary of the microbial conditions for steroids and long-chain adipose acids. Bacteria and fungus both require long-chain adipose acids such as linoleic acid and oleic acid. Microorganisms do not need or use steroids in general, with the exception of cholesterol. Ergosterol serves as a nutritive need in all fungus, including incentive.

Purines and Pyrimidines

It's generally only in bacteria that cases of purine and pyrimidine metabolism have been reported. Algae don't use these composites at all.

Vitamins and growth factors

Depending on their species, other bacteria have varied vitamin and related factor requirements. In the vast majority of situations, vitamins A, C, D, and K are not necessary for growth**Amino acids**

Although certain algal species are capable of using amino acids, they are not normally required for algae. All amino acids can be exercised by other microbes, with the exception of incentives, where there is no evidence of critrulline utilisation. The L-form of the acids is normally biologically active, although some bacteria, unlike higher mammals, can use the D-amino acids as well.

Sources of Nitrogen

It is important to note that not all species bear or employ these composites; rather, some species have been identified as being suited for their usage. Ammonia, nitrate, and nitrite are all found in fungi.

Sources of Sulphur

Essential sulphur and sulphate can be used by some incentive species. In general, incentives do not bear or employ organic composites that contain sulphur. Incentives have sulphonic acid amides, thioacetate, thiocarbonate, thioglycolate, and glutathione, while bacteria have glutathione and thio-acetic acid. Chemical elements and inorganic ions

Mineral nutrients required by microorganisms are species dependent but consists generally of Fe, K, Mg, Mn. Sometimes S, N, Ca, Co, Cu, P, Zn is required.

5.5   Systems of Fermentation

Microbial fermentation can be thought of as a three-phase system, including liquid-solid, gas-solid, and gas-liquid interactions.

Dissolved nutrients, substrates, and metabolites are all found in the liquid phase.

Individual cells, bullets, undoable substrates, and precipitated metabolic products make up the solid phase.

The gaseous phase serves as a reserve for both the oxygen pool and CO2 disposal.

Mixing and Stirring

A appropriate mixing device is required to transmit energy, nutrients, substrate, and metabolite within the bioreactor. The effectiveness of any one nutrient could be critical to the overall fermentation's efficiency

The stirring of a bioreactor causes the following effects in each of the three phases.

- Air dispersion in the nutrient result
- Homogenization to equalise temperature and nutrient concentration throughout the fermentor
- Microorganisms and solid nutrients suspension

- Immiscible liquids dissipation Between the nutrient result and the particular cell, the relative haste should be around 0.5 m/ sec. The way nutrients behave when stirred can be separated into two groups: thick results with Newtonian and non-Newtonian properties, and viscoelastic outcomes, in which regular liquid-state properties are not found in stirred vessels. The most important property impacting the inflow behaviour of a fluid is density, which is defined as a material's ability to resist deformation. Pumping, mixing, heat transmission, mass transfer, and aeration are all affected by similar behaviour. There are just a few examples that fall into the other category, such as polysaccharides and specific antibiotic controversies. The majority of fermentation outcomes fall into the first order. The behaviour of uninoculated results and bacterial societies is common as simple Newtonian liquids.

The provision of tolerable gas exchange is one of the most important aspects of a fermentor's operation. The most essential gaseous substrate for microbial metabolism is oxygen, and the most important gaseous metabolic product is carbon dioxide. When oxygen is required as a microbial substrate, fermentation becomes a limiting issue. Only 0.3 mM O_2, which is original to 9 mg/ l, dissolves in one litre of water at 20 degrees Celsius due to its low solubility. An aggressive and concentrated microbial population will drain this amount of oxygen in a matter of seconds unless oxygen is continuously supplied. In contrast, the amount of other nutrients consumed during the same time period is small compared to the focus of attention. Thus most aerobic microbial processes are oxygen limited.

This is why, although though other gases such as carbon dioxide, hydrogen, methane, and ammonia might be involved in bioprocesses, the idea of gas-liquid mass transfer in bioprocesses is based on oxygen transfer. The minimum oxygen content is actually lower than it would be in pure water because of the influence of the culture nutrients. In the gas pressure range over which fermentors are operated, feast solubility is determined by Henry's law. This indicates that as oxygen concentration in the gas phase rises, the nutrient's O_2 fraction rises as well. As a result, during pure oxygen aeration, the highest O_2 partial pressure is achieved.

When pure oxygen is compared to the value in air (9 mg O_2/ l), 43 mg O_2/ l dissolves in water. The solubility of oxygen reduces as the temperature rises. At 33 degrees Celsius, for example, the solubility is mg O2/l.

Several independent partial resistances must be overcome before oxygen can be transferred from a gas bubble to a single cell.

* Penetration of the phase barrier between the gas bubble and the liquid

* Transfer from the phase boundary to the liquid

* Movement within the nutrient result

* Transfer to the cell's face

The resistance at the phase boundary between the gas bubble and the liquid is the most critical element controlling the rate of transfer in fermentations carried out with single celled organisms such as bacteria and incentive's. Microbial cells in close proximity to gas bubbles may absorb oxygen straight across the phase barrier, resulting in a faster rate of gas transfer to neighbouring cells. The O2 transport within the agglomeration or bullet can be a limiting factor in cell agglomerates or bullets. The mass transfer of oxygen into liquid can be characterized by the oxygen transfer rate (OTR) or by the volumetric oxygen transfer measure. These values have been completely examined as a critical parameter for bioreactor function. The oxygen transfer rate and the volumetric oxygen transfer measure are dependent on the following parameters:

❖ mixing parcels power, impeller configuration and size, baffles.

❖ vessel figure periphery, capacity.

❖ Rate, figure, and position of aeration system sparger

❖ Composition, viscosity, and density of nutritional results

❖ The morphology of the microorganism, and its importance.

❖ The temperature of the antifoam agent

The baffles are used to break up the vortex pattern that forms around a single-shaft impeller spinning in a fluid with no restrictions. The baffles generate a large planar liquid face and a livery input pattern, as well as more liquid hold-up for a given fermentor volume. The rate of oxygen transport is slowed by antifoam agents and other face-active substances. The bubble face in clean water is continuously refreshed by vibration and oscillation. As soon as surface-active chemicals are applied, bubble movement ceases to renew the bubble surface.

Microorganisms affect the rate of oxygen transport by functioning as a barrier, preventing O_2 transfer. Depending on While the rate of oxygen transmission falls progressively as the size of the pellets grows larger, the rate of oxygen transfer in loose forms reduces substantially faster. Where there is negative pressure in the bioreactor, such as behind the agitator blades, the gas bubbles are replenished. Various circumstances can be identified when the rate of aeration rises. Large gas bubbles occur behind individual turbine blades at low aeration rates, and smaller bubbles are centrifugally spun off and into the nutritional solution.

Gas bubbles gather before all turbine blades as the aeration rate is increased, and they continue to accumulate. In unaerated systems, the energy input is one-third lower. Gas dispersion is the vogue in this middle stirring range. When aeration rates are really high, a lot of big gas bubbles stick together and the impeller becomes swamped with gas, resulting in significantly reduced gas dispersion. The term "critical oxygen attention" refers to the amount of oxygen intake rate or oxygen immersion rate that allows for uninterrupted breathing.

In most cultures, critical oxygen concentrations range from 5 to 25% of the oxygen saturation value. Respiration rate is connected with the O2 attention in the result when oxygen immersion rates are lower than crucial limits. There is no correlation between respiration rate and dissolved oxygen above this amount. The critical oxygen concentration in Newtonian fluids, such as those found in yeast and bacterial fermentations, is constant and unaffected by fermentation conditions. The critical oxygen concentration in non-Newtonian systems has been demonstrated to be dependent on fermentation conditions.

Heat Production

Fermentations must be carried at a consistent temperature in order to achieve optimal yields. The heat balance of a fermentation process is now discussed in detail. Heat production from moving, gassing/aeration, and metabolic exertion of microorganisms must be balanced by heat loss through evaporation and radiation, as well as heat removal by the cooling system.

The thermodynamics of the entire microbial exertion cause heat elaboration during metabolism. Apart from anaerobic digestion and a few other thermophilic microbial activities, the quantity of heat produced is usually so great that if it isn't eliminated, the temperature of the contents of the fermentor rises above the system's optimum range. The consumption of carbon and the energy source affects the production of heat during metabolic effort. When the carbon source is laboriously integrated into biomass by anabolism during growth, around 40-50 percent of the available enthalpy in the substrate is preserved in the biomass, with the remainder being lost as heat. All the enthalpy associated with the oxidation of the substrate is released as heat when the carbon source is catabolized to provide energy for cell conservation. If a biochemical product is created, the heat generated is somewhere between that of maintenance and that of active development. The amount of heat released is proportional to the stoichiometry of growth and product creation, but the rate of heat release is proportional to the rate of microbial activity.

5.6   Sterilization

Having impurity-free seed societies at all phases of the fermentation process, from the primary culture to the fermentor, is required in nearly all of them. A fermentor can be sterilised by either killing the microorganisms using a lethal agent such as heat, radiation, or a chemical, or by physically removing the viable germs using filtration.

To ensure sterility during fermentation, keep the following criteria in mind.

- The cultural media's sterility

- Application of bioreactor construction for sterilisation and impurity prevention

- Sterility of incoming and leaving air.

Sterilization of the culture media

According to the contents of the culture medium, the water, and the vessel, nutrient media originally contained a variety of vegetative cells and spores. Before inoculation, these must be removed using a proper method. Sterilization can be accomplished in a variety of ways, although heat is the most commonly utilised method.

The quantity and type of microorganisms present, the composition of the culture medium, the pH value, and the size of the suspended particles are all parameters that influence the success of heat sterilisation. Vegetative cells are promptly rejected at temperatures as low as 60 degrees Celsius for 5-10 minutes, whereas spores must be destroyed at temperatures as high as 121 degrees Celsius for 15 minutes.

The danger of damaging components in the medium during heat sterilising is always there.

The loss of nutritional quality during sterilisation is caused in part by the decline of heat-labile components. The occurrence of Maillard-type browning responses, which result in medium abrasion as well as nutrient quality loss, is a common miracle. Carbonyl groups from reducing sugars, in particular, interact with amino groups in amino acids and proteins to generate these reactions. Similar results may need separate sterilisation of the carbohydrate component of the media. For all heat-sensitive nutrient outcomes, sludge sterilisation is commonly utilised. Heat-labile factors such as sugars, vitamins, antibiotics, and blood factors are examples of heat-labile factors that must be castrated through filtration. At 121 degrees Celsius, the bioreactor is currently castrating maximum nutritional media in batch sizes. The nature of the medium and the size of the fermentor can be used to calculate approximate sterilisation times. The fittings, faucets, and electrodes of the fermentor must all be castrated, in addition to the nutrient material. As a result, real sterilisation periods are much longer than recommended bones, and must be calculated empirically for the individual nutritional results in the fermentor. Lower fermentors are autoclaved, whereas bigger fermentors are castrated by circular or direct steam injection.

Sterilization of fermentation air

The air supplied to the fermentor must be disinfected, as most fermentations require a lot of aeration. The number of particles and bacteria in the air varies significantly depending on location, air flow, and previous air treatment. The average amount of particles per m3 and microorganisms per m3 found in out-of-door air is ten. Fungus spores account for half of the total, while Gram-negative bacteria account for the other half. Aeration rates of 0.5-2 vvm (air volume/liquid volume per nanosecond) are commonly used in fermentation. Filtration, gas injection (ozone), gas scrubbing, UV radiation, and heat are some of the methods for sterilising gases. Filtration and heat are the only two options that are feasible.

5.7 Appropriate Construction of the Fermentor

To maintain sterility, the fermentor should have the fewest possible openings. O-rings are required for small holes, and flat gaskets are required for wider ones. Special sterility preservation issues should be addressed whenever a moving shaft penetrates the fermentor wall.

Fermentation processes

The following is a general outline of how a fermentation process works:

* Stage 1: inoculum storage

* Stage 2: inoculum build-up

* Stage 3: fermentor culture

Stage 1: inoculum preservation

The goal of preservation is to keep strains alive without cell division for as long as feasible. For each strain, the best technique of storage must be determined. The three most regularly utilised techniques are:

* Frozen storage

* Low-temperature storage (2-6 degrees Celsius) (-18, -80 or -196 degrees Celsius)

    Lyophilization is a term used to describe the process of preserving

    The least safe storage temperature range is 2-6 degrees Celsius; there is a substantial risk of contamination and reverse mutation due to frequent transfers. The most common method of storage is freezing, and frozen cultures can last for years. Because up to 95% of microorganisms are killed during freezing and thawing, the number of survivors is crucial. Lyophilization is the greatest way to keep your strains safe (freeze-drying).

Stage 2: growth of inoculums

Originally, the culture was revived by growing it in an erlenmeyer flask on a natural shaker or on a solid media (if spore formation is needed). In order to obtain enough inoculum for small fermentors, a succession of shake cultures in additional flasks is usually performed. Inoculum growth takes 4-10 days from lyophilized strains, 4–48 hours for bacteria, and 1–7 days for fungus from frozen cultures. Inoculum growth takes 4-24 hours for bacteria and 1-5 days for fungi once they have been removed from cooled cultures.

Stage 3: fermentor culture

The product's nutrient media must be optimised not only in terms of the materials utilised, but also in terms of how the medium is set and sterilised, as well as the pH value before and after sterilisation.

Temperature, aeration, and stirring are the most crucial factors to consider during fermentation.

5.7.1   Study of Production of Penicillin Fermentation (fed-batch) Method

Chapter 1 The process flow begins from the basic raw materials to the downstream processes resulting in the final product. This description is a typical bioprocess flow of any penicillin production facility, it is important to note that in reality, companies generally have their own specific set of standards and hence modification of the process flow is necessary to meet their demands also to optimise quality and quantity.

The actual General Process flow diagram (Fig. 5.3) use in the production of penicillin.

In bioprocess facility, there will be an upstream and downstream process, the upstream processes in this case are referring to processes before input to the fermenter, while the downstream processes refers to the processes that are done to purify the output of the fermenter until it reaches to the desired product.

Medium for *Penicillium*

Medium preparation is necessary in bioprocesses which as it generally involves the use of micro-organism to achieve their products. In the case of the *Penicillium* fungus, the medium usually contain its carbon source which is found in corn steep liquor (a byproduct of starch manufacture) and glucose. Medium also consist of salts such as Magnesium sulphate, Potassium phosphate and Sodium nitrates. They provide the essential ions required for the fungus metabolic activity.

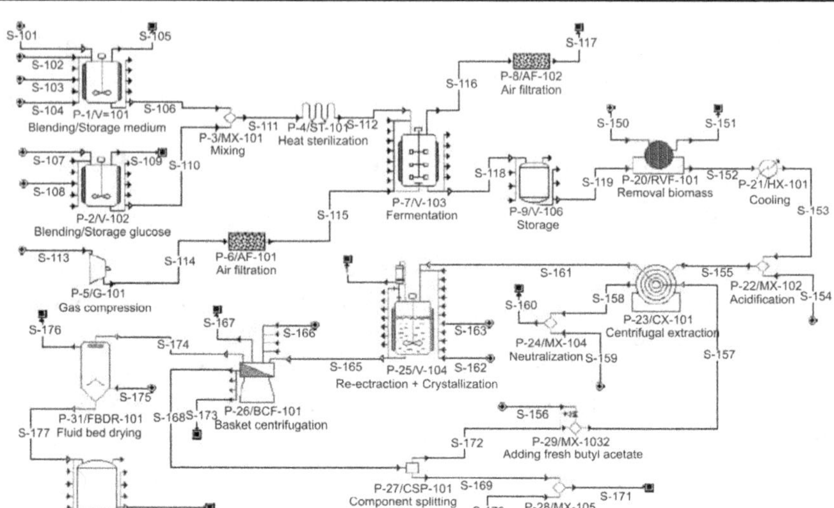

Fig. 5.3 General process flow diagram of penicillin production

Heat Sterilization

Medium is 330tilized 330r at high heat and high pressure usually through a holding tube or sterilsed together with the fermenter. The pressurized steam is used usually and the medium is heated to 121 °C at 30 psi or twice of atmospheric pressure. High temperature short time conditions are used to minimize degradation of certain components of the media.

Fermentation

Fermentation for penicillin is usually done in the fed-batch mode as glucose must not be added in high amounts at the beginning of growth which will result in low yield of penicillin production as excessive glucose inhibit penicillin production. In addition to that, penicillin is a secondary metabolite of the fungus; therefore, the fed-batch mode is ideal for such products as it allows the high production of penicillin. The typical fermentation conditions for the *Penicllium* mold, usually requires temperatures at 20-24 °C while pH conditions are kept in between 6.0 to 6.5. The pressure in the bioreactor is usually much higher than the atmospheric pressure (1.02 atm) this is to prevent contamination from occurring as it prevents external contaminants from entering. Sparging of air bubbles is necessary to provide sufficient oxygen for the viability of the fungus. Depending on the volume of medium, for 2 cubic metres of culture, the sparging rate should be about 2.5 cubic metres per minute. The impeller is necessary to mix the culture evenly throughout the culture medium, fungal cells are much hardy and they are able to handle rotation speed of around 200 rpm.

Seed Culture

The seed culture is developed first in the laboratory by the addition of *Penicillium* spores into a liquid medium. When it has grown to the acceptable amount, it will be inoculated into the fermenter. In some cases, the spores are directly inoculated into the fermenter. After 40 hours penicillin begins to be secreted by fungus.

Removal of Biomass

Filtration is necessary at this point of the bioprocess flow, as bio separation is required to remove the biomass from the culture such as the fungus and other impurities away from the medium which contains the penicillin product. There are many types of filtration methods available today, however, the Rotary vacuum filter is commonly employed as it able to run in continuous mode in any large scale operations. Add this point non-oxidizing acid such as phosphoric acid is introduced as pH will be as high as 8.5. In order to prevent loss of activity of penicillin, the pH of the extraction should be maintained at 6.0-6.5.

Adding of Solvent

In order to dissolve the penicillin present in the filtrate, organic solvents such as Amyl acetate or butyl acetate are used as they dissolve penicillin much better than water at physiological pH. At this point, penicillin is present in the solution and any other solids will be considered as waste.

Centrifugal Extraction

Centrifugation is done to separate the solid waste from the liquid component which contains the penicillin. Usually a tubular bowl or chamber bowl centrifuge is use at this point. The supernatant will then be transferred further in the downstream process to continue with extraction.

Extraction

Penicillin dissolve in the solvent will now undergo a series of extraction process to obtain better purity of the penicillin product. The acetate solution is first mixed with a Phosphate buffer, followed by a Chloroform solution and mixed again with a Phosphate buffer and finally in an Ether solution. Penicillin is present in high concentration in the Ether solution and it will be mixed with a solution of Sodium bicarbonate /potassium bicarbonate to obtain the penicillin-sodium salt/penicillin-potassium salt, which allows penicillin to be stored in a stable powder form at room temperature. The penicillin-sodium salt/penicillin-potassium salt is obtained from the liquid material by basket centrifugation, in which solids are easily removed.

Fluid Bed Drying

Drying is necessary to remove any remaining moisture present in the powdered penicillin salt. In fluid bed drying, hot gas is pumped in from the base of the chamber containing the powdered salt inside a vacuum chamber. Moisture is then removed in this manner and this result in a much drier form of penicillin.

Storage

Penicillin salt is stored in containers and kept in a dried environment. It will then be polished and package into various types of products such as liquid penicillin or penicillin in pills. Dosage of the particular penicillin is determined by clinical trials that are done on this drug.

Industrial uses of bacteria: Lactic acid production, Vinegar production, Amino acid production, L-Lysine production, L-Glutamic acid production

Industrial uses of yeasts: Alcohol production, Baker's yeast, Food yeast

Industrial uses of molds: Penicillin production, Citric acid production, Enzyme production.

5.7.2   Study of Production of Citric Acid

Lemons were the first to contain citric acid. Citric acid is currently 332tilized332r as a component of the ubiquitous Krebs cycle (citric acid cycle), and it is thus found in all living organisms. Citric acid was protected against failures (that contain 7-9 citric acid) in the early days, and today, microbial fermentation produces around 99 percent of the world's citric acid.

Applications of Citric Acid

1. Citric acid is employed as a flavouring agent in foods and beverages, such as logjams, jellies, delicacies, sweets, frozen fruits, soft drinks, and wine, because of its pleasant taste and palatable nature. Citric acid is an antioxidant that protects the 332tiliz of foods in addition to brightening their colour.

2. It's employed as an antifoam agent in the chemical industry, as well as for fabric treatment. Pure essence is confused with citrate in essence assiduity, and essence citrates are formed.

3. It's employed as a blood preservative in pharmaceutical assiduity as trisodium citrate. Citric acid is often used to keep cosmetics and ointments fresh. It's a good source of iron because it's iron citrate.

4. Citric acid can be used as a fat, canvas, or ascorbic acid 333tilized333r333 agent. It binds to essence ions (iron, bobby) and hinders essence-catalyzed reactions. Citric acid is also 333tilized in the treatment of garbage as a mix 333tilized333r.

5. Citric acid has gradually supplanted polyphosphates in soap/cleaning assiduity.

Microbial Strains for Citric Acid Production

Citric acid is produced by a wide range of bacteria. For industrial synthesis of citric acid, the fungus Aspergillus Niger is most commonly 333tilized. A. clavatus, A. wentii, Penicillium luteum, Candida catenula, Candida guilliermondii, and Corynebacteriumsp. Are among the other species found.

Mutant strains of A. Niger have been created for increased citric acid production in industry. Industrially relevant strains include those that can withstand high sugar concentrations and low pH while producing less unwanted derivatives (oxalic acid, isocitric acid, and gluconic acid).

Microbial Biosynthesis of Citric Acid

In the tricarboxylic acid (Krebs) cycle, citric acid is an immediate metabolic product (primary metabolism). Citric acid synthesis relies heavily on glucose as a carbon source. Glycolysis, which converts glucose into two molecules of pyruvate, is part of the metabolic process for citric acid product. Pyruvate then breaks down into acetyl CoA and oxaloacetate, which finally condense to create citrate shown in Fig.5.4.

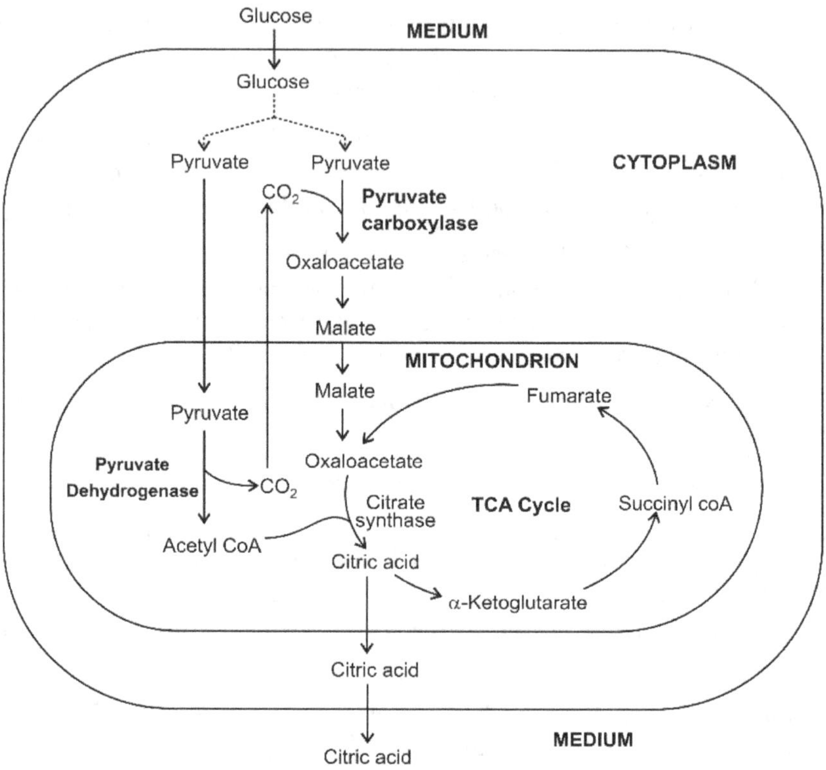

Fig. 5.4 An outline of metabolic pathway for the biosynthesis of citric acid (TCA cycle-Tricarboxylic acid cycle)

Enzymatic regulation of citric acid production

The activity of the enzyme citrate synthase increases tenfold during the manufacture of citric acid, but the activity of enzymes that breakdown citric acid (aconitase, isocitrate dehydrogenase) decreases. Nonetheless, new evidence contradicts the idea that tricarboxylic acid declination (i.e. citric acid buildup) is caused by a reduction in tricarboxylic acid operation.

Enhanced biosynthesis, rather than inhibited decline, is more likely to be the cause of higher citric acid levels. There are also anaplerotic reactions that replenish TCA cycle interceders in order to keep the cycle running. A important enzyme in citric acid synthesis is pyruvate carboxylase, which converts pyruvate to oxaloacetate.

Yield of citric acid

The production of citric acid from sugar, the most often used substrate, has been determined theoretically. It has been calculated that one hydrate can be produced from 100 g sucrose, 112 g anhydrous citric acid, or 123 g citric acid. The yield of citric acid is, however, lower than estimated due to the oxidation of sucrose to CO_2 during trophophase.

Citric acid production is regulated by a number of factors

For maximum citric acid generation, it's critical to keep the nutritional conditions under tight control. The ideal conditions for the synthesis of citric acid by A. Niger have been identified.

Table 5.2 Optimal parameters/conditions for citric acid production

Condition/parameter	Optimum
Sugar concentration	10-25%
Trace metal concentration Manganese Zinc Iron	 $<10^{-4}$ M $<10^{-7}$ M $< 10^{-4}$ M
pH	1.5-2.5
Dissolved O_2 tension	150 mbr
Ammonium salts concentration	>0.2%
Time	150-250 hours

Carbohydrate source

For carbohydrate supply, a wide range of basic materials can be used. Cotton wastes, molasses (sugar beet or sugar cane), date syrup, pineapple waste water, starch (from potatoes), banana extract, sweet potato pulp, and brewery waste are all examples of these. When carbohydrates that are quickly metabolised are employed, such as glucose, sucrose, and maltose, a significant output of citric acid is produced. Molasses from cane and beets are currently the most common. For citric acid production to be optimised, fluctuations in molasses composition (seasonal and product position) must be taken into account.

Citric acid production is influenced by carbohydrate content. The sugar percentage should be between 12 and 25 percent. At sucrose concentrations less than 5%, the production of citric acid is insignificant.

It's thought that a high sugar level causes higher glucose uptake and, as a result, increased citric acid synthesis

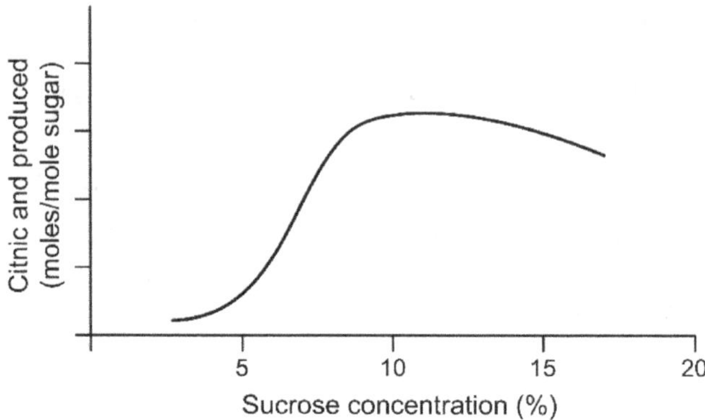

Fig. 5.5 Effect of sugar concentration on citric acid production

Trace metals

The growth of A. Niger requires certain trace elements (Fe, Cu, Zn, Mn, Mg, and Co). Citric acid output is increased by trace metals such as Mn^{2+}, Fe^{3+}, and Zn^{2+}. Manganese ions and their effects have been studied to some extent. These ions increase glycolysis while inhibiting respiration, increasing citric acid synthesis in the process.

For the enzyme aconitase, iron is a cofactor (of TCA cycle). For optimal citric acid synthesis, Fe concentrations of 0.05-0.5 ppm are thought to be desirable. The profits are reduced with greater Fe concentrations, which can be partially reversed by introducing copper.

pH

Citric acid gain is influenced by the pH of the medium, and it is greatest when the pH is less than 2.5. Oxalic acid and gluconic acid synthesis are inhibited at this pH. Citric acid transport is also significantly increased at low pH. If the pH rises over 4, gluconic acid replaces citric acid. Oxalic acid builds as the pH rises over 6. Low pH also reduces the risk of contamination because many organisms cannot grow at this pH.

Dissolved O_2

When the dissolved O2 tension is larger, the yield of citric acid synthesis increases dramatically. Strong aeration or sparging with pure O2 can be used to achieve this. It has been discovered that unexpected disruptions in O2 supply (such as those seen during power outages) result in a significant drop in citric acid production without affecting the organism's growth.

Nitrogen source

Nitrogen sources used in the medium for citric acid production include ammonium salts, nitrates, and urea. As long as they don't change the pH of the medium, all three composites are equally good sources. If molasses is used for nutrient supply, the addition of a redundant nitrogen source is not required. Exogenous addition of ammonium ions has been demonstrated to enhance citric acid synthesis by some researchers.

Production Processes for Citric Acid

The surface process and the submerged process are the two methods for manufacturing citric acid in the industrial setting.

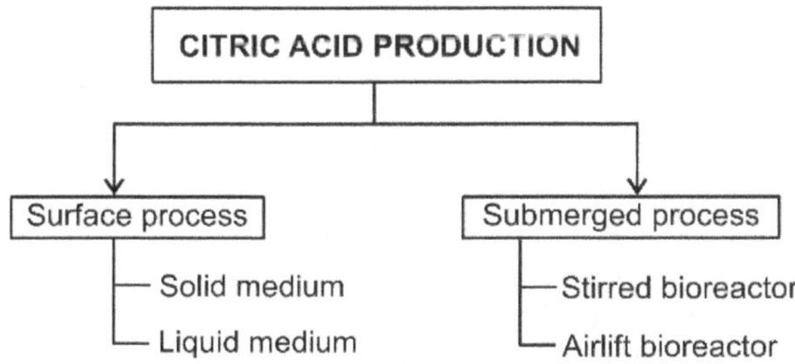

Fig. 5.6 The industrial processes for the production of citric acid

The surface process

The microorganisms are grown as a layer or film on a surface in contact with the nutrient medium, which can be solid or liquid. As a result, supported-growth systems have emerged from the surface process.

The submerged process

The organisms are submerged in the nutritional media or spread throughout it in this situation. Stirred bioreactors and airlift bioreactors are the two types of submerged fermenters (bioreactors) available.

Surface Processes

Solid surface fermentation

Surface activities on solid substrates are particularly common in some Asian countries' underdeveloped fields. As culture media, solid substrates such as wheat bran or sweet potato pulp are utilised. After sterilisation, the medium's pH is adjusted to 4-5. The inoculum, which is in the form of A. niger spores, is now spread out in layers (3-6 cm thick) and incubated at 28 °C.

By adding -amylase to the mix, the organisms' growth can be sped up. The generation of citric acid from solid-state fermentation takes about 80 to 100 hours. Citric acid can be extracted and isolated using hot water at the end of the procedure.

Liquid surface fermentation

The oldest approach for producing citric acid uses surface fermentation with liquid as the feed media. Due to its simple technology, low energy costs, and high reproducibility, it is still in use today. Furthermore, trace essence and dissolved O_2 pressure are insignificant hindrances. However, because the labour force needs for drawing the systems are larger, the labour expenses are higher. Surface techniques deliver roughly 20% of the citric acid produced worldwide.

Typically, beet molasses is used to provide nutrients for surface fermentation. Fermentation is usually done in sterile nutrient medium in aluminium trays. The inoculum is sprayed over the medium in the form of spores. A sterile air stream is circulated to provide O_2 and chill the area. During fermentation, the temperature is kept at about 30°C.A layer of mycelium is developed over the media as the spores germinate (this occurs within 24 hours of inoculation). As the mycelium develops in, the pH of the nutritional media decreases to below 2.

A layer of mycelium forms over the media as the spores germinate (which happens within 24 hours of inoculation). As the mycelium increases in size and forms a thick layer on the surface of the nutrient solution, the pH of the nutrient media falls below 2. After 7-15 days, the fermentation process comes to an end. The mycelium is removed from the nutrition solution. To obtain the most amount of citric acid, the mycelium is mechanically squeezed and thoroughly washed. Citric acid is recovered from the nutritional solution through processing. The final gain of citric acid per gram of sugar is in the range of 0.7-0.9.

Submerged Processes

Submerged operations provide around 80% of the world's citric acid supply. Due to its high efficacy and ease of robotization, this method is the most popular. Submerged fermentation has a number of drawbacks, including the negative impact of trace metals and other contaminants, changes in O_2 pressure, and advanced control technology that need highly skilled workers.

Stirred tanks and aerated towers are two types of bioreactors used. The bioreactors' vessels are composed of stainless steel of the highest quality. From the bottom of the fermenter, air is sparged.

Citric acid synthesis success and yield are mostly determined by mycelium structure. Citric acid production is suitable for mycelium with forked and bulbous hyphae and branches that collect into pellets. When the mycelium is loose, filamentous, and has few branches, no citric acid is produced. Citric acid synthesis requires a sufficient supply of oxygen (20-25 percent saturation value). Aeration rates of 0.2-1 vvm (vol/vol/min) are ideal.

The difficulty of froth generation in submerged fermenters is that it can use up to a third of the bioreactor space. Foaming is prevented by using antifoam substances (such as lard oil) and mechanical antifoam devices. In the industrial manufacture of citric acid, nutrient concentration is particularly significant. Under ideal conditions, 100-110 g/ l citric acid can be produced from 140 g/ l sucrose with a biomass (dry weight) of 8-12 g/l in roughly 250-280 hours.

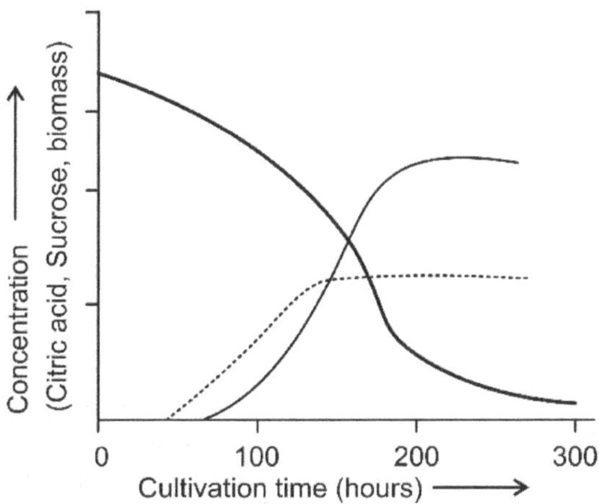

Fig. 5.7 Cultivation time verses Concentration of citric acid

Production of Citric Acid from Alkanes

The use of yeasts and bacteria in the production of citric acid from n-alkanes is possible (C9-C23 hydrocarbons). Hydrocarbons produce more citric acid than carbohydrates, with paraffin producing 145 percent citric acid. The most usually utilised organism is Candida lipolytica. There are three fermentation modes: batch, semi-continuous, and nonstop. It's important to keep an eye on the pH if it's higher than 5. The exceedingly low solubility of alkanes and the increased production of unwanted isocitric acid are the two biggest obstacles to making citric acid from them.

Recovery of Citric Acid

The recovery of citric acid by surface or submerged processes follows a similar path. Filtration of the culture broth and mycelium washing are the first steps in the recovery (which may contain about 10 of citric acid produced). Oxalic acid is an undesirable byproduct that can be precipitated by adding lime to a pH of 3.

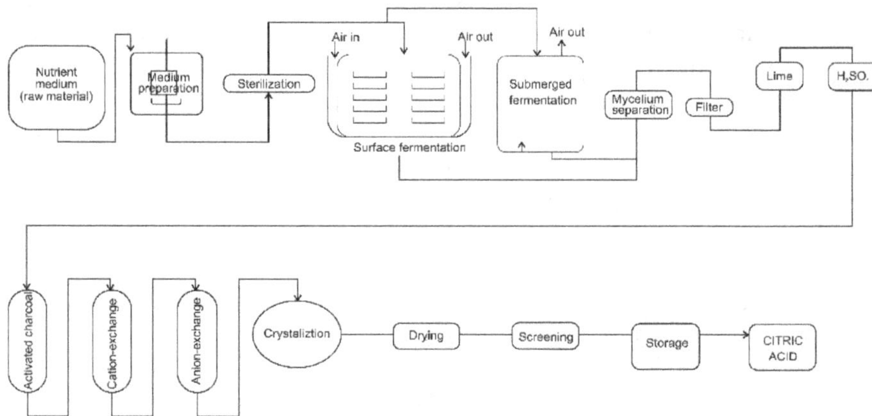

Fig. 5.8 Flow chart for industrial production of citric acid by surface or submerged processes

To precipitate citric acid, the culture broth is also exposed to a pH of 7.2 and a temperature of 70-90 °C. Citric acid is dissolved in sulfuric acid for further purification (calcium sulphate precipitate separates). Treatment with activated charcoal, cation and anion-exchangers, and crystallisation are the ultimate methods for recovering citric acid.

The major commercial product is citric acid monohydrate, which is generated below 36 °C. Citric acid crystallises in anhydrous form above 40°C. The purity of citric acid produced is determined by the function for which it is used.

5.7.3   Study of Production of Vitamins Production

Vitamins are organic compounds that have certain natural activities in an organism's regular conservation and growth. The vitamins can be synthesised by microorganisms. Many vitamins, such as thiamine, folic acid, pyridoxine, riboflavin, pantothenic acid, biotin, vitamin B_{12}, pro-vitamin A, ascorbic acid, and ergosterol, can be successfully produced commercially using microorganisms (pro-vitamin D). However, from an economic standpoint, microbes can create riboflavin, vitamin B_{12}, and ascorbic acid.

Vitamin B_{12}

Introduction

Pernicious anaemia, which is characterised by low haemoglobin levels, a decreased number of erythrocytes, and neurological symptoms, has been known for decades. Employees claimed that liver extracts may cure pernicious anaemia in 1926. Vitamin B_{12}, a water soluble B-complex vitamin, was eventually identified as the active ingredient.

Vitamin B_{12} is found in extremely small amounts in animal tissue (e.g. 1 ppm in the liver). Methylcobalamin and deoxyadenosylcobalamin are the two most common coenzyme types. Vitamin B_{12} is extremely valuable and time-consuming to isolate from animal tissues.

Vitamin B_{12} (cyanocobalamin) has a complicated structure and is a water soluble vitamin. $C_{63}H_{90}N_{14}O_{14}PCO$ is the empirical formula for cyanocobalamin. Vitamin B_{12} is made up of a corrin ring with a cobalt atom in the middle. The tetrapyrrole ring structure observed in other porphyrin compounds such as heme (with Fe) and chlorophyll is almost identical to the corrin ring structure (with Mg).

There are four pyrrole units in the corrin ring. The four pyrrole nitrogens are bonded to the cobalt in the corrin ring's centre. Dimethylbenzimidazole and amino isopropanol also bind to cobalt. As a result, the cobalt atom in vitamin B_{12} has a coordination state of six.

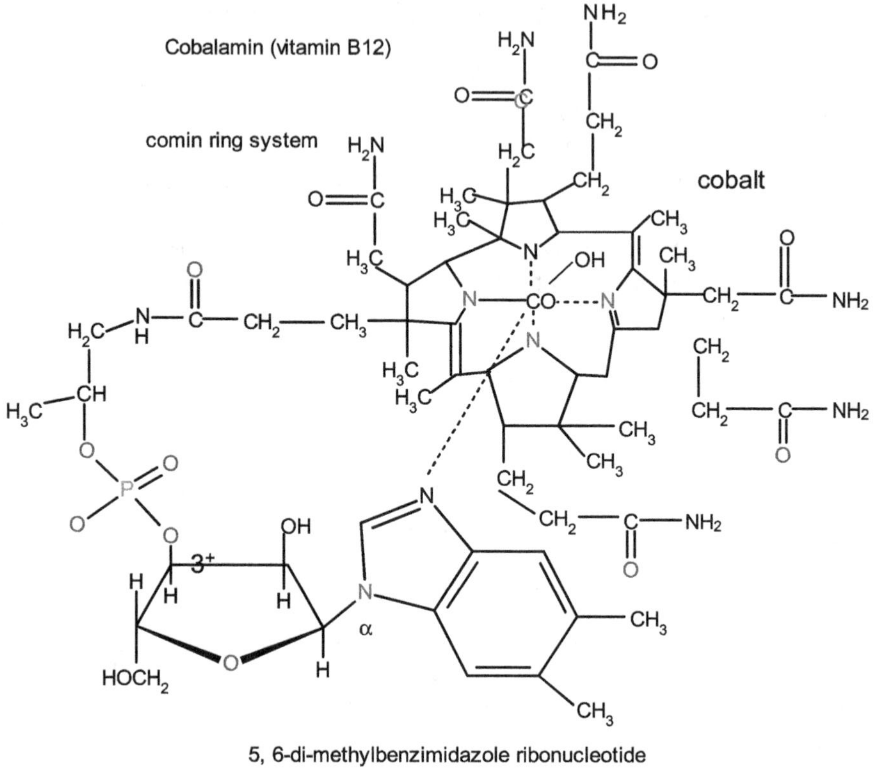

Fig. 5.9 Structure of Vitamin B_{12}

Acetobacterium, Aerobacterium, Agrobacterium, Alcaligenes, Azotobacter, Bacillus, Clostridium, Corynebacterium, Flavobacterium, Lactobacillus, Micromonospora, Mycobacterium, Nocardia, Propionibacterium, Protaminobacterium, Proteus, Pseudomonas, Streptomyces, Streptococcus, Streptomyces

B_{12} is produced in industrial quantities by fermenting chosen bacteria. For many years, Streptomyces griseus, a bacterium that was originally assumed to be a yeast, was the commercial source of vitamin B_{12}. Pseudomonas denitrificans and Propionibacterium shermanii are two of the most often used bacteria nowadays.

Table 5.3 Types of Culture media

Species of Microorganisms	Main Component of Culture Medium	Conditions of Fermentation		Vitamin B12 production /(mg/L)
1	Proplonibacterium freudenreichit	Glucose	Anaerobiosis benzimidazole 5,6-dimethyl	206
2.	Rhodopseudomonas protamicus	Glucose	5,6-dimethyl benzimidazole	135
3	Propionibacterium shermanil	Glucose	5, 6-dimethyl benzimidazole	60
4.	Pseudomonas denitrificans	Sucrose	Aerobiosis, betainc	60
5.	Nocardiarugosa	Glucose	Aerobiosis	18
6.	Rhizobium cobalaminogenum	Sucrose	Aerobiosis	16.5
7.	Micromonospora sp.	Glucose	5,6-dimethyl benzimidazole	11.5
8.	Streptomyces olivaceus	Glucose	5,6-dimethyl benzimidazole	6
9.	Nocardiagardneri			
10.	Butyribacterium methylotrophicum	Hexadecane Methanol	Aerobiosis Anaerobiosis	4.5 3.6
11.	Pseudomonas sp.			
12.	Arthrobacter hyalimus	Methanol Isopropanol	5, 6-dimethyl benzimidazole 5, 6-dimethyl benzimidazole	3.2 1.1

Commercial Production of Vitamin B$_{12}$

Fermentation is used in the commercial production of vitamin B$_{12}$. It was first discovered as a byproduct of Streptomyces fermentation in the manufacture of antibiotics (chloramphenicol, streptomycin or neomycin). However, the profit was insignificant. Later on, high-yielding strains appeared. Vitamin B$_{12}$ is currently generated exclusively through fermentation. The global annual output of vitamin B$_{12}$ is estimated to be 15,000 kg.

In sewage-sludge solids, high levels of vitamin B$_{12}$ have been found. Microorganisms are responsible for this. In some locations of the United States, vitamin B$_{12}$ was recovered from sewage sludge. Unlike most other vitamins, vitamin B$_{12}$ cannot be synthesised chemically because it requires approximately 20 complex reaction steps.

Production of Vitamin B$_{12}$ Using *Propionibacterium sp*

Propionibacterium freudenreichii and Propionibacterium shermanii, as well as mutant strains of these bacteria, are extensively utilised to produce vitamin B$_{12}$. Cobalt is added in two stages to complete the process.

Anaerobic phase

This is a preliminary stage that could take 2-4 days to complete. The anaerobic phase is dominated by the production of 5'-deoxyadenosylcobinamide.

Aerobic phase

In this phase, riboflavin is converted to 5, 6-dimethylbenzimidazole, which is then integrated to make the vitamin B-p coenzyme, 5'-deoxyadenosylcobalamin.

In recent years, some fermentation technologists have effectively combined the anaerobic and aerobic phases in two reaction tanks to carry out the operation continuously.

Submerged bacterial fermentation using beet molasses medium supplemented with cobalt chloride produces the majority of vitamin B$_{12}$.

Recovery of vitamin B$_{12}$

Fermentation produces cobalamins that are primarily attached to the cells. Heat treatment at 80-120°C for 30 minutes at pH 6.5-8.5 will solubilize them. The fermentation broth is collected after the sediments and mycelium have been filtered or centrifuged. Cobalamins can be transformed to cyanocobalamins, which are more stable. This vitamin B_{12} is approximately 80% pure and can be used directly as a feed additive. However, vitamin B12 should be refined further for medical usage (especially in the treatment of pernicious anaemia) (95-98 percent purity).

Production of Vitamin B_{12} using *Pseudomonas sp*

Pseudomonas denitrificans is also utilised to produce vitamin B_{12} in big quantities at a low cost. Starting with a poor yield (0.6 mg/l) two decades ago, many improvements in P. denitrificans strains have resulted in a massive increase in production (60 mg/l). Cobalt and 5, 6-dimethyl Benz imidazole must be added to the medium. When the medium is treated with betaine, the yield of vitamin B_{12} increases (usual source being sugar beet molasses).

Carbon Sources for Vitamin B_{12} Production

The most prevalent carbon source for large-scale vitamin B_{12} production is glucose. Other carbon sources with varying yields can be employed, such as alcohols (methanol, ethanol, isopropanol) and hydrocarbons (alkanes, decane, hexadecane). In a fed-batch growth method, the bacterium Methanosarcina barkeri produced 42 mg/l of vitamin B_{12} using methanol as the carbon source.

Table 5.4 Carbon Sources for Vitamin B_{12} Production

Species	Medium	Aeration	Temp. (^{O}C)	Time (hr)	Yield (mg/ltr)
B. megaterium	Molases, mineral salts, cobalt	Aerobic	30	18	0.45
P.Shermanii	Glucose. corn steep, ammonia, cobalt pH 7.0	Anaerobic (3 days), aerobic (4 days)	30	150	23
B. Coagulants	Citric acid, teiethanolamine, corn-steep, cobalt	Aerobic	55	18	6.0
P.denitrificans	Oxalic acid, betaine cobalt, mineral salts	Aerobic	-	-	10

5.7.4   Study of Production of Glutamic Acid

Dr.K. Ikeda, a Japanese scientist, discovered glutamic acid from kelp, a marine alga, in 1908. He also observed that after neutralising glutamic acid with castic soda, it took on a completely new, pleasant flavour.

Monosodium glutamate (MSG) was first used as a flavour enhancer about this time. The isolation of a separate soil-inhabiting gram-positive bacterium, Corynebacterium glutamicum, by Dr. S. Ukada and Dr. S. Kinoshita in 1957 was a milestone in the manufacture of MSG. The successful commercialization of monosodium glutamate (MSG) with this bacterium boosted amino acid production, which was then replicated with other bacteria such as E. coli.

Commercial Production of Glutamic Acid

Commercial glutamic acid production through microbial fermentation meets 90 percent of global demand, with the remaining 10 percent met by chemical techniques. Microbial strains are produced in fermentors as large as 500 m3 for the actual fermentation. Carbohydrates (glucose, molasses, sucrose, etc.), peptone, inorganic salts, and biotin are among the raw materials used.

The amount of biotin in the fermentation medium has a big impact on the glutamic acid yield. The fermentation takes 2-4 days to complete, and the broth contains glutamic acid in the form of its ammonium salt at the conclusion.

The bacterial cells are isolated and the broth is passed through a basic anion exchange resin in a typical downstream process. Ammonia is released when glutamic acid anions bind to the resin. This ammonia can be collected and utilised in the fermentation process through distillation.

Purification and recovery

Elution with NaOH is used to remove monosodium glutamate (MSG) from the solution while also regenerating the basic anion exchanger. MSG can be crystallised directly from the elute, followed by additional conditioning operations such as decolorization and serving to produce a food-grade MSG.

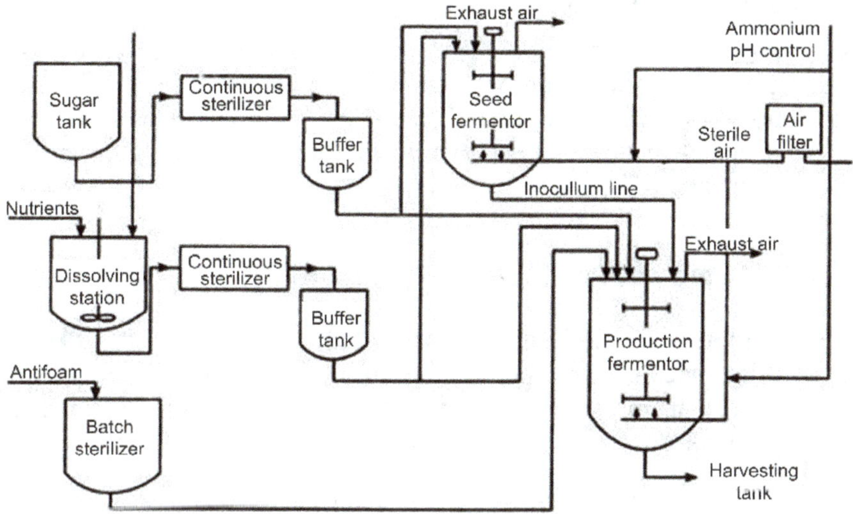

Fig. 5.10 A flow diagram of commercial production method of glutamic acid (glutamate)

The precursor of glutamic acid is -ketoglutaric acid, and the enzyme glutamic acid dehydrogenase is required for the conversion of - ketoglutaric acid to glutamic acid. It has been discovered that adding penicillin to the medium increases glutamic acid synthesis by a factor of ten.

$$
\begin{array}{ccc}
\text{COOH} & & \text{COOH} \\
| & & | \\
\text{C} = \text{O} & & \text{CHNH}_2 \\
| & \xrightarrow[\text{dehydrogenase}]{\text{Glutamic acid}} & | \\
\text{CH}_2 + \text{NH}_3 & & \text{CH}_2 + \text{H}_2\text{O} \\
| & & | \\
\text{CH}_2 & & \text{CH}_2 \\
| & & | \\
\text{COOH} & & \text{COOH} \\
\alpha\text{-ketoglutaric acid} & & \text{L-Glutamic acid}
\end{array}
$$

Uses of Glutamic Acid

Glutamic acid is frequently used in the manufacture of MSG, often known as "seasoning salt." Glutamic acid is produced at a rate of 800,000 tonnes per year around the world. MSG is a condiment and flavour enhancer that is most commonly found as a frequent ingredient in convenience foods.

5.7.5   Study of Production of Griseofulvin

Griseofulvin is an antifungal antibiotic that was discovered in 1939 in a Penicillium species. The fungus Penicillium griseofulvum produces it as a secondary metabolite. Water is insoluble, while ethanol, methanol, acetone, benzene, ethyl acetate, and acetic acid are slightly soluble.

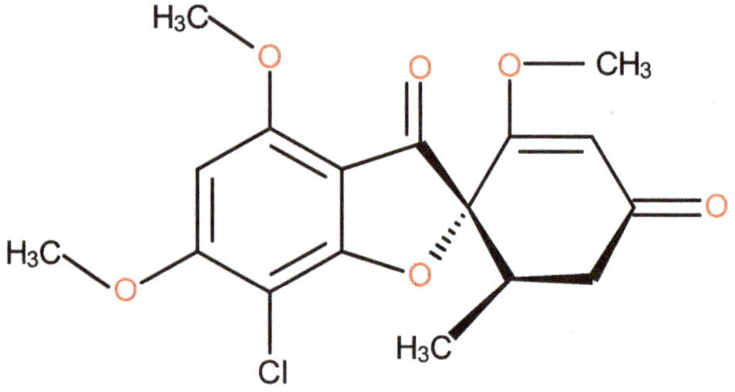

Mode of Action

Griseofulvin suppresses mitosis and nuclear acid production in fungi. It also binds to alpha and beta tubulin, interfering with the function of spindle and cytoplasm microtubules. It attaches to keratin in human cells before binding to fungal microtubules at the fungal site of action, causing the fungal process of mitosis to be disrupted.

Uses

It's used to treat Ringworm infections, Nail Fungal Disease, and Athlete's Foot.

Side effects

Nausea, vomiting, diarrhoea, heartburn, flatulence, and cracking at the side of the mouth are the most prevalent adverse effects.

Soreness and/or blackening of the tongue, thirst, and headache are some of the symptoms.

Preparation of Media

Medium: Czapek Dox Medium

Glucose- 5%

Sodium Nitrate- 0.2%

Potassium Hydrogen Phosphate- 0.1%

Magnesium Sulphate 7H$_2$O- 0.05%

Industrial preparation of Griseofulvin by submerged fermentation

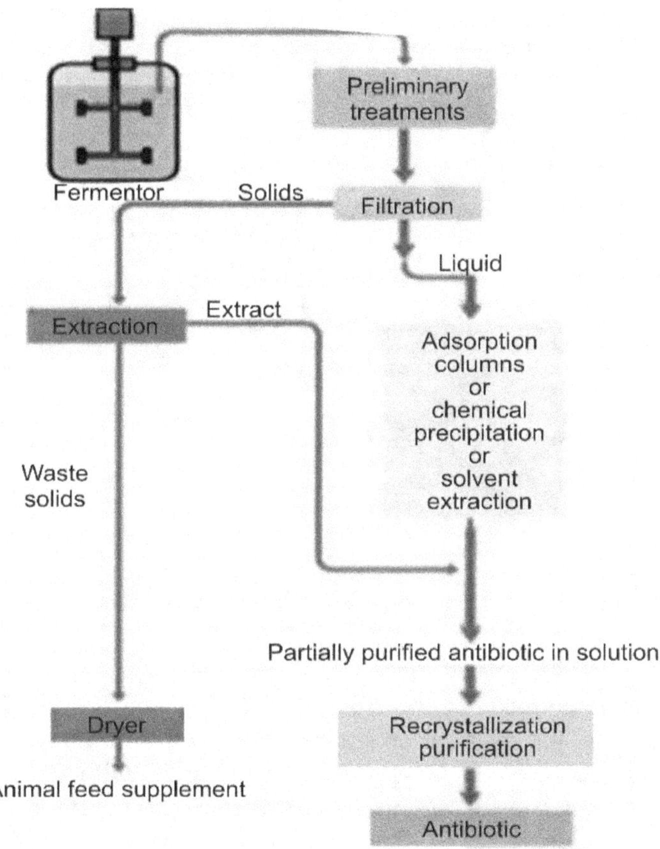

Fig. 5.11 Industrial preparation of Griseofulvin by submerged fermentation

The following Steps are involved in the manufacturing process

Fermentation

Czapek-Dox medium's pH was changed to 6.0-7.2. In the fermenter, the medium was added.

On raper steep agar (CzapekDox medium + corn steep+ agar), a new sample of mycelial suspension of the fungus Pencillium griseofulvum was collected from a fresh slope. The solution was autoclaved for 200 minutes at 120°C under 15 pounds of pressure before being fermented for 14 days at 24

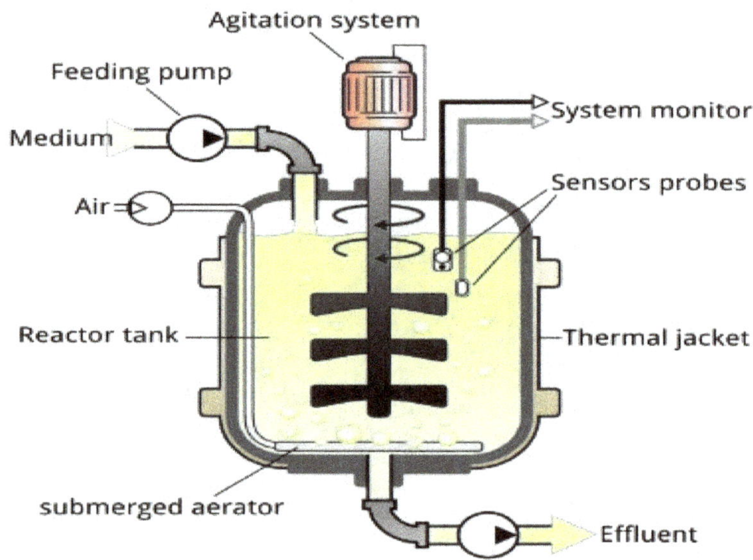

Fig. 5.12 Fermenter

Pretreatment of fermentation broth

The broth is cooked for 20- 30 minutes at a temperature above 60°C. After heating, the material coagulates sufficiently to improve the broth's separation qualities. Heating time can be brief, with 5-10 minutes at 80°C providing a sufficient improvement in filtration rate.

Filtration

Drum half-filled with diatomaceous earth materials and allowed to revolve under vacuum in the slurry tank. A small amount of coagulation agent was added to the soup and then poured into the slurry tank. A thin coating of clotted patches adheres to the drum as it rotates in the slurry tank under vacuum. The layer thickens to the point where it looks like cake. The cake portion in the drum is cleaned with water and dewatered incontinently by blowing air over it as it reaches the higher region not immersed in the liquid. The dried section is also chopped off from the drum by a cutter before it is re-fascinated into the liquid shown in Fig.5.13.

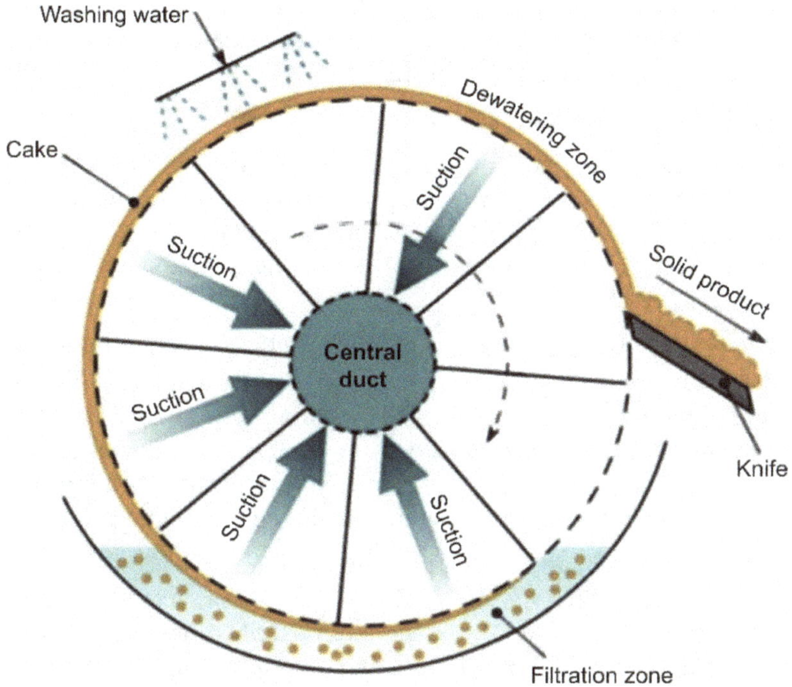

Fig. 5.13 Filtration drum

Extraction

When it's utilised as a breeding agent, griseofulvin is extracted using cold acetone. Cold acetone lines can have efficiencies ranging from 75 to 96 percent, and even up to 99 percent. In large-scale production, the volume of solvent required in extraction should be limited to a bare minimum. Acetone should be 3-5 times the volume of the mycelial sensed.

Decolorization

Calcium hydroxide, usually 2.5-50 g/ litre rather than 5-30 g/ litre, can be added to improve the colour of the extract. The extract's pH must be greater than 10. By removing the lime or applying mineral acid, it can be neutralised.

Isolation and Fractionation

Contaminations or waxy beings are eliminated by washing the extract in a solvent that is immiscible for the extract and insoluble for griseofulvin. In general, aliphatic hydrocarbons similar to hexane or petroleum with a high hexane content are ideal for this stage.

Precipitation and purification

Griseofulvin can be precipitated in a variety of ways from the solvent passage. The use of a liquid solvent, in which griseofulvin is mostly insoluble, is one of the methods. Water is the Griseofulvinnon-solvent. Alkaline water is more successful in removing coloured impurities from griseofulvin crystals.

Ammonia, alkali essence carbonate, or alkali essence hydroxide are used to make water alkaline. The ideal pH is around 8.5. The purity of the precipitate is often improved by washing with a solvent to remove any remaining contaminants. Dry or wet acetone, as well as a lower alkanol such as methanol or butanol, are appropriate washing medium. The use of methanol for this stage results in marked purification.

Blood is a constantly circulating fluid that nourishes, oxygenates, and removes waste from the body. Blood flows via vessels in the body (arteries and veins). Blood products are described as blood factors (red cells, platelets, fresh frozen plasma, and cryoprecipitate) manufactured in a blood transfusion centre or plasma derivates created in plasma separation centres from pooled plasma donations (similar as albumin, coagulation factors and immunoglobulins). The Medicines Act regulates plasma derivations, which, like any other medicine, must be prescribed by a licenced practitioner. Transfusions with whole blood are becoming less common. Because most instances contain a single element of blood, such as red cells or platelets, blood element therapy makes clinical sense, and the treatment may be tailored.

Each component is kept in optimal conditions (red cells must be refrigerated, platelets do not), allowing for more efficient use of scarce blood donations.

Collection, Processing and Storage

Objectives

1. To keep the viability and functionality of the organisation.

2. To avoid bodily alterations.

3. To keep bacterial contamination to a minimum.

The desired volume of collected blood samples varies depending on a number of parameters, including the length of the study and the anticipated uses for these samples, but can range from 1 mL to 450 mL in repeated collections. If the goal is to harvest plasma and blood cells, the samples must be treated with an anticoagulant to prevent clotting. Stabilizers can be included in the collection device or added to the sample after collection to prevent analytes from breaking down. Blood is generally taken in the absence of anticoagulants when serum is sought.

A blend of cellular essentials, colloids, and crystalloids makes up whole blood. When centrifugal force is used to separate blood components with varied relative viscosity, sediment rate, and size, they can be separated. Plasma, platelets, leucocytes (Buffy Coat (BC)), and packed red blood cells have the highest specific gravity (PRBCs). Each element's functional usefulness is determined by appropriate processing and storage. Element remedy must be adapted widely in order to use one blood unit properly and rationally.

5.8   Concept of Blood Components

Blood is usually transfused to keep tissues oxygenated or to treat bleeding and coagulation problems.

The role of each blood component when transfused

1. When a patient's red cells are lost as a result of bleeding or anaemia, red cells (erythrocytes) keep the oxygen supply to the tissues going.

2. Platelets (thrombocytes) help to treat thrombocytopenia-related bleeding.

3. After a haemorrhage caused by trauma or surgery, plasma is occasionally administered to keep blood volume up.

4. Fresh plasma can be used to replace clotting factors and to help with abnormal bleeding correction.

5. Plasma can be separated to make derivatives that can be used to treat clotting factor abnormalities, offer short-term immunity with immunoglobulins, or treat burns with albumin.

Transfusion of white cells (leucocytes, including granulocytes) is not usual. They may contain TTIs like CMV or cause immunological modulation, both of which are harmful to the patient. Although granulocyte transfusions may have some indications, the goal of component therapy is to limit the number of white cells transfused in general.

Advantages of separation of Whole Blood into components

Blood serves a variety of purposes. There are evident benefits for the patient and the blood transfusion service when a whole blood unit is processed into particular red cell, plasma, and platelet components:

- A single blood donation can help a number of patients. This is the efficient utilisation of a limited resource.

- Patients only get the component(s) necessary to treat their ailment; components not required by the patient are not transfused (such as white cells or plasma proteins when the patient requires only red cells). This lowers the chances of a transfusion response.

- By selecting the right additive, temperature, bag type, and other variables, the storage conditions of the items can be improved to guarantee that each component remains functional for the longest time feasible.

Processing Whole Blood into Components

A basic understanding of the following is necessary to convert whole blood into components:

1. Blood donors are chosen first.

2. System for sterility

3. Bags for collecting blood

4. Centrifugation Principles

5. Blood component preparation

1. **Selection of blood donors:** The criteria used by drug control authorities and the National AIDS Control Organization to determine a willing fit donor for whole blood or apheresis collection are outlined below.

2. **Sterile systems:** All blood bags, anticoagulants, and cumulative findings must be sterile (free of bacteria or contagions) and pyrogen-free, according to blood bag manufacturers (do not hold endotoxins ormicro-organism debris).

All blood bags, anticoagulants, and cumulative findings must be sterile (free of bacteria or contagions) and pyrogen-free, according to blood bag manufacturers (do not hold endotoxins ormicro-organism debris).

The venepuncture spot on the donor's arm is thoroughly drawn and the sterile needle on the blood bag tubing is placed into the vein at the time of blood donation. The donor's bloodstream and the sterile blood bag are thus linked directly. The tube is shut at the end of the donation, and the blood bag's contents should be clear of bacteria. Once the blood bag is sealed, it becomes a 'unrestricted system,' which is ideal because the product's integrity is guaranteed.

However, because the bag has been opened either intentionally or accidently, it is classified as a 'open network' (i,e. environmental air, which contains microbial aerosols, could have entered the bag). When a blood bag is accidentally opened, sterility can no longer be assured, and the blood bag must be thrown. This is due to the fact that microorganisms can get into any product that has been exposed to the environment. A blood bag is occasionally intended to be opened under controlled conditions (for example, using a laminar inflow press) in order to produce a specific blood product. A docked expiry period is applied to the product in these circumstances, which is usually over 24 hours from the moment of opening.

The availability of unrestricted blood bag systems is required for routine factor processing. Individual bags in multiple bag systems are connected by tubing and so form an open system. Because the primary bag is never opened and the entire process takes place in an unconstrained system, the factors can be pushed into the associated bags (after centrifugation) without compromising sterility.

3. **Bag systems for blood collection:** Many suppliers offer a wide range of polyvinyl chloride (PVC) plastic blood bag systems. The type of bag to use is determined by the needs of the specific blood service:

- Cost-effectiveness
- Whether units will be handled manually or mechanically

- The level of product storage that will be reached (additive solutions, special plastic bags for platelets)
- Whether filtration (leucodepletion) is necessary

Single bag systems

This is the most basic bag that may be found. The pilot tube is then shut when the donation is placed in the bag. The unit is transfused as whole blood, with no further processing into components. An anticoagulant solution is stored in the bag (CPDA). Sodium citrate prevents clotting, whereas citric acid (C), monobasic sodium phosphate (P), dextrose (D), and adenine (A) offer buffers and nutrition to help red cells survive.

Double bag (two bag system)

The principal bag in a multiple bag system is the one that contains the anticoagulant and into which the donation is placed. The primary bag is identical to the single unit's, but in the twin bag system, a new empty bag is attached (called a transfer or satellite bag). After centrifuging the whole blood, the plasma can be transferred to the associated transfer bag through the tubing, resulting in two factors: a red cell concentrate suspended in plasma (in the primary bag) and plasma (in the transfer bag).

Triple bag (three bag system)

Only having a fresh transfer bag distinguishes a triple bag from a double bag. There's still another empty transfer bag attached to the first transfer bag once plasma has been separated. This setup is used to collect platelets or make platelet concentrates from platelet-rich plasma. Freshly frozen plasma is cryoprecipitated.

Quadruple (quad) bag (four bag system)

A quadrilateral bag system is similar to a triadic bag system, but it includes a new bag storing the red cell cumulative result, and it is commonly used in automated systems to prepare.

- Red cell concentrates (RCC), which have had the white cells removed and a total result added to them.

Top and bottom bag

This is a three-bag system designed specifically for automated complexes. An empty transfer bag is attached to the top of the primary collection bag, and a transfer bag carrying the cumulative results is attached to the bottom. Following centrifugation, the bag is placed in a blood processing machine, which separates the plasma from the top and the red cells from the bottom, leaving the BC in the primary collection bag. The same three items are produced as in the quadrangle bag system:

- A BC layer of white cells and platelets that stays in the primary bag.

- Red cell concentrates (with buffy coat removed and suspended in additive solution) in the bottom transfer bag This BC can either be thrown away or used to make platelet concentrate.

The transfusion service's management team should make the decision on whether or not to remove BCs from RCCs.

Removing the BC has several advantages:

- The procedure lowers micro-aggregate formation during storage and makes RCC leucocytes deficient (not the same as leucocyte-depleted).

- All of the plasma is extracted and preserved as fresh frozen plasma, which can either be used as is or as a starting material for fractionated products.

- The red cells can be resuspended in a solution, such as saline adenine-glucose-mannitol, that is designed to provide optimal conditions for red cell storage (SAGM).

- Platelet concentrates can be made with the BCs.

A quad or top and bottom blood bag system, as well as automated processing equipment, are typically required to create these advanced goods. Where collection and demand are not high enough to justify the system, the cost of bags and machinery may make these processes hard to execute. In these circumstances, simpler double or triple bag systems might be more viable.

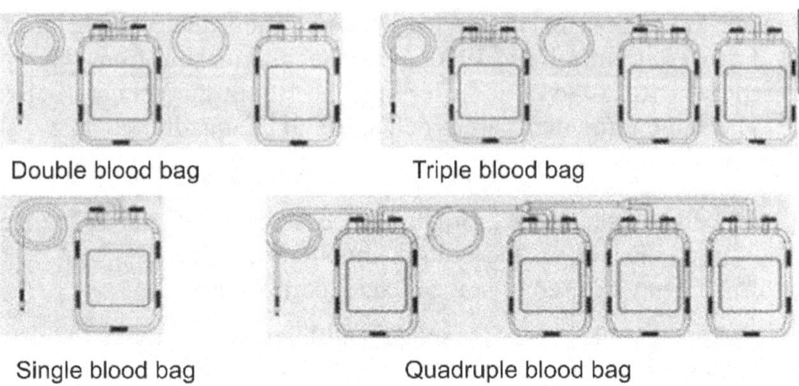

Fig. 5.14 Types of Bag systems for blood collection

4. **Principles of centrifugation:** Because the white cells and platelets are thinner, they take longer to settle and remain in suspense. The white cells precipitate above the red cells as centrifugation continues, and the platelets solidify a layer above the white cells, leaving the original suspending fluid (now clear plasma plus anticoagulant) at the top. The separation of components following moderate or hard centrifugation of a unit of whole blood is depicted in Figure 11 • 6. The speed and duration of centrifugation to be 358tilized to separate the desired element are the decisions to be made. If platelet-rich plasma is required, centrifugation should be halted before platelet sedimentation occurs, for example.

It would be easier to choose the time to stop if the centrifugation speed was lower for a longer period. However, cell-free plasma is required. If you centrifuge at a high speed for a long enough time, you'll get clear tubes with densely packed red cells. To obtain the requested factors, it is critical that the optimal conditions for a satisfactory separation be exactly determined for each centrifuge.

After centrifugation, the bag system is precisely withdrawn from the centrifuge (to aid mixing) and the primary bag is partitioned in a plasma extractor or an automated processing equipment. The element layers are transferred in order into one of the transfer bags connected in the unrestricted system under pressure.

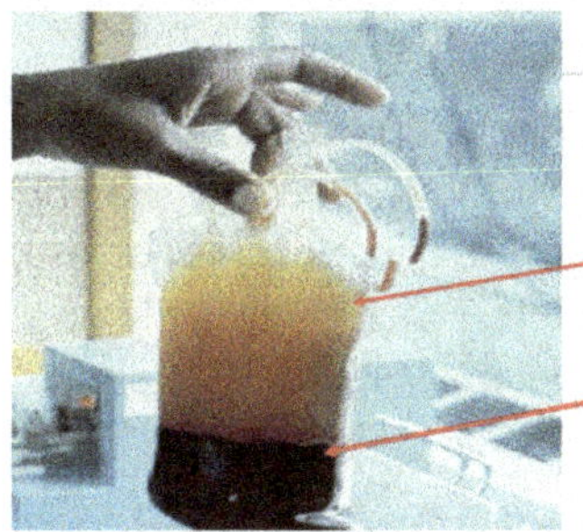

Fig. 5.15 Whole blood Unit

5. **Preparation of specific blood components:** Blood components can be manufactured in a variety of methods, depending on the transfusion service's needs and the resources available (donors, personnel, disposables, funding and space).

WHOLE BLOOD

Whole blood is the starting point for making blood components, and it keeps its qualities for a limited duration if it isn't treated any further.

The term "storage lesion" refers to a series of alterations that occur after around 5 days of blood storage.

- Coagulation factor activity (including factor VIII) degrades rapidly, especially during the first 24 hours of storage, making this product unsuitable for treating haemostatic diseases.
- Platelets in whole blood soon lose their viability and functioning, making them unsuitable for use in platelet therapy patients.
- Red blood cells lose viability when their oxygen affinity increases.

The release of leucocyte proteases causes leucocytes to degrade. Microaggregates form as a result of the formation of the microaggregates.

- The red blood cells discharge potassium.

RED CELL CONCENTRATES

Red cell concentrates in plasma

Red cell concentrates in plasma are prepared by removing part of the plasma from centrifuged whole blood. Enough plasma is removed to reduce the haematocrit (packed red cell volume) to between 0·65 and 0·75, and white cells and platelets remain with the red cells. This is a simple separation of whole blood that is usually collected into a double bag.

Red cells in plasma are used for replacement of blood or red cell loss. As white cells are not reduced and the storage medium for the red cells is not improved by the use of additives, they do not offer much advantage over whole blood other than reduced volume in the transfusion. However, the separated plasma may be used as another component or forwarded to a fractionation facility

Red cell concentrate (RCC), Buffy coat (BC) removed, in additive solution (RCC, leucocyte-reduced)

By adding additive solutions (ADSOL) or saline, adenine, glucose and mannitol solution (SAGM) PRBC can be stored for 42 days. Since BC contains most leucocytes, during the preparation of components by BC method, if entire BC is discarded then each PRBC and PLTC unit will have leucocytes $<1·2 \times 10^9$. Such products are called leucocyte reduced but not leucocyte depleted. Leucocyte depletion is achieved only by filtration.

The main advantage of BC removal is that the microaggregate formation during storage is greatly reduced (compared to whole blood or RCCs stored with BC) and the incidence of recipient febrile reactions is reduced. Storage in additive solution can support red cell viability and function if stored at $+4°C \pm 2°C$ for up to 42 days from the date of donation.

Red cell concentrate, filtered (RCC, leucocyte-depleted)

Each leucocyte depleted blood product viz-PRBC or single dose platelet or adult therapeutic dose platelet should contain leucocytes $<5 \times 10^6$ per unit to prevent alloimmunisation to leucocyte antigens in patients where transfusions are likely to be ongoing. This is achieved by following methods:

i) **Pre storage filtration:** This process includes immediate filtration within 48 h from collection before or after component separation.

Advantages:

- Complete quality assurance

- Process is done when leucocytes have not dissociated or broken or cytokine released. Hence expected benefits are almost 100%

- No storage lesions and shelf life is unchanged.

Disadvantages:

- Leucodepletion irrespective of demands adds to cost and time

- Need well-trained dedicated technical staff.

- On demand also called as Lab side-This is done only on demand. Bags with built in filters ensure a closed system when used with sterile connecting device (SCD) and are also easy to operate

- Pre transfusion also called as bedside: This is done by spiking blood component bag with a specialized transfusion set having leucocyte filter with continuous leucoreduction during transfusion. Here the effect of cytokines cannot be avoided.

Recommended indications for leukoreduction (groups/principles)

- Patients needing transfusion and had at least two episodes FNHTR in previous transfusion

- In haematopoietic stem cell transplant recipients requiring transfusions

- To avoid post transfusion CMV infection in immunocompromised patients

- All neonatal and paediatric transfusions for children less than a year.

Prestorage in line products are used in two ways:

1. A filter is located in the tubing between the whole blood donation bag and a second transfer bag. On receipt in the components laboratory, the whole blood is filtered into the transfer bag, which then becomes the new primary container of filtered whole blood. Red cell and plasma components made from this filtered whole blood are leucocyte-depleted. Most whole blood filters also remove platelets so the method is unsuitable for making buffy coat platelets (although some new generation filters claim not to remove platelets).

2. A filter is located in the tubing between the primary bag and an additional attached transfer bag. On receipt at the components

laboratory the whole blood is processed as usual into components (RCC, plasma, Buffy coat). The Buffy coat reduced RCC is then filtered through to the additional transfer bag that is then appropriately labelled leucocyte-depleted RCC.

Prestorage add on systems require a sterile transfer bag with a leucocyte filter in line. This is sterile welded to a BC reduced RCC prepared from quad or top and bottom bags in a routine separation procedure. The red cells are then allowed to flow through the filter and into the transfer bag, which must be correctly numbered and labelled as leucocyte depleted RCC. A transfusion service may benefit from the flexibility of this system. With proper management, selected amounts and blood groups can be processed with little wastage resulting from expiry.

On demand systems generally meet the need for filtration in situations where prestorage products are not available.

ii) On demand filtration

A transfusion service may apply an on demand policy, filtering units only when requested. This has obvious cost saving advantages as filters are generally considered to be expensive and there is little wastage because of expiry.

In line filter systems are supplied with a filter built into the closed system to ensure sterility and ease of operation. The system may be designed to filter the whole blood donation prior to further processing or to filter the red cell concentrate after removal of the plasma and BC.

Add on filter systems involve a separate bag with integral filter that is attached to the unit to be filtered by pushing the spikes (cannulas) into its port or by connecting it using an SCD. If the connection is made using an SCD then the shelf life of the component is unaffected. Other methods require that the product is used within 24 hours of the 'add on'.

On demand filtration has several disadvantages:

- The unit can be at any stage of its shelf life at the time of filtration.

- A larger number of personnel in various laboratories and hospital wards need to be trained to perform the procedure.

- It is likely that personnel performing the task do so only infrequently, and competency may be reduced as a result of lack of practice.

- Good laboratory practice (GLP) is difficult to apply to a procedure performed in multiple centres.

- Taking the required number of quality testing samples in the correct way to obtain accurate counts is difficult if not impossible in some areas.

- White cell fragmentation occurs as a result of extended storage prior to filtration.

On demand processing of filtered red cells in the components laboratory is the most practical way to supply the component when usage is low and only occasionally requested. In this instance the technologists who are most familiar with component production perform the filtration in a laboratory setting where GLP may be applied. Quality testing is possible because personnel are familiar with quality testing requirements and how to take the samples for testing. Connection of the filter/transfer bag can be achieved using an SCD (expiry date of component therefore unaffected) or by using the cannula (open system – expiry reduced to 24 hours).

On demand processing by blood bank technologists in a cross matching laboratory may be practical in some situations. Connection of the filter/transfer bag is likely to be made using the cannula just before issue (open system – expiry reduced to 24 hours). As the number of individuals performing the procedure is limited to blood bank trained personnel, there is some quality control and measure of GLP. It is likely that personnel performing the task do so only infrequently and competency may be reduced because of lack of practise.

On demand bedside filtration is achieved by using a transfusion set with an in line white cell filter, and the red cell product is filtered as it is being transfused. The transfusion service is not involved in the filtration process, training or quality control as this responsibility has shifted to the hospital personnel responsible for setting up the transfusion.

Red cell concentrate (RCC), pediatric

Neonates and very young children have a smaller circulating blood volume, generally higher haematocrit values, reduced metabolic capacity and immature immune systems. These factors need to be taken into consideration when preparing components for their use. A pediatric dose of RCC is prepared either from RCC with BC removed, or filtered RCCs by dividing the adult unit into quantities suited to the smaller patient's needs (usually from 25–100 ml).

Additional bags may be built into the blood bag system used to take the donation to ensure that sterility is maintained during transfer of red cells (closed system). To use this method the need for the product must be identified at the outset and the special bag must be committed to the process at the time of blood collection. Care must be taken to ensure that separated paediatric doses of RCC are identified with unique numbers that can be clearly linked to the original donation. When a paediatric patient requires blood over several days, all the split units should be reserved for that patient to limit the number of donor exposures received.

Red cell concentrate, cryopreserved (frozen)

When frozen, the shelf life of red cells can be extended up to 10 years and more if the units are correctly protected during freezing, and ultra-low freezing temperatures (colder than –65°C) are maintained during the entire storage period.

The following damage to red cells occurs if frozen without protective solutions:

Red cell dehydration: This occurs when extracellular water freezes before intracellular water, creating a difference in osmotic pressure between red cells and their surroundings, and resulting in intracellular water diffusing out of the red cells, collapsing them.

Intracellular ice: The red cells rupture from mechanical trauma caused by ice crystals that form inside the cells.

The most commonly used cryoprotective solution is a high concentration of glycerol (40%). Other protective solutions such as low concentrate glycerol and hydroxyethyl starch are less frequently used. Glycerol consists of a small molecule that can cross the red cell membrane and this is known as a penetrating cryoprotective agent. After entering the red cell it provides an osmotic force that will stop the migration of water from the cell as ice is formed outside it. The high concentration of glycerol also prevents the formation of intracellular ice crystals and thus prevents cell membrane damage.

Frozen storage of red cells is used mainly to preserve units of blood with rare blood types. It can be used to stockpile blood for emergency use in disasters, but the high cost and short shelf life after recovery from the frozen state make it impractical as a routine tool to manage inventory.

Procedures for glycerolization of cells vary. Usually, all plasma and/or additive solution is removed from whole blood or RCC within 6 days of collection. The glycerol solution must be added slowly with adequate, constant mixing to allow equilibration of solution and cells. Failure to equilibrate during addition results in a high degree of cell damage that is seen as excessive haemolysis and poor red cell recovery when the unit is thawed.

The original blood collection bag can be used for frozen storage, but the volume capacity is rather small to facilitate mixing of cells and glycerol so it may be preferable to use a larger volume bag (800 ml). Some polyvinyl chloride (PVC) bags can cause cellular damage during the freeze/thaw process so these larger bags are usually made of polyolefin plastic that minimizes cell damage. Polyolefin bags are also less brittle when frozen to the very low temperatures required and are less likely to break during storage and transportation.

Donations destined for freezing can be collected into special primary packs with these specifications, but it is also possible to connect a suitable freezing bag to any stock donation. Automated equipment and disposables that perform the entire freezing and thawing operation in a closed system are available.

Freezing and thawing technique

- Red cells prepared with a final glycerol concentration of 40% (weight to volume) are placed in metal or cardboard protective canisters to minimize breakage during the long period of frozen storage during which they might be handled or transported several times.

- The canisters and units are placed in a mechanical freezer capable of operating at $-80°C$. Although the freezer can run at this temperature, it is more likely to run at about $-70°C$ to maintain the temperature of the cells below the required $-65°C$.

- If temperatures are maintained continuously below $-65°C$ the units have an expiry date set at 10 years from date of donation.

- Most donations that are stored frozen are rare blood types, so when this type of donation reaches expiry it is not discarded. Scientific evidence indicates that cell recovery and viability from units stored for up to 21 years is acceptable, so if a frozen rare donation is required after its official expiry, it may be used as long as the reasons are clearly documented (e.g. no frozen units less than 10 years in storage and no other compatible donations or donors available).

- When frozen cells are to be recovered (deglycerolized) the unit is thawed with gentle agitation at +37°C for about 20 minutes.

- The thawed cells contain a high concentration of glycerol that should be removed gradually by washing with sterile saline solutions of decreasing osmolarity to avoid red cell haemolysis.

- Using a typical three wash procedure, the cells are diluted with 12% saline for the first wash, with 1.6% saline for the second wash and finally with 0.9% (normal) saline for the third wash. After the addition of each wash solution and gentle mixing, the bag is centrifuged, and then the supernatant removed from the red cells and discarded. The solutions are always added slowly with mixing and plenty of time for osmotic equilibration.

- The technique used should be properly validated for local conditions, and the final product should be free of cryoprotective agent, show minimal signs of haemolysis and yield at least 80% of the cells originally frozen.

- The freeze/thaw process involves adding solutions and extra bags and as this is usually performed using an open system it is carried out using a laminar flow cabinet. The red cells have a post thaw shelf life of 24 hours at +4°C ± 2°C.

- Automated equipment, disposables and solutions that perform the thaw operation in a closed system are commercially available and provide a post thaw shelf life of up to 14 days at +4°C ± 2°C

Red cell concentrate, Saline washed

Saline washed red cells are a specialised element prepared only on demand for patients with antibodies to plasma protein (e.g.,anti-IgA) and those who have severe allergic responses when transfused with blood products. This is a cheaper method than both Leuco and Plasma depletion.

Washed red cells are usually prepared by further processing of RCC, Buffy coat removed, in additive solution. Some transfusion services use filtered RCC as the starting material. Approximately 250 ml of cold (+4°C ± 2°C), sterile, isotonic saline is added to the RCC and the contents are gently and thoroughly mixed. The saline bag can be attached to the RCC bag using an SCD. In this way it is possible to maintain a closed system throughout the process. If saline is added by making connections using the spikes (cannulas) on transfer bags and transfusion sets, then the connections should be made under laminar flow conditions, and the expiry time of the product reduced to 24 hours.

After centrifugation in a refrigerated centrifuge set at approximately +4°C, the supernatant saline is removed and discarded. This is referred to as the first wash. The wash process (of adding saline, mixing and centrifuging) is usually repeated three or four times, with each wash resulting in the removal of more plasma protein from the product and finally producing washed red cells suspended in saline with less than 0.5 g protein per unit.

PLASMA

The first step in component processing is to remove the plasma from a centrifuged unit of whole blood. Fresh plasma contains proteins such as albumin, coagulation factors (most notably Factor VIII), and immunoglobulins. It is not practical to store plasma in liquid form as some fractions deteriorate rapidly, even if stored at refrigerator temperature (+4°C ± 2°C). Liquid plasma stored for more than a few days at this temperature is suitable only as a blood volume expander. To preserve labile fractions, plasma must be stored frozen and then becomes known as fresh frozen plasma (FFP). Blood donations to be processed into FFP or cryoprecipitate should not take longer than 15 minutes as poor flow during donation leads to consumption of clotting factors. FFP is used therapeutically, or is a starting material for the preparation of plasma derivatives in a fractionation facility.

- Freezing must be carried out within a maximum time of 24 hours from time of collection.

- From the time of donation to the time of freezing, the donation must be kept at controlled room temperature (+22°C ± 2°C).

- The time taken to freeze the plasma to a core temperature colder than −30°C must not exceed 1 hour from the time freezing is commenced. Core temperature refers to the temperature in the centre of the unit − the warmest part of the plasma pack during the freezing process.

FRESH FROZEN PLASMA (FPP)

FFP for therapeutic use is prepared by snap freezing the plasma component of whole blood as soon as practicably possible after collection. Specifications require that this time should not be longer than 18 hours from time of collection.

Once frozen, units are best stored at temperatures consistently colder than –25°C, and under these conditions have an expiry date of up to 3 years after date collected. The shelf life when stored at temperatures of –18°C to –25°C is 3 months only. Because FFP stored below –25°C has a long shelf life, the risk to recipients can be minimized by instituting a quarantine system (also known as a 'donor retest' programme). The plasma from donations found to be nonreactive for viral markers to HBV, HCV, and HIV is stored until the donor makes a subsequent donation that is also nonreactive, meaning that his/her stored plasma is safe for use. However, if the subsequent donation is found to be reactive, the stored plasma is discarded and the donor excluded from further donation. The quarantine period is designed to eliminate window period donations (donated during the latent period of immunosilence).

FFP is often stored in cardboard or polystyrene protective containers that minimize the risk of breakage of the brittle frozen product during storage, handling and transportation. Labelling of frozen bags of plasma is difficult because stick-on labels will not adhere securely. Units are either labelled before freezing, and a rigorous checking system put into place to verify safe donations once TTI testing results become available, or donations are labelled using tie-on tags. In all instances the use of computer records to identify safe donations is essential. Manual tracking of donations in a quarantine system is not recommended.

Fresh frozen plasma for fractionation

Plasma not used therapeutically may be supplied to a fractionation facility for the extraction of clotting factors, albumin and immunoglobulins. Fractionation facilities require bulk lots consisting of several thousand units of 'safe' plasma frozen within 24 hours of collection. Fresh plasma is preferred as albumin, immunoglobulin and clotting factor concentrates can be made from the same pool.

Plasma that is separated and frozen after the deadline of 24 hours from collection is considered to be 'outdated' plasma. Separation of this type of plasma may continue for up to 1 week after the expiry date of the whole blood provided that it was stored within the prescribed temperature range (+4°C ± 2°C).

Any supplier of 'safe' plasma as a raw material to a fractionation facility must comply with legislation and the fractionator's guidelines. 'Safe' plasma implies that collection, processing, storage and testing criteria met the same standard as that required for FFP. The records of plasma forwarded to a fractionation facility must be supported by a comprehensive data capture system to ensure quality and traceably of every unit in the batch.

FREEZE-DRIED PLASMA

A suitable product for use in outlying rural hospitals and emergency rooms can be manufactured using a process of freeze-drying (lyophilization). By this method the clotting factors present in fresh plasma can be preserved in powder form, and stored at ambient temperature (usually at +25°C or less).

A measured amount of distilled water (the same amount as was lost during drying) is added to reconstitute the powder just before use. Fresh plasma is transferred to a glass bottle under laminar flow conditions and then frozen by rolling the bottles in a bath of alcohol and dry ice, which when mixed, results in a temperature of colder than –60°C. This process is called 'shell freezing' as the plasma freezes in a thin layer over the inner surfaces of the bottle so that a large surface area is made available for evaporation when the product is in the process of being dried.

After freezing, each shell frozen plasma bottle has its rubber bung replaced with a sterile vapour-permeable membrane, also under laminar flow conditions. The bottles are then loaded onto the shelves of a refrigerated freeze-drying machine, the door is sealed and a vacuum is created in the chamber. In the presence of a vacuum, the plasma releases its water in the form of vapour, without passing through a liquid phase – the product does not melt. This process of sublimation (changing from a solid directly to a vapour) is called lyophilization. The drying process is accelerated by mildly heating the shelves on which the bottles are placed. The vapour migrates from the plasma shell, through the permeable membrane positioned over the neck of the bottle, to the coldest area in the freeze-drier (the condenser) where it forms ice again.

Freeze-dried plasma in single donation units is not as commonly used as in the past. It has been superseded by pooled fresh plasma that is solvent/detergent treated and dried in a fractionation facility.

CRYOPRECIPITATE

When the plasma of freshly donated blood is frozen shortly after collection, and later slowly thawed at +4°C ± 2°C, a white precipitate (called cryoprecipitate) may be seen in the plasma. This cryoprecipitate contains most of the factor VIII, von Willebrand factor and fibrinogen that was present in the original fresh plasma. After hard centrifugation at a cold setting (the precipitate will go back into solution if the plasma is warmed) the precipitate is concentrated in the bottom of the plasma bag. The cryoprecipitate-poor ('cryo-poor') supernatant plasma is then removed into an attached bag leaving only about 40 mL for resuspension of the cryoprecipitate. This product is also called wet cryoprecipitate or 'wet cryo'.

Cryoprecipitate contains concentrated clotting factor VIII, the factor lacking in patients with haemophilia A. Cryoprecipitate is also called anti-haemophilic factor (AHF). Cryoprecipitate isolated from fresh plasma may be stored frozen for up to 3 years at temperatures colder than –25°C or for 3 months at temperatures of between –18°C and –25°C. Alternatively, it may be freeze-dried and stored for at least 1 year.

Wet cryo is also used as a source of fibrinogen and is indicated for the treatment of bleeding conditions such as disseminated intravascular coagulation (DIC). Factor VIII concentrate, prepared within a fractionation facility by cryoprecipitation of large pools of fresh plasma, is solvent/detergent treated to inactive viruses. This is therefore the product of choice for the safe treatment of haemophilia.

PLATELET CONCENTRATE

Blood donations for the preparation of platelet concentrates should not take longer than 12 minutes as poor flow during donation leads to consumption of platelets. Blood should be collected only from individuals who have not taken aspirin. (If drugs containing aspirin were used in the previous 72 hours, platelet function is adversely affected.)

Whole blood used for the preparation of platelets should not be refrigerated, which would initiate clumping of platelets and reduce their functionality. Suitable donations should be stored in conditions validated to cool donated blood to +22°C ± 2°C as rapidly as possible after donation and then maintain this temperature range for up to 24 hours. This is usually achieved using an insulated transport box and coolant packs (or plates) filled with a specially selected coolant that has an appropriate melting point (e.g. butane diol).

The treatment of patients requiring platelets cannot be effectively achieved by using platelets in whole blood, RCCs or plasma because the number of platelets in such components prepared from a single donation is insufficient to be therapeutically effective. A standard adult therapeutic dose is generally considered to be the platelets derived from 4–6 whole blood donations, and clearly patients needing platelets only do not need that volume of red cells or plasma.

The yield of platelets from a single donation of whole blood (approximately 50–70 × 109) can be recovered and concentrated in a small volume (50–60 mL) by various techniques. Five platelet concentrates (an adult therapeutic dose) can then be administered to a patient in a 250–300 ml volume.

Platelet yield is the total number of platelets present in the final storage bag and is calculated using the platelet count per liter and adjusting it according to the total volume in which the platelets are suspended.

Platelet concentrates (PCs) may be issued for therapeutic use as individual units, or they may be pooled into a single bag to provide the therapeutic dose in a convenient package for easier administration.

When pooled in the components laboratory the connections are performed using an SCD and product sterility and expiry time are not compromised. It is also possible to use a leucocyte filter during pooling and provide filtered (leucocyte-depleted) platelet concentrate pools.

The storage conditions

- The PC must be continually stored at a controlled room temperature (+22°C ± 2°C). This temperature is best maintained in a temperature controlled room or cabinet. Though this is the best temperature for platelet storage, it is also a warmer temperature that will encourage rapid growth of bacterial organisms that may contaminate the donation from the phlebotomy site or the donor's circulation. For this reason the maximum storage period for PCs is only 5 days. The expiry time could be extended to 7 days if appropriate contamination reduction measures are implemented by performing bacterial detection tests on each unit (or pool).

- The PVC bags used for platelet storage differ from collection and transfer bags in that they are made from special plastics that are permeable to gases and guarantee availability of oxygen to the platelets, thus preventing a drop in pH. The bags are large; a bag of approximately 1000 ml is used for the storage of 300 ml of pooled platelets, to enhance oxygen transfer over a bigger surface area. The amount of oxygen required depends on the number of platelets in the bag – more platelets need more oxygen. Bag manufacturers usually give guidelines on the capability of their products.

- During storage, gentle and continuous agitation on a flat bed agitator rotating at approximately 70 cycles per minute is essential to prevent clumping of the platelets and to enhance oxygen transfer

Methods of preparation: platelets

The two main procedures of preparing PLTC are either by platelet-rich plasma (PRP) method or BC method. PRP method is simple, easily done manually and comparatively cheaper, but platelet and plasma yield is less. BC is a better method but complicated if done manually and hence needs automation.

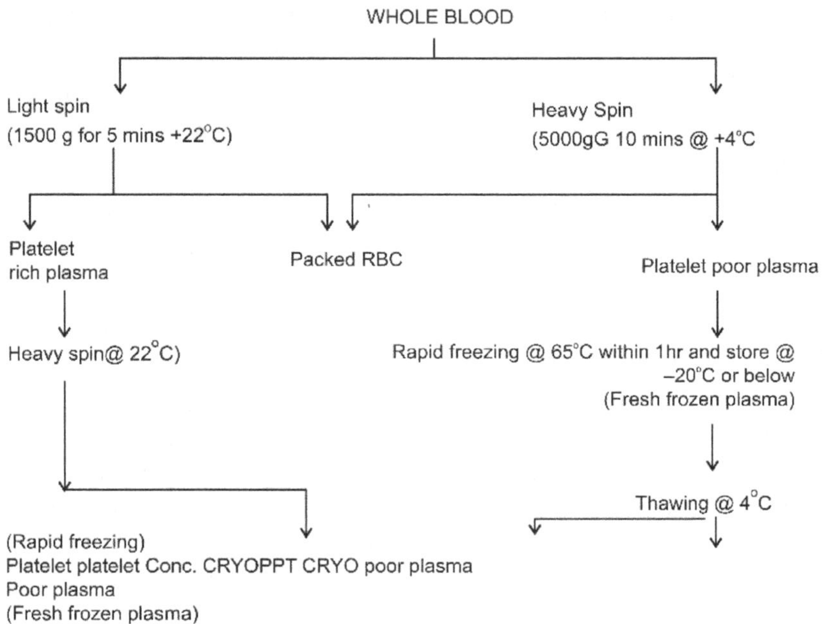

Fig. 5.16 Preparation method for platelets

Principles of platelet components preparation

The Whole blood is collected as 350 ml or 450 ml in double/triple/quadruple/penta bags with CPDA-1 or additive solution. After blood collection, components should be separated within 5 - 8 hours. Component room should be a separate sanitised room. All precautions to avoid red cell contamination have to be taken such as tapping the segment ends, proper balancing of opposite bags, following standard programs and protocols described in the manual of refrigerated centrifuge manufacturer. The programme is run with mainly two spins-heavy spin (e.g., 5000 G for 10-15 min) and light spin (e.g., 1500 G for 5-7 min). The heavy and light spin configuration varies with manufacturer and model. Here 'G' is relative centrifugal force calculated using revolutions per minute and rotor length. Use of totally automated component separator instrument will allow for the preparation of low volume BCs with a recovery of 90% of whole blood platelets.

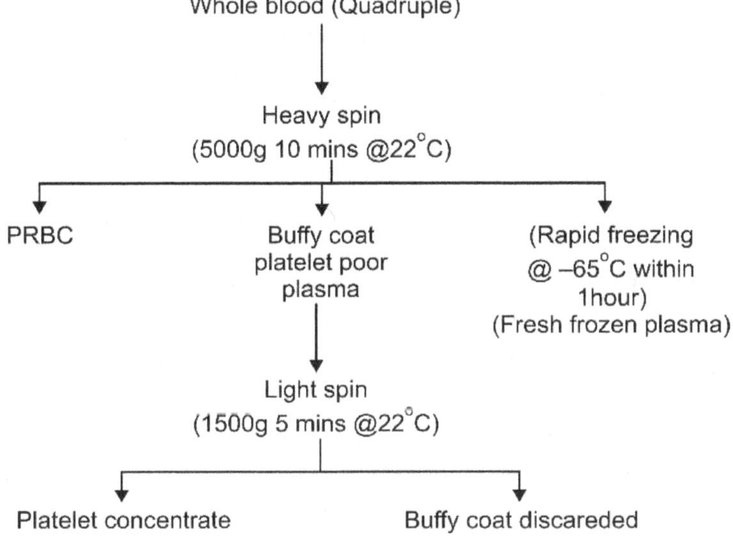

Fig. 5.17 The platelet-rich plasma (PRP) method

'Random donor platelets'

Random donor (or recovered) platelets refer to individual or pooled platelet products made from whole blood donations. Platelets from 4–6 donations are required to prepare a therapeutic dose and they therefore pose a greater risk to the patient of TTIs and alloimmunization to HLA antigens than apheresis platelets

Apheresis platelets

Apheresis is an operation where required single or further than one component is collected, and the rest of blood factors are returned back to the donor.

The working principle of apheresis equipment is either by centrifugation (different specific gravity) or by filtration (different size). The most generally used equipments use the centrifugation principle and also give leucodepleted products. In this method, fixed quantity of blood is collected in a bolus called as Extracorporeal volume (ECV) and the required element (e.g. Platelets) is separated and collected in the collection bag and the other factors (e.g. red blood cells, leucocytes and plasma) are returned back to the donor. Centrifugation apheresis equipments are classified as ' intermittent and continuous working'.

The *Intermittent equipment* uses single vein access for both collection and return. One cycle consists of-one ECV whole blood collection in kit bowl, centrifugation of bowl to separate factors, collection of needed element (platelets) in collection bag and eventually return other ingredients like red cells, leucocytes and plasma to donor. This cycle is repeated till therapeutic cure is attained.

In continual working equipment, two contemporaneous phlebotomies are done One for the collection and other for the return. The collection, centrifugation, element collection and return do continuously and contemporaneously. Each type has its own advantage and limitation.

The ultimate aim of the procedure isn't to overshoot ECV collection further than 15 of total blood volume (TBV). To avoid hypovolemia at any point ECV shouldn't reduce beyond 20 of TBV and the final product shouldn't exceed 15% ECV of TBV.

The various factors that can be collected are-double unit red cell collection (red cells), single donor platelet (SDP) harvesting platelets, leucapheresis (harvesting granulocytes, supplemental blood haematopoietic stem cell), plasmapheresis (collecting normal plasma) and remedial plasma exchange (for swapping with normal plasma after collecting and discarding patient's plasma).

General guidelines

Apart from being fit as per the whole blood donation criteria, additional criteria to be met for apheresis donors include prominent accessible vein for withstanding apheresis procedure and weight more than 55 kg.

In spite of strict guidelines for donors of apheresis procedures, advanced equipments like continuous apheresis equipment have allowed complicated procedures (like therapeutic erythrocytapheresis and leucapheresis of small children for thalassemia and leukaemia respectively) to be performed safely in children weighing 11-25 kg without increased morbidity

The donor should be asked to sign a consent form in the language which he understands after being explained the procedure and the risks involved.

Certain investigations should be done and all parameters should be within the acceptable range prior to subjecting the donor for apheresis procedure such as complete blood count, total proteins including albumin, globulin, same ABO grouping. (if necessary same Rh typing and negative atypical antibody status), transfusion transmitted disease screening (mandatory and to be non reactive), minor cross match (to be compatible, If necessary major should be compatible in case of red cell contaminated product).

The various Blood components that can be prepared from component preparation or apheresis procedures are as follows:

- PRBCs, double unit red cell (apheresis)

- PLTC or RDP, SDP (apheresis)

- Granulocyte concentrates (now very uncommon), autologous or allogeneic peripheral blood hematopoietic stem cell collection-PBHSCT (apheresis)

- FFP, cryoprecipitate

Plasma Fractionation

Plasma for fractionation is obtained either as 'recovered' plasma from whole blood donations, or as 'source' plasma from apheresis donations. If such plasma is frozen to a core temperature below –25°C within 24 hours of donation, labile clotting factors may also be harvested; if plasma is frozen after 24 hours of donation, labile clotting factors can no longer be extracted.

Fractionation process

The most widely used method of separation is cold ethyl alcohol fractionation. This was developed by Cohn-Oncley in the USA (1940s), and Kistler-Nitschmann in Switzerland (1964). Both methods involve the addition of ethanol at varying concentrations, to a large pool of plasma while simultaneously cooling it and controlling the temperature, pH and ionic strength. The methods rely on the different solubility of the protein fractions in plasma, and their behaviour when subjected to varying concentrations of alcohol, degree of acidity or alkalinity (pH), temperature and salt concentration (ionic strength).

Cold ethanol fractionation results in the desired protein fraction being isolated, either by precipitation as a paste, or by retention in solution, while other protein fractions are precipitated. This is achieved without destroying their biological function by processing at cold temperatures so that in the final form they remain efficacious, suitable for infusion (non-toxic, non-pyrogenic) and remain stable when stored.

The yield for the different clotting factors and protein fractions is not the same for each; some are more abundant in unprocessed plasma than others, and this affects the yield, as does the actual process. Albumin is the most abundant and FVIII gives the lowest yield. The process of fractionation is time-consuming; it takes days to isolate a fraction and weeks or months before the final product is bottled and available for therapeutic use.

The first stage of fractionation is concerned with the isolation of coagulation factors, notably factor VIII and fibrinogen (factor I) in cryoprecipitate and factor IX or prothrombin complex from the cryo-poor plasma. FFP from the blood transfusion service is control-thawed to isolate cryoprecipitate in bulk, using a process of continuous flow centrifugation. This is normally carried out prior to commencing fractionation with ethanol, because of the labile nature of the coagulation factors.

After these clotting factors have been separated, the residual plasma pool is cold ethanol fractionated to extract the predominantly protein groups; gamma globulin (immunoglobulins) and albumin. This is a sequential process using conditions that will precipitate groups of proteins that are required and may then be isolated, or that are contaminants and must be removed, or that remain in solution for subsequent precipitation into a more concentrated form (paste). Once isolated into these groups other techniques are used to ultimately produce the final products.

Other processing techniques used in the fractionation of plasma

Although cold ethanol fractionation is the foundation of fractionation, refinements in protein separation techniques have added new benefits. These include new products from the plasma or plasma fractions, improved yields, increased safety, higher purity and enhanced stability. Of these, the developments in chromatography (such as size exclusion, anion exchange and immunoaffinity) and filtration (such as membrane filtration, ultrafiltration and nanofiltration) have had the biggest impact. This has enabled a better utilization of the plasma and plasma fractions obtained from ethanol fractionation. The development of these techniques also facilitated the introduction of viral inactivation processes that significantly further enhance the safety of fractionated products.

Human Plasma Protein Fraction

It is a solution of the proteins from liquid plasma or serum containing albumin and globulins. The protein content is not less than 4.3% w/v and the product exerts a colloidal osmotic pressure approximately equivalent to that of pooled liquid plasma containing 5.2%w/v of protein. It must be stored between 5 to 20 degrees centigrade and protected from light. Its use remains the same as dried plasma. Addition of a stabilizer such as sodium caprylate or acetyltryptophan allows the prevention of denaturation of proteins in the solution during heating. Sodium chloride is added to make the preparation approximately isotonic. The solution must be sterilized by filtration, aseptically distributed into blood bottles and to destroy the viruses of infective hepatitis and homologous serum jaundice it was heated at 60 +/- 0.5 degrees centigrade for ten hours. Dried human plasma protein fraction is prepared by freeze-drying human plasma protein fraction. Its use is also the same as that of dried plasma

Human fibrinogen

Fibrinogen is the soluble constituent of plasma, which on addition of thrombin will convert to fibrin (which is insoluble). After separation from plasma by fractionation, the precipitate is collected by centrifugation, dissolved in citrate-saline, and freeze dried. The air in the containers is displaced by nitrogen. The citrate prevents automatic clotting when the substance is reconstituted. Fibrinogen dissolves sluggishly. Still, like numerous other protein solutions, it froths a lot if shaken and the solid - stabilized foam is very slow to disperse, therefore agitation should be limited to rocking. The solution should be used as soon as possible and not later than three hours after preparation. The fibrinogen must be stored under dry conditions, protected from light and at a temperature below 20 degrees centigrade. The other storage conditions are similar to that of dried serum.

Human Thrombin

Thrombin is an enzyme that converts fibrinogen to fibrin. The prothrombin attained from the separation of plasma is washed with distilled water, dissolved in citrate saline and is converted to thrombin by adjustment of pH to 7 by adding thromboplastin and calcium ions. The solution is filtered and indurate- dried, and the air in the holders replaced by nitrogen. It's reconstituted with saline when required. The fibrin clot produced when thrombin is mixed with fibrinogen is used in surgery to suture severed nerves and to assist adhesion of skin grafts. The clot also acts as a haemostat.

Human fibrin foam

This is prepared by whipping a solution of fibrinogen into froth by mechanical means and then adding thrombin. The product is poured into trays and freeze-dried, then cut into pieces of convenient size and sterilized by dry heat at 130 degrees centigrade for three hours. The froth must be stored under dry conditions, protected from light and at a temperature below 20 degrees centigrade. The other storage conditions are analogous to that of dried serum except that fibrin froth needs not to be stored under nitrogen. Generally, Human fibrin foam is used as haemostatic agent to arrest bleeding by dipping it in thrombin solution and applying locally. The combination of thrombin and the large rough surface provided by the sponge causes the blood to clot. The foam can be left in situ, where it will be absorbed because it is entirely of human origin.

Human normal immunoglobulin injection

Immuno- or gamma globulin can be obtained from the globulins fraction separated in stage 3 of the fractionation of plasma. The ionic strengths are critical and further fractionation is done as follows:

The immunoglobulins are dissolved in a good solvent, generally0.8 sodium chloride solution, and a preservative.,e.g. 0.01% thiomersal, is added. The solution sterilized by filtration, packed in single - dose containers and stored at 4 to 6 degrees centigrade, with protection from light. Typically a pool of not lower than 1500 donations is used to ensure a satisfactory representation of the various types of adult antibodies. However, as in the preparation of antivaccinia and antitetanus immunoglobulins, which is obtained from the blood of recently immunized donors, the pools of blood can be smaller.

Uses of Immunoglobulins

* Used to prevent or attenuate diseases such as Measles, Rubella, infectious hepatitis, hepatitis B, Chickenpox, Hypogammaglobulinaemia (deficiency in gamma globulins)
* It is used to prepare specific immunoglobulins such as:
– Human Anti-Vaccinia Immunoglobulin – for small pox
– Human Anti-Tetanus Immunoglobulin

- Human Anti-D Immunoglobulin – used to suppress sensitization of Rh –ve mothers to the Rh(D) antigen (Rh +ve infant)
- Anti-HBs Immunoglobulin – this is still under investigation. It is an immunoglobulin for Hepatitis B surface antigen.

STORAGE

General Requirements for Storage of Blood Products

As per standard guidelines, the storage temperature for

- red cells are between +2°C and +6°C,
- Platelets and leucocytes-between +20°C and +24°C and
- plasma products, below −18°C

All ingredients are to be kept in three chambers or equipments, the untested components, the Tested and safe to be issued components and the Tested unsafe or quarantined constituents for discarding.

In addition separate equipment is needed for keeping safecross-matched units if obtainable. During the transport, the ingredients can be stored for an outside of 24 h if maintained at suggested temperatures. PRBC must be maintained between 2 °C to 10 °C. All factors are routinely stored between 20 °C and 24 °C and also packed at same temperatures. All frozen factors should be transported in a manner to maintain their frozen state. The temperature changes can be covered and proved either through pointers fixed on units or checking each element manually for any deterioration. The cold chain conservation for all blood factors should extend to the point of transfusion.

The storage and transport equipments used are:

Refrigerators (+4 ± 2°C): For storage of whole blood and PRBC and for storage of thawed FFP and other plasma products.

Platelet incubator-agitators (+22 ± 2°C) with agitation speed at 60 cycles per minute: For storage of all type of platelet products

Deep freezers (−80°C): For freezing FFP or frozen blood constituents. Rapid freezing can be achieved by Mechanical blast freezers and storage of frozen PRBC or Platelets below −65°C or even colder

Freezers (−40°C): Storage of all plasma products below −30°C or even colder

Transport boxes: Transport boxes are used for transportation of blood or blood components for a short duration between two storage sites.

Even blood mobiles have built in cold chain storage devices with backup power.

Table 5.5 Blood Component Storage conditions

Product	Description	Storage °C	Expiration
Whole Blood Red Cells	All components of donor blood plus anticoagulant CPD, CPDA-1 whole blood with 200-250 plasma removed; final volume- 300 ml, Hct < 80% AS : with most plasma removed And 100 ml additive soln. added; Final volume - 350 ml Hct 55-65%	2-6 ml 2-6	CPD - 21 days CPDA-1 - 35 days Closed system - see whole blood Open system - 24 hr. AS additive - 42 days
Red Cells - Leucocytes Reduced	R.C. modified by centrifugation removing buffy coat or filtration to remove >70% leucocytes while retaining >70% of original R.C.	2-6	Closed system - see whole blood/Red cells Open system - 24hr.
Red Cells Washed	R.C. washed with normal saline;	2-6	24 hr
Red Cells Frozen- Deglycerol	R.C. frozen with glycerol,	Frozen at - 65 (high glycerol) - 120 (low glycerol) Deglycerol ized-at 2-6	10 yr 3 yr 24 hr
Platelets	>5.5 x 10^{10} in 40-70 ml plasma	20 - 24 with agitation	3 or 5 days depending on storage bag 4 hr after pooling
Platelets, pheresis	>3.0x 10" in about 200 ml plasma	20 - 24 with agitation	5 days

Table 5.5 *cont...*

Product	Description	Storage °C	Expiration
Granulocytes	About 1×10^{10} in 200-250 ml plasma	20 - 24 without agitation	24 hrs
FFP	200-250 ml with anticoagulant	Frozen -18 or below Thawed 2-6	1 yr 12 hr
Plasma	200-250 ml with anticoagulant Liquid plasma	Frozen -18 or below Thawed 2-6	5yr 5 days after whole blood expiration
Cryo precipitated AHF	80-120 units Factor Vlll 40-70% von Willebrand factor	Frozen < -18 Thawed 2-6 After pooling	1 yr 6 hr 4 hr

PLASMA SUBSTITUTES

Any liquid used to replace blood plasma, generally a saline solution, frequently with serum albumins; dextrans or other medications are the plasma backups. These substances don't enhance the oxygen- carrying capacity of blood, but simply replace the volume. They're also used to treat dehumidification.

The limited inventories of plasma, the cost of producing the dried form and the threat of transmitting serum hepatitis stimulated attempts to find backups of non - human origin that could be used to restore the blood volume temporarily while the recipient replaced the lost protein.

Properties of an Ideal Plasma Substitute

- The same colloidal osmotic pressure as whole blood.

- A viscosity similar to that of plasma.

- A molecular weight such that the molecules do not easily diffuse through the capillary walls.

- Eventual and complete elimination from the body.

- Freedom from toxicity, e.g. no impairment of renal function.

- Freedom from antigenicity, pyrogenicity, and confusing effects on important tests such as blood grouping and the erythrocyte Sedimentation rate

- Isotonicity, in solution, equal to that of blood plasma.

- High stability in liquid form at normal and sterilizing temperatures and during transport and storage.

- Ease of preparation, ready availability and low cost.

GUM SALINE

This is a synonym for Injection of Sodium Chloride and Acacia, which was official in the 1932 British Pharmacopoeia. In the First World War Bayliss experimented with soluble starch, dextrin, and gelatin as plasma substitutes and finally used 6% acacia in 0.9% Sodium Chloride solution. It was transfused extensively until signs of liver dysfunction disclosed that the gum was not metabolized but stored in various organs.

POLYVINYLPYRROLIDONE

In the Second World War, the Germans presented a man-made colloid, polyvinylpyrolidone, for the treatment of shock. It was retailed in the 1950s but was latterly dropped back because of assumed carcinogenicity.

DEXTRAN

Dextran is a complex radiated glucan (polysaccharide made of numerous glucose molecules) composed of chains of varying lengths (from 3 to 2000 kilodaltons). It's used medicinally as an antithrombotic (antiplatelet), to reduce blood viscosity, and as a volume expander in hypovolaemia. The straight chain consists of α-1, 6 glycosidic association between glucose molecules, while branches begin from α-linkages. Dextran is synthesized from sucrose by certain lactic acid bacteria, Leuconostoc mesenteroides and Streptococcus mutans. Dental plaque is rich in dextrans.

Louis Pasteur as a microbial product in wine first discovered dextran. Dextran 70 is on the WHO Model List of Essential Medicines, the most important drugs necessitated in a introductory health system.

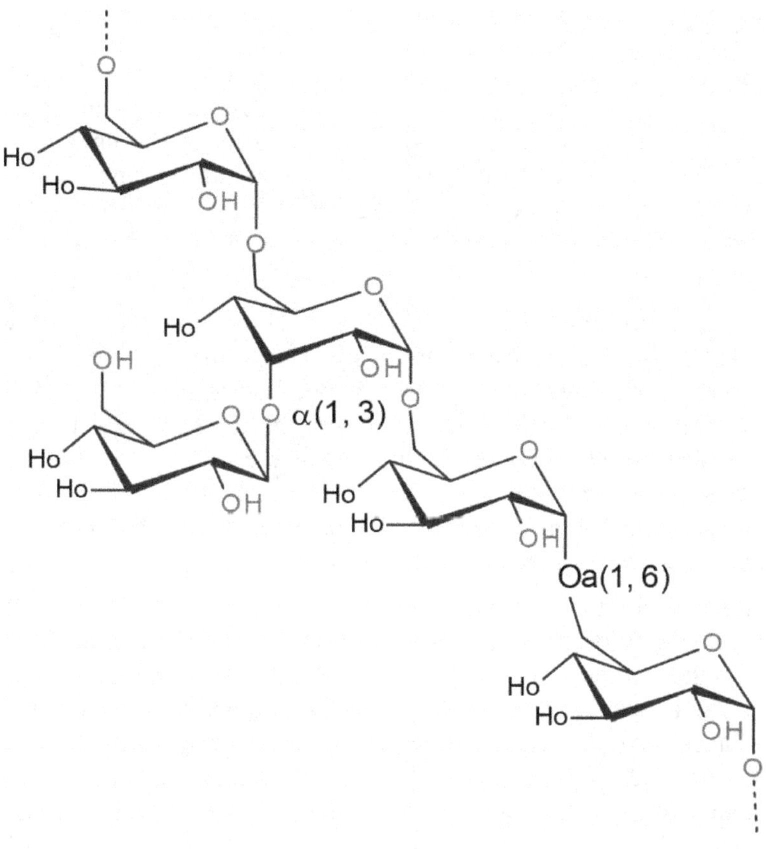

Fig. 5.18 A fragment of the Dextran structure

Dextran Characteristics

- Dextran fractions are characterized by their average molecular weights and molecular weight distributions.

- Dextran is used in various fields such as pharmaceutical, photographic, and agricultural industries.

- The versatile use of Dextran products relates to the favorable properties

- Dextran is neutral and water-soluble.

- Dextran is biocompatible and biodegradable.

- Dextran is stable for more than 5 years.

Production

The product procedure involves laboratory culture followed by growth in seed tanks in the factory and then in 4500 cubic dm fermenters (Similar process to antibiotic production). The synthesis of the enzyme and its action on the sucrose are rapid-fire, the high degree of asepsis maintained in antibiotic fermentation isn't necessary. In addition, the process is inhibited by aeration; there's no need for a expensive force of sterile air.

Another special feature is the need to prevent the hydrolysis of sucrose to glucose and fructose during sterilization of the culture media. However, dextran won't be produced because in nature the conversion doesn't involve inversion but is a straight transglycosidation, If this occurs. Preventive measures include adjustment of the media to neutral pH before sterilization, and the avoidance of overheating. When maximum conversion to dextran has been obtained, it's precipitated by adding a suitable organic solvent

Natural dextran consists of chains of about glucose units with molecular weights up to about 50 million. Veritably large molecules i.e. those with a molecular weight above about have serious disadvantages They yield veritably thick solutions that are sensitive to administer. They may cause renal damage and allergic reactions. They interfere with blood matching and sedimentation tests by causing rouleaux formation. Rouleaux are summations of red cells that act piles of plates. They produce colloidal osmotic pressures that are lower than those of small molecules. Therefore, to produce a material suitable for medical use it is necessary to reduce the size of the natural molecules. This can be accomplished in several ways:

- Acid Hydrolysis (the method most widely used)
- Thermal Degradation
- Ultrasonic Disintegration
- Seeding the Fermenter

Acid Hydrolysis

The pH of dextran is adjusted to a pH of 2 a is heated at 90 degrees centigrade. As hydrolysis proceeds, the preparation becomes less viscous and the reaction is stopped at the required viscosity. Acid hydrolysis is the method most often used. The hydrolyzed product contains molecules ranging from 10,000 to 1 million in molecular weight.

Thermal Degradation

A solution of dextran is heated under pressure at 160 degrees centigrade in the presence of sodium sulphite, to prevent oxidative deterioration, and calcium carbonate, to neutralize acidity. The method is slower than acid hydrolysis but the yield of the preferred molecules is better and fewer reducing groups are produced

Ultrasonic Disintegration

Bombardment with ultrasonic waves splits the molecules into fragments of approximately the same size and the product is clinically acceptable, unlike the material from the previously mentioned methods, which requires considerable fractionation. Unfortunately, this technique is much more expensive to use.

Seeding the Fermenter

If a low molecular weight dextran is added in the culture medium before fermentation, the organism will use it as a template on which to build more glucose molecules. The average molecular weight of the product is much lower than if no template dextran is provided. The very small molecules, i.e. those of below a molecular weight of about 60,000 also have disadvantages

– They are rapidly excreted in the urine.

– They pass into the tissue fluids causing an adverse osmotic pressure

- Therefore, the product should contain the minimum of molecules of molecular weight less than 60,000 (i.e. the number of molecules with a molecular weight of less than 60,000 should be kept to a minimum)

  The opted fraction still requires significant sanctification to remove –

- Reducing Sugars – by further solvent precipitation. The main adulterant is fructose, the derivate of fermentation.

- Separation detergents – by evaporation under reduced pressure.

- Inorganic mariners – by demineralization in a mixed bed ion exchanger. It's particularly important to remove phosphates because they cause precipitation during sterilization and storehouse.

- Colour – by adsorption on to actuated charcoal.

- Pyrogens – by adsorption on to asbestos, or cellulose derivations.

- Micro - organisms – by filtration. Between each treatment, the medication is passed through a fibrous pad and just before bottling a membrane filter is used.

The result is diluted to a concentration of 5 in either 5 Dextrose Injection or Sodium Chloride Injection, packed in sulphur treated soda - lime bottles, and closed with lacquered rubber plugs also eventually, it's sterilized, generally by heating in an autoclave.

Control for Dextran

The following tests from the sanctioned specification for Dextran 110 Injection illustrate the preventives taken to confirm that the product is suitable as a plasma substitute. Chemical techniques limit the quantity of lead, acetone and alcohol, reducing sugars, nitrogen (from culture medium) and acid and alkali. Biological styles show that the preparation isn't pyrogenic, is sterile, and is free from proteins that could cause anaphylaxis. This involves the injection into rabbits; the urine collected throughout the succeeding 48 hours mustn't contain more than 30 of the injected dose. (as small molecules are excreted in the urine).

The dextran content is determined by polarimetry and there are limit tests for small and large molecules. It necessitates precipitation of the top 10 of the fraction with alcohol and determining its intrinsic viscosity; this mustn't be greater than0.4, which is equivalent to an average molecular weight of about. The intrinsic viscosity of the fraction as a total is also found and must indicate an average molecular weight of about 110,000.

Dextran 40 Injection

A number of conditions, including severe burns, crush injuries and acute peritonitis, are accompanied by a severe degree of sludging in the blood. This can be reduced by the administration of Dextran 40 injection, which, because it contains polymers of low molecular weight, lowers plasma viscosity and improves capillary inflow. Both changes reduce cell aggregation and this in turn, further improves the inflow. A crude dextran of low molecular weight is manufactured by including very small template molecules in the fermentation medium. Also fractionation is used to produce the clinical material, which has an average molecular weight of 40,000.

Dextran 70

Dextran is a representative plasma replacement. Various medications can serve as choices Infusion (Result for infusion), dextran70.6 in glucose intravenous infusion 5 or sodium chloride intravenous infusion0.9%

Uses Short- term blood volume expansion

Contraindications Severe congestive heart failure, renal failure; bleeding complications similar as thrombocytopenia and hypofibrinogenaemia

Precautions

Cardiac disease or renal impairment; monitor urine output; avoid haematocrit falling below 25–30%; where possible, monitor central venous pressure; can interfere with blood group cross-matching and biochemical tests—take samples before start of infusion; monitor for hypersensitivity reactions; pregnancy

Dosage

Short- term blood volume expansion, by rapid-fire intravenous infusion, adult 500 – 1000 ml originally, followed by 500 ml if necessary; total lozenge shouldn't exceed 20 ml/ kg during the original 24 hours; if needed 10 ml/ kg daily may be given for a further 2 days (treatment shouldn't continue for longer than 3 days); child total lozenge shouldn't exceed 20 ml/ kg

Adverse effects

Hypersensitivity reactions including fever, nasal congestion, joint pains, urticaria, hypotension, bronchospasm—rarely severe anaphylactoid reactions; transient increase in bleeding time

POLYGELINE

Polygeline is a representative partially degraded gelatin. Various preparations can serve as alternatives: Infusion (Solution for infusion), polygeline 3.5% with electrolytes, 500-ml bottle

Uses:

Correction of low blood volume

Contraindications

Severe congestive heart failure; renal failure

Precautions

Blood samples for cross-matching should be taken before infusion; haemorrhagic diasthesis; congestive heart failure, renal impairment, hypertension, oesophageal varices.

Dosage:

Correction of low blood volume, by intravenous infusion, initially 500–1000 ml of a 3.5% solution

Adverse effects

Hypersensitivity reactions including urticaria rarely severe anaphylactoid reactions; transient increase in bleeding time

ABSORBABLE HAEMOSTATS

These materials are used to control bleeding when it cannot be checked by means that are more conventional. The tissue gradually absorbs them and, therefore, if used during surgery can be left in the body when the incision is closed, and if applied to a surface wound need not be removed when the dressing is changed.

There are four important types:

- Human Fibrin Foam
- Gelatin Sponge
- Oxidized cellulose
- Calcium Alginate

Gelatin Sponge

This is prepared by adding a small percentage of formaldehyde to a warm solution of good quality gelatin, which is whisked and freeze-dried

Oxidized cellulose

Cellulose can be converted into polyanhydro-glucuronic acid, an absorbable haemostatic material, by oxidation with nitrogen dioxide.

Calcium Alginate

This is derived from alginic acid, a colloidal substance obtained from seaweeds *Laminaria digitata* and *Laminaria cloustoni* which grow off the scottish and Irish coasts. Alginic acid is a polyuronide built up from dmannuronic acid units. Its carboxyl groups react with the metallic ions to form alginates and, since the parent acid is unstable, the water-soluble sodium salt is used as the source of other alginates.

HYDROXYETHYL STARCH

An intravenous solution of hydroxyethyl starch is used to prevent shock following severe blood loss caused by trauma, surgery, or other issues. These solutions contain a heterogenous solution of Hydroxyethyl starch molecules with an average molecular weight of 69,000.

PENTASTARCH

The primary intended use of pentastarch is as a substitute for older colloids such as albumin or hetastarch for use in plasma volume expansion.

Questions

1. Explain Bioreactors/ Fermenters in detail, emphasizing their general requirements.
2. Describe the design, types, and methodologies of fermentation techniques, and their control.
3. Add a description of the Penicillin production process.
4. Write a summary of how citric acid is made.
5. Write a summary of Vitamin B12 production.
6. Write a summary on Glutamic acid formation.
7. Make a summary of Griseofulvin's production.